MW00451871

PACIFIC CREST TRAIL

From the California
Border to Canada

Jordan Summers

prior editions by Jeffrey P. Schaffer and Andy Selters

 WILDERNESS PRESS . . . *on the trail since 1967*

PACIFIC CREST TRAIL: OREGON & WASHINGTON
FROM THE CALIFORNIA BORDER TO CANADA

First edition 1974
Second edition 1976
Third edition 1979
Fourth edition 1986
Fifth edition 1990
Sixth edition 2000
Seventh edition 2004
Eighth edition 2020

Cover design: Scott McGrew
Book design: Travis Bryant
Maps: Scott McGrew
Cover photo: Glacier-cloaked Mount Jefferson is a favorite Cascades destination and stands as a landmark just a few miles beyond Russell Lake.
Frontispiece photo: Mount Winthrop, the last mountain before Canada
Opposite page: Through Indian Heaven Wilderness, Mount Adams Wilderness, and on to Canada, the PCT visits dramatic scenery.
Cover and interior photos: Jordan Summers, unless otherwise noted on page; photos on pages 38–41 by Dan R. Lynch
Index: Potomac Indexing LLC

Library of Congress Cataloging-in-Publication Data

Names: Summers, Jordan, 1951– author.
Title: Pacific Crest Trail. Oregon & Washington (from the California border to the Canadian border / by Jordan Summers.
Description: 8th edition. | Birmingham, AL : Wilderness Press, 2020. | Includes bibliographical references and index.
Identifiers: LCCN 2018037053 | ISBN 9780899978444 (pbk.) | ISBN 9780899978451 (ebook)
Subjects: LCSH: Hiking—Pacific Crest Trail—Guidebooks. | Hiking—Oregon—Guidebooks. | Hiking—Washington (State)—Guidebooks. | Oregon—Guidebooks. | Washington (State)—Guidebooks.
Classification: LCC GV199.42.P3 S854 2018 | DDC 796.510979—dc23
LC record available at https://lccn.loc.gov/2018037053

Published by ℞ WILDERNESS PRESS
An imprint of AdventureKEEN
2204 First Ave. S., Suite 102
Birmingham, AL 35233
800-678-7006, fax 877-374-9016

Manufactured in China
Distributed by Publishers Group West

Visit wildernesspress.com for a complete listing of our books and for ordering information. Contact us at our website, at facebook.com/wildernesspress1967, or at twitter.com/wilderness1967 with questions or comments. To find out more about who we are and what we're doing, visit blog.wildernesspress.com.

DISCLAIMER

Although Wilderness Press and the authors have made every attempt to ensure that the information in this book is accurate at press time, they are not responsible for any loss, damage, injury, or inconvenience that may occur to anyone while using this book. You are responsible for your own safety and health while in the wilderness. The fact that a trail is described in this book does not mean that it will be safe for you. Be aware that trail conditions can change from day to day. Always check local conditions, know your own limitations, and consult a map.

As any hiker knows, nature and our pathways into it are ever-changing; wildfires reshape whole forests and open up views, floods and landslides obliterate long-established routes, roads and trails change as new routes are built and old trails are abandoned, and businesses close. Your comments on recent developments or changes for future editions are always welcome.

While this guidebook revision has been under development for more than four years, at press time in the summer of 2020, COVID-19 is widely spread at critical levels in California, Oregon, and Washington. The Pacific Crest Trail Association is currently only recommending local, fully self-supported trips on the PCT that don't include travel to communities along the trail. Follow local regulations and maintain physical distance between non-family members. Explore the PCT locally or visit other beautiful trails near your home until it's safe to travel more fully. For the latest information on PCT restrictions, visit pcta.org/covid-19.

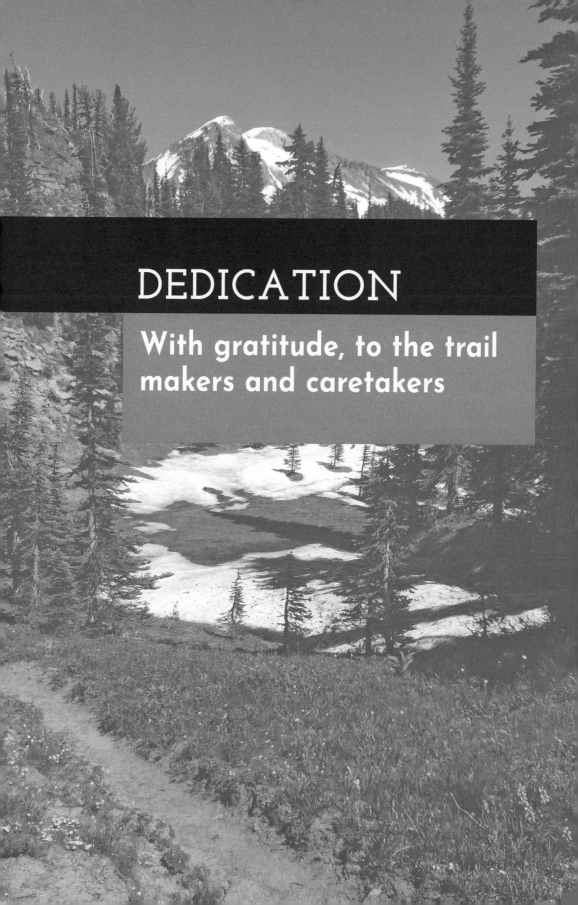

DEDICATION

With gratitude, to the trail makers and caretakers

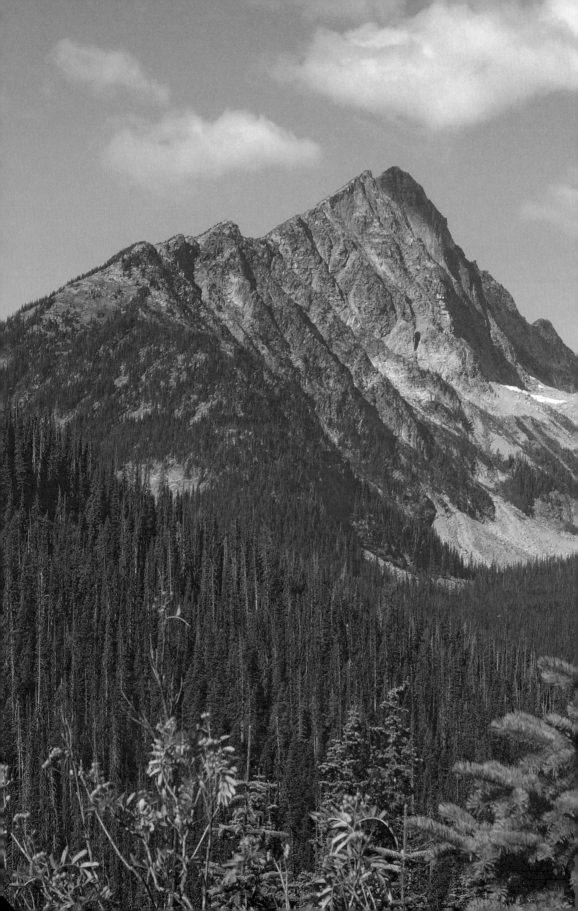

>>>CONTENTS

>>>ACKNOWLEDGMENTS

These precedent-setting volumes, begun nearly five decades ago by fellow hikers and authors Thomas Winnett, Jeffrey P. Schaffer, John W. Robinson, J. C. Jenkins, Andrew Husari, Ben Schifrin, Bev Hartline, Fred Hartline, Ruby Johnson Jenkins, and Andy Selters, have been invaluable to me. Their work still stands as a solid foundation for my observations.

I am grateful for the many special efforts of the professionals at Wilderness Press. Scott McGrew produced the new cartography for these books, and his work has vastly improved the usability of these trail maps. Editors Holly Cross, Amber Henderson, Kate Johnson, Ritchey Halphen, and Emily Beaumont kept me on track grammatically and guided me patiently in the direction of the readers' eye whenever I needed to buy a vowel. They have a tactful way of managing the need for fewer words, more facts, and clearer descriptions. I am continually grateful to Molly Merkle for giving me the opportunity to work on these special volumes. It is due to Molly's generous efforts over the past few years that these guides are maintained in print today. I am proud to work with you all and would not have known which way to turn without you.

I am especially thankful for the kindness of trail angels who picked me up when I hitched or who handed me refreshments when I was hungriest and driest. I can only say it again: thanks for the ride; those cookies were great; sweetest watermelon I ever had; that bottle of water saved me. There are more of you than anyone can know and you are, each one, appreciated.

When friends drive long distances to meet and feast off-trail, it's uniquely special. I am eternally grateful to Dave and PJ Dye; Randy and Mary Peterson; Tim Stumbles; Eddy Malik; Jodi Friedman and her crew, Matt, Kai, and Nicu; and Dan Hyland and Darlene Marcellay-Hyland. All of your rescues are fondly remembered.

Home cooking is often the stuff of dreams on the trail. But when I hike, I truly enjoy eating the nourishing and delicious dishes from Austin-based Packit Gourmet. Loren Mullins-Divino and the Mullins family hand-pack their meals in which every ingredient tastes fresh.

Many thanks to those who watched my route, alert to a lack of check-in or any signal of distress. In successive years, this important role was filled by my son-in-law, Andrew Herum; my Tahoe hiking partner, Wayne McClelland; my Sacramento hiking partner, Trig Rosenblatt; and my son and John Muir Trail hiking partner, Jason. And thanks to my friends for putting up with all of the calls I failed to make and all of the get-togethers I postponed. You were there for me while I walked north, cheering me on, tracking my daily hike, and massaging my spirits with each cheerful message. Then, while I sat at my desk writing for months on end, you would call and pick up as if I had never wandered away.

I owe much appreciation to my research assistant, Taylor Herum, for her web skills, which saved me hours of tediously valuable work. Thanks, as well, to her mother and my daughter, Ashley, for producing my first Pacific Crest Trail (PCT) blog in 2009. My son, Jason, rendezvoused with me at each resupply point throughout Northern California. I am grateful that he could and that he would. Each one was a day of stories and news, laughter, and reflection. I am thankful that my partner, Karin, could be my lifeline for all of my last-minute forgotten items needing delivery by drone, as well as for handling my ever-fluid resupply dates in an indoor voice. I would not have had the meals, the treats, or the zero-day hotel rooms without her.

There isn't a hiker who has set foot on the PCT who hasn't had some positive experience with the Pacific Crest Trail Association (PCTA), beginning with the outstanding work of Jack "Found"

Haskel, the PCTA's trail information manager, who gets us out there and keeps us informed once we're on our way. As usual, Jack got me on the trail with a permit, and when I returned to write these guides, I asked Jack for some feedback. He and several of his colleagues bravely took a deep dive into my final copy. These new volumes are far better because of the kind generosity and tedious work contributed by Jack and PCTA staff members Dana Hendricks, Columbia Cascades regional representative; Ian Nelson, Big Bend regional representative; Michael DeCramer, North Cascades regional representative; Justin Kooyman, associate director of trail operations; and Mark Larabee, associate director of communications and marketing. They took time out of their busy schedules to add clarity, corrections, updates, and insights that benefited these guides immensely. I am decidedly grateful for their involvement.

Each time I'm on the trail, I become a bit more mindful of how deep it is, of what's on and under it. And I have had time to think about what the PCTA means to me and have read or listened to what it means to other hikers. The PCTA has protected the trail for us today, and it works diligently to preserve it for our descendants. For this we are universally grateful. We sincerely appreciate the tireless leadership of Liz Bergeron, executive director and CEO of the PCTA; the entire PCTA staff; the board members; the many partner organizations; the multitude of donors; and the thousands of volunteers who all work on behalf of hikers from everywhere so that we can hike far and return home safely from this most memorable wilderness experience.

—*Jordan Summers, Pioneer, CA*

>>>ABOUT THIS BOOK

Wilderness Press published its first book on the Pacific Crest Trail, *The Pacific Crest Trail, Volume 1: California,* in June 1973, more than 47 years ago. Since then, our PCT guidebook series has earned the reputation as the most essential resources available to anyone who is planning a PCT trek.

That first book is now covered by two books: *Pacific Crest Trail: Southern California (From the Mexican Border to Yosemite's Tuolumne Meadows)* and *Pacific Crest Trail: Northern California (From Tuolumne Meadows to the Oregon Border).* A third book, *Pacific Crest Trail: Oregon & Washington,* first published in 1974, covers the Northwestern part of the PCT. Because only a few users of the Pacific Crest Trail are complete thru-hikers, the division of these texts makes it easier for planning the kind of shorter two- to three-week treks that most hikers do. These new editions feature all new photos and maps. Our detailed maps are based on the most current data available.

We would love to hear your comments or suggestions on how our books can be improved. Contact us at pct.wildernesspress.com, at facebook.com/wildernesspress1967, or at twitter.com /wilderness1967.

Thank you for buying and using this book. We hope it serves you well as you prepare for and set off on an incredible trip along the Pacific Crest Trail.

—*Bob Sehlinger, Publisher, Wilderness Press*

>>>FOREWORD

One of the reasons I love outdoor adventures is because they are largely unscripted. Sure, you plan your precious days off and where you'll go. You meticulously pick your gear, food, and watering holes, and, hopefully, you get in and out of the wilderness without mishap. Life is good.

But the wilderness often throws you a curve, mostly because the backcountry is organized chaos. There may be a trail, even a great one like the Pacific Crest Trail (PCT), but it's often the case that Mother Nature tosses obstructions, such as downed trees, a landslide, a swollen river, a lightning storm, or even a wildfire, in your way. Seasoned veterans of the backcountry have come to expect such obstacles.

Working for the Pacific Crest Trail Association (PCTA), the nonprofit that protects, preserves, and promotes the Pacific Crest Trail, I regularly see firsthand the amazing work that dedicated volunteers do to keep the trail open and passable for hikers and horseback riders. PCTA staff and volunteers often go to the same places year after year to reopen the trail. Imagine what the trail would be like without this gargantuan effort.

All that says nothing of the risks that are still out there. Rattlesnakes, bears, and mountain lions can change things in a hurry. A simple shift in weather can bring snow at higher elevations, making that planned cowboy campout a little uncomfortable to say the least. We've all heard—or lived—stories about someone breaking an ankle or bears stealing food 15 miles from the trailhead. Suddenly, a weekend backpacking trip becomes a survival mission.

This risk comes with the territory. The more we get outside and away from our modern conveniences, the more we become comfortable facing the unknown. I love the anticipation of a

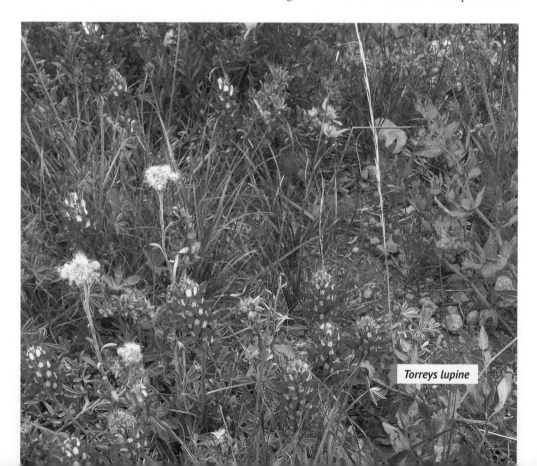

Torreys lupine

backcountry trip. For me, this element of wilderness travel is essential. Rising to meet challenges makes us feel alive. This guidebook will help show you the way and work out the logistics, but you never know what the day will bring. That's a good thing.

I can tell you it's always interesting. Personal contact with nature can push us to our limits and challenge our mental capacity to endure and survive. Most times it's tough but still safe and peaceful. But even experts sometimes find themselves in situations so dangerous it's foolish. The thing is, you never see it coming. You can be prepared, but each time out is a roll of the dice. I wouldn't have it any other way.

In testing ourselves outside, we live larger than is possible within the confines of our "real world" existence. Making good decisions about the weather and when to turn back is part of the challenge and the joy. Outside, I learned how to push my limits and when to back off.

It may be dangerous to, say, dodge a car flying though a downtown crosswalk, but that doesn't feed my soul. I want to do more than exist. I want to *really* feel alive. I do this on the trail, slowing down my awareness of time passing, turning minutes into hours, speeding up my heart rate, and sharpening my senses.

Contact with the natural world, wildflowers, flowing streams, wildlife, towering trees, and mountains—large, wild landscapes in general—reveals as much about who we are as it does about the natural world. Outside, we have space and time to look deep inside and reflect. We can put our worldly troubles into perspective and work through whatever it is we need to work through. We spend time in our own heads and realize how little we need to truly live large. On the trail we have time without distraction. We find enlightenment and we emerge stronger.

We build bonds with family and friends over our shared experiences and physical challenges in the wilderness. The friendships I have formed while hiking or climbing mountains are the most meaningful.

It all boils down to this: the trip you are about to take will be life changing. Whether you are going out for 26 miles or 2,650, what you will find on the Pacific Crest Trail will be nothing short of amazing. Most of the people I encounter who've hiked on the PCT—whether they've day-hiked, section-hiked, or thru-hiked—find rewards. They come away with an understanding about what's important in life. They have focus and grit. They learn determination out there. It's worth the price of admission.

The trail can teach us all of these things and more. I have never met anyone who completed a long trip on a trail or river who could not offer some kind of evidence of personal growth. Sure, we complain about the heat, the bugs, the sweat, the stench of our clothes, the dirt under our nails, and the blisters. Oh, the daily suffering! But then we launch with greater passion into the beauty and the grandeur and how small we felt out there. Have you ever seen a mountain lake so blue? A meadow so wonderfully inviting? Has a burger and a beer after a long day's walk ever tasted better? Ask any of them, even in the middle of whining about the switchbacks, and they'll tell you instantly how they would do it all again tomorrow.

This is who we are. This is how we live. We suffer, we grow, we feel alive. Then we rinse and repeat. Life is good. Definitely.

—*Mark Larabee*
PCTA Associate Director of Communications and Marketing

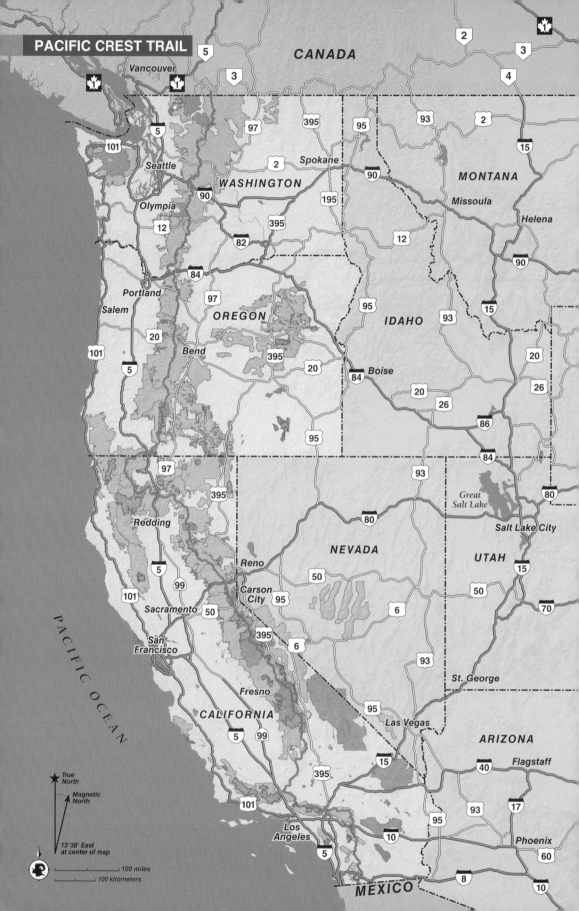

SOUTHERN CALIFORNIA

Section	Starting Mileage	Length
A: Mexican Border to Warner Springs	0.0	109.5
B: Warner Springs to San Gorgonio Pass	109.5	100.0
C: San Gorgonio Pass to I-15 near Cajon Pass	209.5	132.5
D: I-15 near Cajon Pass to Agua Dulce	342.0	112.5
E: Agua Dulce to CA 58 near Mojave	454.5	111.9
F: CA 58 near Tehachapi Pass to CA 178 at Walker Pass	566.4	85.6
G: CA 178 to John Muir Trail Junction	652.0	115.0
H: John Muir Trail Junction to Tuolumne Meadows	767.0	175.5

NORTHERN CALIFORNIA

Section	Starting Mileage	Length
I: Tuolumne Meadows to Sonora Pass	942.5	74.4
J: Sonora Pass to Lower Echo Lake	1,016.9	75.4
K: Lower Echo Lake to I-80	1,092.3	64.4
L: I-80 to CA 49	1,156.7	38.7
M: CA 49 to CA 70	1,195.4	91.5
N: CA 70 to Burney Falls	1,286.9	132.1
O: Burney Falls to Castle Crags	1,419.0	82.2
P: Castle Crags to Etna Summit	1,501.2	98.5
Q: Etna Summit to Seiad Valley	1,599.7	56.2
R: Seiad Valley to I-5 in Oregon	1,655.9	63.0

OREGON & WASHINGTON

Section	Starting Mileage	Length
A: Seiad Valley to I-5 in Oregon	1,655.9	63.0
B: I-5 near Siskiyou Pass to OR 140 near Fish Lake	1,718.9	54.5
C: OR 140 near Fish Lake to OR 138 near the Cascade Crest	1,773.4	74.4
D: OR 138 near the Cascade Crest to OR 58 near Willamette Pass	1,847.8	60.1
E: OR 58 near Willamette Pass to OR 242 at McKenzie Pass	1,907.9	75.9
F: OR 242 at McKenzie Pass to OR 35 near Barlow Pass	1,983.8	107.9
G: OR 35 near Barlow Pass to I-84 at Bridge of the Gods	2,091.7	55.5
H: I-84 at Bridge of the Gods to US 12 near White Pass	2,147.2	147.7
I: US 12 near White Pass to I-90 at Snoqualmie Pass	2,294.9	98.2
J: I-90 at Snoqualmie Pass to US 2 at Stevens Pass	2,393.1	71.0
K: US 2 at Stevens Pass to WA 20 at Rainy Pass	2,464.1	127.0
L: WA 20 at Rainy Pass to BC 3 in Manning Provincial Park	2,591.1	70.3

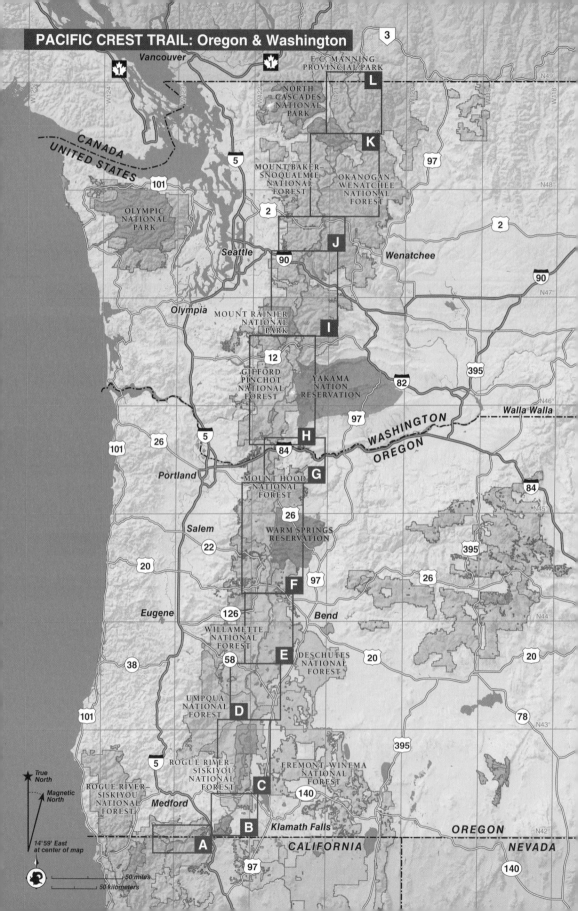

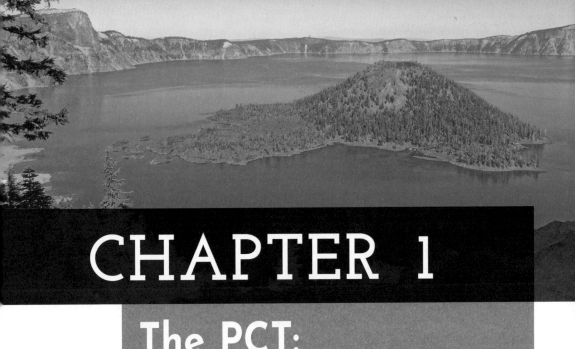

CHAPTER 1

The PCT:
Its History and Use

During the 1800s Americans traveling west toward the Pacific States were confronted with mountain barriers, such as the Cascades and the Sierra Nevada. The idea of making a recreational trek along the crest of these ranges probably never entered anyone's mind and most likely did not occur until the 1880s. However, relatively early in the 1900s, a party did make a recreational, multiday crest traverse of a part of the Sierra Nevada. From July 8 to July 25, 1913, Charles Booth, accompanied by his wife, Nora, and two friends, Howard Bliss and Elmer Roberts, made a pack trip from Tuolumne Meadows north to Lake Tahoe. Today's Pacific Crest Trail (PCT) closely follows much of their trek. (*Note:* For brevity in this book, we refer to the Pacific Crest Trail as the PCT. The official name is the Pacific Crest National Scenic Trail, abbreviated PCNST. However, that abbreviation is more cumbersome, and essentially no one uses it.)

CONCEPTION OF THE PCT

One of the earliest proposals for the creation of a Pacific Crest Trail is contained in the book *Pacific Crest Trails* by Joseph T. Hazard (Superior Publishing Co., 1946). He writes that, in 1926, Catherine Montgomery, an avid outdoorswoman and teacher at the Western Washington College of Education in Bellingham, suggested to him that there should be:

> A high winding trail down the heights of our western mountains with mile markers and shelter huts—like these pictures I'll show you of the "Long Trail of the Appalachians"—from the Canadian Border to the Mexican Boundary Line!

Above: Wizard Island stands near the western shore of Crater Lake in Section C.

Hazard writes that, on that very night, he conveyed Montgomery's suggestion to the Mount Baker Club of Bellingham, which was enthusiastic about it. He says that soon a number of other mountain clubs and outdoors organizations in the Pacific Northwest adopted the idea and set about promoting it.

More recent research has unearthed evidence that the first written record of the idea for the PCT occurred even earlier than Montgomery's plea. In 1918 a U.S. Forest Service (USFS) ranger in Oregon named Fred W. Cleator led a six-man crew in routing and posting a road from Mount Hood to Crater Lake. However, the budget was cut and so the road was left as a trail. Named the Oregon Skyline Trail, it was one of the early links of the PCT. Cleator's pencil-scrawled field diary, discovered by academic researchers in 2014, includes an August 20, 1918, entry in which he speculates "that a Skyline Trail the full length of the Cascades in Washington and Oregon, joining a similar trail in the Sierras of California, would be a great tourist advertisement" and "fine to plan upon." In 1928 Cleator became supervisor of recreation for Region 6 (Oregon and Washington) of the USFS. He established and began to develop the Cascade Crest Trail, a route down the spine of Washington from Canada to the Columbia River. Later, he extended the Oregon Skyline Trail at both ends so that it, too, traversed a whole state. In 1937 USFS Region 6 developed a design for PCT markers and posted them from the Canadian border to the California border.

But USFS Region 5, which includes California, did not follow this lead. Eventually, a private citizen provided the real spark, not only for a California segment of the PCT but indeed for the PCT itself. In the early 1930s the idea of a Pacific Crest Trail entered the mind of Clinton C. Clarke of Pasadena, California, who was then chairman of the executive committee of the Mountain League of Los Angeles County. A graduate of

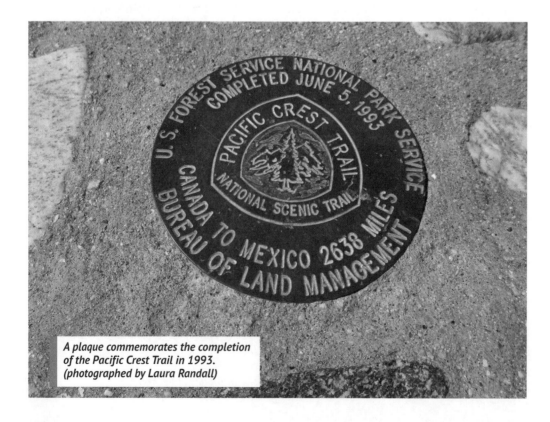

A plaque commemorates the completion of the Pacific Crest Trail in 1993. (photographed by Laura Randall)

Harvard who moved west and spent summers trekking the high Sierras, Clarke launched a passionate one-man letter-writing campaign, urging the heads of the USFS, Sierra Club, and other outdoors clubs to consider a supertrail from Mexico to Canada.

"In March, 1932," writes Clarke in *The Pacific Crest Trailway* (The Pacific Crest Trail System Conference, 1945), he "proposed to the United States Forest and National Park Services the project of a continuous wilderness trail across the United States from Canada to Mexico. . . . The plan was to build a trail along the summit divides of the mountain ranges of these states, traversing the best scenic areas and maintaining an absolute wilderness character." For years, Clarke insisted on calling his proposed wilderness corridor the John Muir Trail, but eventually relented to protests that the name belonged exclusively to the High Sierras area where Muir's legacy is so distinguished. When Harold C. Bryant, acting director of the National Park Service, wrote to Clarke in 1934 with several other name suggestions, Clarke gave in and embraced one of them, the Pacific Crest Trail.

The proposal included the formation of additional Mountain Leagues in Seattle, Portland, and San Francisco by representatives of youth organizations and hiking and mountaineering clubs, similar to the one in Los Angeles. These Mountain Leagues would then take the lead in promoting the extension of the John Muir Trail northward and southward to complete a pathway from border to border. When it became evident that more than Mountain Leagues were needed for such a major undertaking, Clarke led the formation of the Pacific Crest Trail System Conference, with representatives from the three Pacific Coast states. He served as its president for 25 years.

As early as January 1935, Clarke published a handbook/guide to the PCT, giving the route in rather sketchy terms: "The Trail goes east of Heart Lake, then south across granite fields to the junction of Piute and Evolution Creeks." This covers about 9 miles.

In the summer of 1935—and again the next three summers—groups of boys under the sponsorship of the YMCA explored the PCT route in relays, proceeding from Mexico on June 15, 1935, to Canada on August 12, 1938. This exploration was under the guidance of a YMCA secretary, Warren L. Rogers, who served as executive secretary of the Pacific Crest Trail System Conference from 1932 to 1957, when Clarke died (at age 84) and the conference dissolved. (Rogers was an enthusiastic hiker—and mountaineer—despite a bout with polio as a child that left him with a limp.) On his own, Rogers more or less kept the idea of the PCT alive until hiking and trails began receiving national attention in the 1960s. He launched a determined campaign to take possession of Clarke's papers after his death and continued to promote the trail and its joys through correspondence, camping magazines, and radio shows almost to the time of his death in 1992 at age 83.

National Trails System

In 1965 the Bureau of Outdoor Recreation, a federal agency, appointed a commission to conduct a nationwide trails study. The commission, noting that walking for pleasure was second only to driving for pleasure as the most popular recreational activity in America, recommended establishing a national system of trails of two kinds—long National Scenic Trails in the hinterlands and shorter National Recreation Trails in and near metropolitan areas. The commission recommended that Congress establish four scenic trails—the already existing Appalachian Trail, the partly existing Pacific Crest Trail, the Potomac Heritage Trail, and the Continental Divide Trail. Congress responded by passing, in 1968, the National Trails System Act, which set the framework for a system of trails and specifically made the Appalachian and Pacific Crest Trails the first two National Scenic Trails.

Today, there are 11 National Scenic Trails, totaling more than 18,000 miles, within the National Trails System. They are long-distance trails (more than 100 miles long) and are recreational in nature. Just as wonderful for a short day visit as a long-distance backpacking adventure, these trails call to all who want to explore America's natural landscapes.

The Proposed Route

Meanwhile, in California, the USFS in 1965 had held a series of meetings about a route for the PCT in the state. These meetings involved people from the USFS, the National Park Service, the State Division of Parks and Beaches, and other government bodies charged with responsibility over areas where the trail might go. These people decided that so much time had elapsed since Clarke had drawn his route that they should essentially start all over. Of course, it was pretty obvious that segments like the John Muir Trail would not be overlooked in choosing a new route through California. By the end of 1965 a proposed route had been drawn onto maps. (We don't say *mapped* because that would imply that someone had actually covered the route in the field.)

When Congress, in the 1968 law, created a citizens' advisory council for the PCT, it was the route devised in 1965 that the USFS presented to the council as a first draft of the final PCT. This body of citizens was to decide all the details of the final route; the USFS said it would adopt whatever the citizens wanted. The advisory council was also to concern itself with standards for the physical nature of the trail, markers to be erected along the trail, and the administration of the trail and its use.

In 1972 the council agreed on a route, and the USFS put it onto maps for internal use. Because much of the agreed-upon route was cross-country, these maps were sent to the various national forests along the route, for them to mark a temporary route in the places where no trail existed along the final PCT route. This they did—but not always after fieldwork. The result was that the maps made available to the public in June 1972 showing the final proposed route and the temporary detours did not correspond to what was on the ground in many places. A common flaw was that the USFS would base a segment on a preexisting USFS map that was incorrect, showing a trail where there was none.

Perfect or not, the final proposed route was sent to Washington for publication in the *Federal Register,* the next step toward its becoming official. A verbal description of the route was also published in the *Federal Register* on January 30, 1973. But the material in the register did not give a precise route that could be unambiguously followed; it was only a general outline, and the details in many places remained to be settled.

Private Property Glitches

As construction on PCT segments began, many hikers were optimistic that the entire trail could be completed within a decade. Perhaps it could have, if it weren't for private property located along the proposed route. While some owners readily allowed rights-of-way, many others did not, at least initially, and years of negotiations passed before some rights were finally secured. While negotiations were in progress, the USFS sometimes built new trail segments on both sides of a parcel of private land, expecting to extend a trail segment through it soon after. At times this approach backfired, such as in the northern Sierra Nevada in the Gibraltar environs (Section M, *Pacific Crest Trail: Northern California*). The owners of some property never gave up a right-of-way, and so a new stretch of trail on Gibraltar's south slopes was abandoned for a snowier, costlier stretch on its north slopes, completed in fall 1985. But at least the stretch was built.

The major obstacle to the trail's completion had been the mammoth Tejon Ranch, which began in Civil War days as a sheep ranch, then later became a cattle ranch, and in 1936 became a public corporation that diversified its land use and increased its acreage. This "ranch," about the size of Sequoia National Park, straddles most of the Tehachapi Mountains. An agreement between the ranch's owners and government representatives was finally reached, and in 1993 this section of the PCT was completed. However, rather than traversing the length of the Tehachapi Mountains as intended by Congress, the PCT for the most part follows miles of roads along the west side of the high desert area of Antelope Valley before ascending to the edge of ranch property in the north part of the range. This part of the trail is described in Section E, *Pacific Crest Trail: Southern California.*

In 2008 Tejon Ranch Company unveiled a landmark conservation and land-use agreement providing the framework for conserving up to 90% of Tejon Ranch—about 240,000 acres. In keeping with the original vision for the PCT, a significant part of the plan includes a set of easements that will protect the trail corridor and allow the PCT to be relocated from the floor of the Mojave Desert to the crest of the Tehachapi Mountains, following the route agreed upon by the USFS, the Pacific Crest Trail Association (PCTA), and the Tejon Ranch Company.

In May 2014, The Tejon Ranch Conservancy received the final paperwork for a 10,000-acre conservation easement from the Tejon Ranch Company, protecting habitat for the endangered California condor and other threatened, endangered, and sensitive plant and animal species and associated habitats, as well as vistas visible from a proposed new section of trail. This is the first tangible act in relocating 37 miles of the PCT from the Mojave Desert to the Tehachapi Mountains, the largest relocation project since the trail's official completion in 1993. The PCT easement still needs to be finalized, setting the route for the trail through Tejon Ranch and identifying off-trail campsites and access to critical water sources. The actual trail construction and realignment is still years away.

In 2016 an opportunity arose allowing the PCTA to acquire 245-acre Landers Meadow in Kern County, California, which was transferred into public ownership and incorporated into the Sequoia National Forest in 2018. Through member and community donations, the PCTA was able to protect this wet meadow and keep the trail uninterrupted along the route.

Also in 2016, thanks to a supporter's generosity, the PCTA was able to acquire 160-acre Donomore Meadows in Siskiyou County, California, near the Oregon border, as it was suddenly available for immediate sale. For about 0.5 mile, the PCT borders this lush habitat, home to rare plant species, northern spotted and great gray owls, deer, elk, and wolves. In 2017 the property was transferred to the USFS for inclusion into the Rogue River–Siskiyou National Forest for permanent protection.

Finally, there is another stretch in Northern California, covered in Section Q of *Pacific Crest Trail: Northern California,* where the route uses existing roads. To get the trail off a dangerous road walk, a new footbridge would need to be built across the Klamath River, an expensive and time-consuming project with little energy behind it. The lack of the bridge means that PCT travelers must tread 7.3 miles along the road. While a new bridge would cross the Klamath River just downstream of Seiad Valley, the town would remain an important resupply point for PCT hikers and horseback riders regardless.

Golden Spike Dedication

The Pacific Crest National Scenic Trail was officially dedicated on National Trails Day, June 5, 1993, a lengthy 25 years after Congress passed the National Trails System Act that had mandated it. The dedication was touted as the Golden Spike Completion Ceremony, in which a "golden" spike was driven into the trail, a reenactment of the 1869 ceremony at Promontory Point near Ogden, Utah, where the Central Pacific and Union Pacific railroad companies converged to complete the transcontinental railroad. For the PCT, there were no competing trail crews, so a PCT site close to metropolitan Southern California was chosen because it was the final easement acquired: a flat at the mouth of a small valley on the north side of Soledad Canyon (Section D, map 6, *Pacific Crest Trail: Southern California*). Protected under a canopy to shelter them from the unseasonably cold, windy, drizzly weather, Secretary of the Interior Bruce Babbitt and others spoke to an unsheltered audience of about 300 hearty souls (and a dozen or so others protesting various unrelated environmental issues). The trail was proclaimed to be 2,638 miles long officially, though the accuracy of this mileage is questionable because this number existed as early as 1990, before the completion of several stretches in Southern California and in the southern Sierra Nevada, and before the major relocation of the Hat Creek Rim stretch north of Lassen Volcanic National Park.

Future relocations are likely, and so the authors of the Pacific Crest Trail books, following the lead of our fellow hikers, have used the 2020 version of Lon "Halfmile" Cooper's trail mileage for all locations.

SOME WHO WALKED AND RODE

No doubt hikers in the 19th century did parts of the PCT, though that name didn't exist back then. It may be that someone walked along the crest from Mexico to Canada or vice versa many years ago. The first documented hiker to complete the entire three-state trek was Martin Papendick (1922–2000), who did so in 1952, when a tristate trail was still a dream and the PCT was decades away. It was his second attempt, and it took him 149 days to backpack from E. C. Manning Provincial Park south to Campo. The first person to receive official acknowledgment from the U.S. Forest Service for hiking the actual PCT route in one continuous journey (that is, a thru-hike)—in 1970—was Eric Ryback, who described his north-to-south trek in *The High Adventure of Eric Ryback*. This was quite a feat for anyone, much less a 130-pound 18-year-old, hiking solo in the more difficult north-to-south direction without a guidebook or detailed maps. His 1971 book focused attention on the PCT, and other people began to plan end-to-end treks. In 2009 Ryback became a PCTA board member and designed and funded the PCT completion medal.

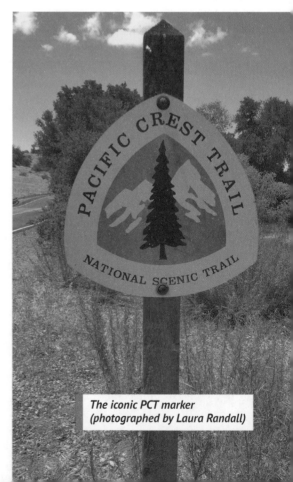

The iconic PCT marker (photographed by Laura Randall)

As mentioned earlier, in June 1972, the USFS maps of the PCT route became available to the public, and the race was on. The first person to hike this entire route from south to north was Richard Watson, who finished it on September 1, 1972. Barely behind him, finishing four days later, were Wayne Martin, Dave Odell, Toby Heaton, Bill Goddard, and Butch Ferrand. Very soon after them, Henry Wilds went from Mexico to Canada solo. In 1972 Jeff Smukler did the PCT with Mary Carstens, who became the first woman to make it. The next year, Gregg Eames and Ben Schifrin set out to follow the official route as closely as possible, whether by trail or cross-country. Schifrin—who would go on to coauthor early editions of the California volume of this guidebook—had to drop out with a broken foot at Odell Lake, Oregon (he finished the route the next year), but Eames got to Canada and is probably the first person to have walked the official route almost without deviation.

In 1975 at least 27 people completed the PCT, according to Chuck Long, who was one of them and who put together a book of various trekkers' experiences. Perhaps as many as 200–300 hikers started the trail that year, intending to do it all. In 1976 one who made it all the way was Teddi Boston, the first woman to solo the trail. Like Ryback, the 49-year-old mother of four made the trek the hard way, north to south.

Fascination with the trail steadily dropped, so that by the late 1980s, perhaps only a dozen or so thru-hikers completed the entire trail in a given year. However, as completion of the trail approached, interest in it waxed, and some notable hikes were done. As enthusiasm for the trail continued to grow, so did a thirst for chronicling the personal stories and adventures of individual hikers. Countless PCT memoirs can be found on bookstore shelves and blogs these days, providing both useful data for serious hikers and enjoyment for armchair adventurers.

However, in a trail guide, space is limited, so we will mention only a select few who set "higher" goals. In the past we recommended

that the thru-hiker allow five to six months for the entire PCT. No more, thanks to ultralight backpacking first espoused by Jenny and Ray Jardine. In 1991 the couple completed the entire trail (their second thru-hike) in only three months and three weeks, and Ray subsequently wrote a how-to book (see page 11) based on the accomplishment.

A few thru-hikers not only did the PCT but also did the two other major north–south National Scenic Trails, the Continental Divide Trail (CDT) and the Appalachian Trail (AT). The first triple-crown hiker may have been Jim Podlesney, hiking the AT in 1973, the PCT in 1975, and the CDT in 1979. Back in 1975 many new stretches of the PCT had yet to be built, and in 1979 the CDT's route was still largely a matter of whatever you chose it to be. By 1980 the PCT was essentially complete, except for gaps between the Mexican border and the southern Sierra and the initial southern Washington stretch. And with the PCT mostly complete, the first person who hiked it plus the AT and CDT may have been Lawrence Budd, who did all three in the late 1980s. Starting earlier but finishing later was Steve Queen, who hiked the PCT in 1981, the AT in 1983, and the CDT in 1991. The first woman may have been Alice Gmuer, who hiked the PCT in 1987 and 1988, the AT in 1990, and the CDT in 1993. Close behind was Brice Hammack, who over eight summers completed the last of the three trails in 1994—at the very respectable age of 74.

In the 21st century, some outstanding hiker-athletes have posted speed records and other fantastic on-trail accomplishments. A PCT thru-hike can take up to six months for most hikers. In 2006 triple-crown hiker Scott Williamson made it to Canada in three months and then turned around to return to the Mexico border, which he reached in three more months. This was his second yo-yo hike (back-to-back thru-hike) on the PCT and his ninth PCT thru-hike. (His first yo-yo was completed two years before on his fourth PCT thru-hike.)

In 2013 Heather Anderson traversed the route in 60 days, 17 hours. This was her second PCT thru-hike, and as of 2020, she holds the record for women on the trail. More recently, in 2016, 26-year-old Belgian dentist Karel Sabbe completed the trail with a new fastest-known-time record of 52 days, 8 hours, and 25 minutes. (There is no official record of PCT speed records; these numbers rely on verified GPS tracks and the honor of those making the claims.)

While there have been thousands of successful thru-hikers on the PCT, very few equestrians have matched this feat. Often, thru-hikers are unable to hike every foot of the trail (because of fire closures, snowpack, stream crossings, tree fall, or resupply exits), and for thru-equestrians, this feat has so far proved extremely challenging due to icy snowfields impassable for stock.

Perhaps the first equestrians to do the trail were Don and June Mulford in 1959. Barry Murray and his family rode it in two summers in the early 1970s. Much later, in 1988, Jim McCrae became the first thru-equestrian, completing the entire trail in just under five months. Retired veterinarian and former PCTA president Ben York rode the entire PCT on horseback in 1992 and again in 1996.

THE PCT IN THE 21st CENTURY

The escalation of social media and the internet had an unprecedented effect on the PCT in the last decade, creating new channels for hikers to stay connected and driving the increased popularity of the trail. Thru-hikers can now "meet" one another ahead of their starts through PCT Facebook groups, share information and ask questions on the discussion boards of Reddit, and post photos and videos from the trail on Instagram. The PCTA shares important updates and other data on its Twitter feed, @PCTAssociation, using the hashtag #PacificCrestTrail.

Cheryl Strayed's best-selling 2012 memoir *Wild* and the subsequent film of the same name, starring Reese Witherspoon, also had an impact on the PCT in the 21st century. Strayed recounted her 1,100-mile solo hike in 1995, weaving personal struggles with descriptions of stunning scenery and all the bruises, aches, and lost toenails that come with long-distance hiking. Strayed used a previous version of this guide, *Pacific Crest Trail, Volume 1: California* (before it was split into two), to navigate the first part of the trail. *Wild* won multiple awards and inspired many people to get on the trail.

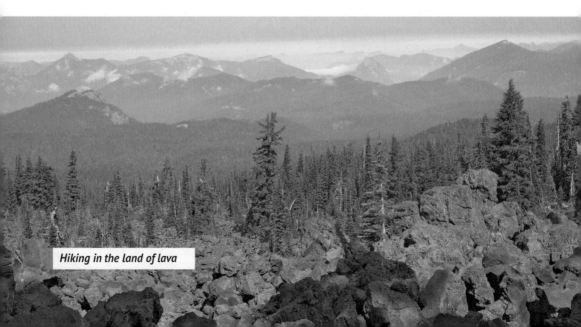

Hiking in the land of lava

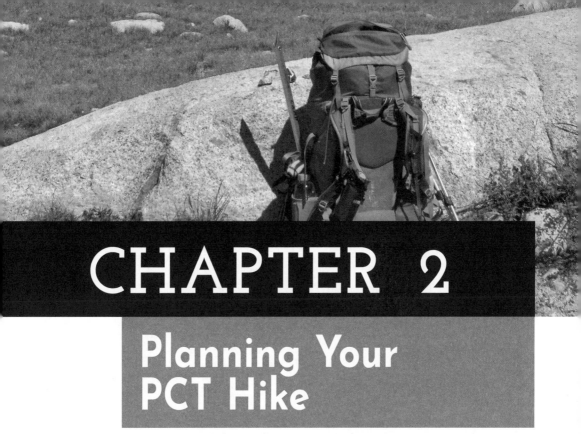

CHAPTER 2

Planning Your PCT Hike

TREKKING DAYS OR WEEKS VERSUS TREKKING MONTHS

On the basis of our limited research, we have concluded that the majority of those who buy this book will do parts of the Pacific Crest Trail (PCT) as a series of short excursions, each lasting about two weeks or less. More than 90% of all backpackers take a weekend to hike about 6 miles in from a trailhead to a known beauty spot—lake, mountain, stream—and return with memories of a wonderful trip. Others may venture out for a couple of weeks, seeing several beauty spots along the route.

For these hikers, less logistical planning is necessary than for thru-hikers, but there are still considerations. Depending on your goal, you may need to resupply once or twice. If so, identify the location—grocery store, post office, hostel—where you intend to resupply, and plan to carry sufficient food to reach the next resupply point, plus food for one extra day. Also consider what gear you will need. Will you be traveling solo, with a partner, or in a group? Going solo requires greater attention to gear weight than if you're sharing equipment with a partner or group. How long will you be gone? And what is your experience level? The answers to these questions will help you decide which items to pack. On the next page is a checklist to help with your packing. You may want to carry more or less, but regardless of your preferences, be prepared for potentially bad weather. Without food, your backpack should weigh only about 15–20 pounds; allow an additional 2 pounds per person

Above: The average backpack, without food, weighs 15–20 pounds.

ITEMS TO CONSIDER FOR YOUR HIKE

day pack/backpack (plus pack cover/pack liner)	biodegradable soap
PCT permit (must carry a paper copy at all times)/wilderness permit/CA campfire permit	quick-dry towel and/or washcloth
emergency contact information	trowel
paper maps; digital maps stored on your smartphone are a bonus	toilet paper
compass	zip-top bags for used toilet paper
GPS/tracking/emergency signal device	hand sanitizer
guidebook(s) (This one!)*	first aid kit and first aid notes*
emergency whistle	molefoam/blister kit
shelter (tent/tarp/mid/hammock/bivy sack)	mosquito repellent
sleeping bag	bear repellent (pepper spray)
sleeping pad or air mattress	headlamp and batteries
nylon or Tyvek ground cloth	smartphone
stuff sacks	watch
50 feet of 3-millimeter nylon cord (shelter guy outs/laundry line)	keys
hiking shoes or boots	wallet/cash/credit card/ATM card
socks (wool)	water bottle(s)/hydration bag
lightweight camp shoes or sandals	water purification system
shorts	mini lighter or matches in waterproof container
pants	stove/fuel/pot
T-shirt or short-sleeved shirt	bowl/cup
long-sleeved shirt	spoon/fork
wind shirt/sweatshirt	food/beverage mixes
thermal top/bottom	salt/pepper/spices
underwear	1-gallon odor-proof zip-top freezer bags (for food and trash)
swimsuit	bear-proof food-storage container
raingear or poncho (the latter can double as a ground cloth)	small pocketknife/small multitool
down puffy (vest/hoodie/jacket)	camera and accessories
warm cap/brimmed hat	micro-tripod
lightweight gloves	compact binoculars
bandanna	trekking poles
glasses/contact lenses	ice ax
sunglasses (polarized)	microspikes/crampons
sunscreen and lip balm (with sunscreen)	fishing gear and fishing license
personal-hygiene items	duct tape for emergencies (for example, broken pack, tent pole, or shoe)
prescription medications, plus list*	

*may be stored on smartphone

per day for food. If you are out for a week, your pack initially should be under 35 pounds. One thing is certain in backpacking: when the weight goes up, the fun goes down. When day or section hiking, it is easier to pinpoint your clothing requirements for that specific time of year. However, a lot can happen between point A and point B, so it is important to research what you might encounter in each section or state that you choose to hike. Ultimately, your preparations must include, at the least, a way to return to your car or reach home at the end of your hike.

Much of the PCT in Oregon and Washington can be day hiked, averaging about 15 miles a day. Over some sections you'll do less than 5 miles, while over others you'll do more than 25 (but less than 30). There are at least five advantages to day hiking. First, access is easier and less complicated. The national parks and the popular wilderness areas require wilderness permits for overnight stays, and some popular PCT stretches even have trailhead quotas for overnighters, but fewer areas require permits for day hikers. Second, day hiking does not require in-depth planning or preparation—though you should always be prepared for changing weather, carry the Ten Essentials, and know your limitations. Have a plan for emergencies—inform a trusted friend of your whereabouts and leave a list of what to do if you don't return as promised. Third, because your pack is lighter, you may enjoy the hike more because you'll expend less effort and suffer less wear and tear on your body, especially your feet. Day hikers can usually get by with running shoes or cross-training boots, which are much lighter than hiking boots and cause less wear on the trails. Fourth, you can easily carry a day's supply of water, so you won't have to worry about finding or purifying water. And finally, day hikers have less impact on the environment, as they usually use toilets near trailheads rather than along the trail. Particularly around a popular lake, excrement can affect the water quality; for instance, excrement from humans infected with *Giardia lamblia*,

discussed under "Waterborne Microscopic Organisms" (page 35), can lead to the establishment of these microorganisms in a previously untainted lake or stream.

If you prefer shorter outings, consider obtaining Wilderness Press's Day & Section Hikes series on the PCT. The series is divided by region and sold in four guides: Southern California, Northern California, Oregon, and Washington. (For books on or related to the PCT, see the "Pacific Crest Trail" section under "Recommended Reading and Source Books" [page 339]. For books on general hiking or riding, see the "Backpacking, Packing, and Mountaineering" section.)

At the other end of the spectrum of PCT trekkers are the growing number of thru-hikers (919 in 2019) who attempt to do the entire trail in one multimonth effort. Before the early 1990s there was a rather high attrition rate among these thru-hikers—typically 50%–80% didn't complete it. This need not be so. Today, there are great books and online resources available to prepare you mentally, physically, and logistically for this odyssey, as well as free smartphone apps and crowd-sourced water reports to guide you every step of the way.

Jenny and Ray Jardine were instrumental in a long-distance backpacking revolution with their 1992 how-to book *The Pacific Crest Trail Hiker's Handbook*, published by AdventureLore Press (unfortunately, out of print since the late 1990s). The Jardines' book advocated ultralight backpacking. If you have only 20 pounds on your back, you'll be able to traverse more miles per day than if you have 60. No longer do you have to take five-and-a-half to six-and-a-half months for a thru-hike; traveling light, you can do it in five months or less (the Jardines did it in less than four months). Ultralight gear has gained popularity since then and is championed by big and small outfitters alike. Richard A. Light's *Backpacking the Light Way* (Menasha Ridge Press, 2015) takes a thorough look at packing lightly and efficiently without compromising safety or comfort. Geared to both beginner and advanced hikers, it is packed with tips on planning, specific gear options, helpful techniques, and winter conditions.

There are several advantages to ultralight backpacking. A lighter pack is easier on your joints and muscles, making the excursion more pleasurable. Furthermore, by traveling light, you are less likely to have an injury because 1) your body isn't overstressed; 2) you're less likely to fall; and 3) if you do, the impact isn't as great. Traveling light, you'll perspire less, which is a plus on the long dry stretches. Additionally, you'll burn fewer calories, getting by with less food and, hence, less weight. By reducing your pack's weight to less than 20% of your body weight (that is, about 25–35 pounds for most hikers), you can probably get by with lightweight running or walking shoes, or even high-quality hiking sandals, making you less prone to the painful blisters synonymous with almost all boots. Both lighter packs and lighter footgear increase your daily mileage, providing an advantage other than comfort. You can start later and finish earlier, thereby encountering fewer storm-and-snow problems in the High Sierra early in your trek and in Washington near completion.

However, there is a drawback to ultralight backpacking. If you're caught in a blizzard or some other adverse condition, you may not have sufficient gear to survive; indeed, some ultralighters on long-distance trails have died. Light's book offers specifics on dealing with winter conditions, including shelter and food considerations and contingency planning. Also—and this applies to everyone, whether you take four or six months for a thru-hike—foremost on your mind will be keeping to your schedule, but because unexpected events or trail conditions can delay you and force you to make up for lost time, you likely won't have the time or energy to stop and smell the flowers. For this reason alone, our suggestion to those intent on doing the entire trail is to do it in two to five or more hiking seasons, each trip one

to three months long, taking sufficient time to enjoy your trek. For most hikers, 15 miles per day under optimal trail and weather conditions is far more pleasurable than 25 miles per day under high-pressure conditions.

An excellent book on hiking long-distance trails is Karen Berger's *Hiking the Triple Crown: How to Hike America's Longest Trails: Appalachian Trail, Pacific Crest Trail, Continental Divide Trail* (Mountaineers Books, 2001). Where Light's and the Jardines' books advocate ultralight backpacking, Berger offers a smorgasbord of choices, as each successful thru-hiker has his or her own preferences. The first third of her book is a how-to on long-distance backpacking, while the remainder addresses issues specific to the AT, PCT, and CDT. A more detailed and PCT-specific volume is *The Pacific Crest Trail: A Hiker's Companion* (Countryman Press, 2014) by Berger and Daniel R. Smith; if you plan to be on the PCT for more than a month, read it.

Long-distance backpackers should consider several other books. One that many hikers feel is indispensable is *Yogi's Pacific Crest Trail Handbook* (Yogi's Books, 2019) by Jackie McDonnell, which has detailed advice on the mechanics of keeping supplied and in touch with humanity while hiking long-distance trails. Triple-crowner McDonnell offers details on things one thinks about after deciding to hike, such as resources to consult, logistics of each resupply and what supplies to expect, and services available for most PCT towns or resorts, complete with detailed maps. More than half of the pages are perforated to be sent to resupply points, along with food, maps, and so on.

Paul Bodnar's *Pocket PCT: Complete Data and Town Guide* (2016) also offers detailed accounts of supplies and services available for most PCT towns or resorts, each with a map compatible with the popular Guthooks smartphone app. The book is great for planning and, at under 5 ounces, is easy to carry.

How-to books and reference books are certainly useful in preparing for and planning a thru-hike, but so are personal accounts, and several (both in print and out-of-print) are listed under "Recommended Reading and Source Books" (page 339). Larger libraries may have copies of out-of-print books. There's nothing like firsthand accounts to give you a feel for the thru-hike and its challenges.

Given that few equestrians attempt most or all of the PCT, it is not surprising that a how-to book for them does not exist. However, PCT veterans Adeline and Ben York, who covered the entire trail on horseback twice, recommended earlier editions of the packers' bible, *Horses, Hitches, and Rocky Trails* by Joe Back (Johnson Books, 2018). You will encounter more problems than do backpackers, and so the following caution is even more important: a short horseback trip does *not* qualify you for a lengthy excursion on the PCT.

PHYSICAL FITNESS

Whether you are section hiking or thru-hiking, backpacking is exceptionally hard work. Plan to begin your conditioning long before you think you need to. There are numerous sources for conditioning routines geared specifically for hikers. *Backpacker* magazine features at least one in each issue, often including multipage, full-body routines and strategies to benefit from them. You can also find excellent conditioning advice in *The Joy of Backpacking* (also by Wilderness Press), specifically in the chapter on "Getting Fit for the Trail."

Of course, the best way to get in shape for your PCT hike is to get out and go hiking! Menasha Ridge Press publishes the 60 Hikes Within 60 Miles series for almost 30 metropolitan areas throughout the United States. Snag one of these guidebooks, get out on the trail, and get fit.

If you have any medical concerns, be sure to consult with your doctor and share your backpacking plans before you begin training.

PERMITS

If you will be traveling fewer than 500 miles on the PCT, you will need to obtain your permit from the local agency for the trailhead from which you will start. Check the website of the agency to learn about quotas and other restrictions. Permits and campsite reservations should be investigated well in advance. Increasingly, permits can be acquired on recreation .gov. This is an easy way to obtain your permit, but it is not available in all cases.

In Crater Lake National Park, if you're not thru-hiking, you must obtain a permit at the park visitor center for backcountry camping. PCT thru-hikers do not need a permit but must be sure to sign the trail register as they enter the park. In North Cascades National Park, Pacific Crest Trail Association (PCTA) long-distance permit holders (see below) no longer need to obtain a backcountry camping permit for Six Mile Camp and Bridge Creek Camp. All other hikers must obtain a backcountry permit at designated ranger stations in advance for camping inside the park. Visit nps.gov/noca/planyourvisit/permits.htm   for details. Beginning in 2021, you will need a Central Cascades Wilderness Permit to visit the Mount Jefferson, Mount Washington, and Three Sisters Wilderness Areas. For updated information visit fs.usda.gov/detail/willamette /passes-permits/recreation/?cid=fseprd688355.

Anyone planning to hike or horseback ride 500 or more continuous miles on the PCT should obtain an interagency long-distance permit from the PCTA. Permits are free, but there are limits to the number of permits available.

In an effort to manage the increasing numbers of long-distance hikers hitting the trail, stricter permitting regulations were implemented in 2020 for both north- and southbound hikes. All thru-hikers starting at or near the Mexican border between March 1 and May 31 need to obtain a long-distance permit from the PCTA. Through an agreement with the

U.S. Forest Service (USFS), National Park Service, Bureau of Land Management, and other agencies, the PCTA usually begins accepting permit applications via its website in October for northbound hikers and in January for southbound hikers. The permit must be printed out and carried at all times. The application opening dates are subject to change, and the permits have various terms that you must follow, so be sure to visit pcta.org/discover-the-trail/permits at the start of your planning phase for the most updated information.

Crossing the Border

If you're planning to cross into Canada from the United States, you must obtain permission from the Canada Border Services Agency (CBSA)/Government of Canada and carry a paper copy of your approved Canada PCT Entry Permit with you at all times while in Canada. Apply for this permit at least 8–10 weeks before the start of your hike. Visit pcta.org/discover-the-trail/permits/canada-pct-entry-permit to download the application and get the latest information on this matter. Follow the simple instructions, and then scan and submit your application by email. If your trip is merely one into Canada to E. C. Manning Provincial Park and then a prompt return to the United States by vehicle or other transportation (such as bus), then you won't have to report to Canada Customs.

When you download the application form, you'll also get an information sheet. Basically, you need to know the following: Foremost, you must have photo identification that proves evidence of your citizenship, such as a passport, Enhanced Driver's License, or Nexus Card. Guns and most other weapons are banned, but a hunting knife or pocketknife (no switchblades) is OK. Don't take your dog or fresh fruit and vegetables across the border.

If you're an equestrian, you'll need a USDA Export Health Certificate for your stock. Get this from a USDA accredited veterinarian, who will send it to the USDA veterinary service in Olympia, Washington (360-753-9430). They will return it to your veterinarian. You should do this within 30 days of your border crossing, which is very inconvenient for those planning to spend several months on the trail. Once in Canada, you must take your stock directly to Canada Customs at Huntingdon, B.C., or Osoyoos, B.C.

Note: There is no legal way to enter the United States from Canada (E. C. Manning Provincial Park) on the PCT. Don't try it.

INTERNET RESEARCH AND APPS

In recent years, blogs and social media have changed the way hikers research and plan

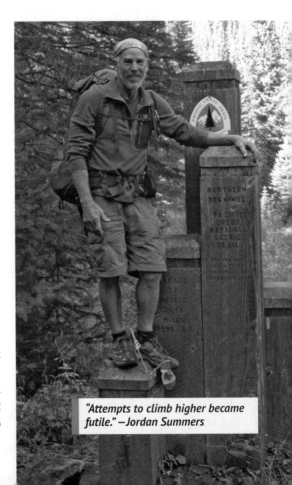

"Attempts to climb higher became futile." —Jordan Summers

their PCT experience. Many hikers chronicle their every step with photos, anecdotes, and advice posted on personal blogs or websites created exclusively for their PCT adventures. (Trailjournals.com and postholer.com are two popular hiking sites with PCT sections.) And don't forget to join the strong PCT-based groups on social media: each year's class of thru-hikers has a Facebook group that serves as a real-time forum to ask questions, offer suggestions and updates, and post photos along the way. One intrepid hiker was even able to regain the phone he forgot at a trail angel property (places that host thru-hikers with tent sites, water, and other amenities) by communicating with fellow trekkers who had stayed behind.

The PCTA does a good job of posting current blog entries for each PCT class on its website. It also posts regular updates and photos on Facebook, Twitter, and Instagram under the moniker PCTAssociation. Favorite hashtags include #pacificcresttrail, #PCTrail, and #PCT2020 (or current year). Some hikers use the PCT's Facebook page, facebook.com /PCTAFan, to connect with others while on the trail. Another rich source of first-person accounts and advice is the PCTA's blog: pcta .org/blog.

The internet is especially helpful in looking for current trail closures and restrictions before each trip. Visit pcta.org/closures for closure information and consult local agency websites (page 26) for permit information and to find out if fire bans are in place.

Also be sure to check the essential PCT water report (pctwater.com), which provides, via hikers reporting from the trail, the most updated information on water sources. It will tell you when water tanks are empty, guzzlers are accessible, and seasonal streams are down to a trickle. Most Southern California PCTers print out a copy before heading out on the trail and keep it with them at all times.

Finally, Guthook Guides provides trail location and campsite data in a simple smartphone app that is compatible with both iPhone and Android devices.

Staying Wired

Hikers with electronics (such as smartphones, GPS, or personal location devices) can keep their batteries juiced up if they carry battery packs or solar chargers. Hikers can also use the charging blocks and cables at on- and off-trail hospitality or resupply stops, though such charging stations are sporadic. Often there is a choice of power strips, but at the least, duplex outlets are always available for hikers' use. Some trail angel properties have them, while others don't. Observant hikers look for open outlets to use while eating in restaurants, doing laundry, buying groceries, drinking cool beverages, and any other temporarily sedentary activity where the lights are on. However, always be sure to ask businesses before charging and use common courtesy. Don't linger for hours at a restaurant charging your devices and taking up a table unless you've been given permission to do so. And don't expect that free power will always be available; if you really want power, consider paying for a hotel room.

Keeping your batteries charged does not imply that you'll have a signal when you most need one. Most hikers look forward to unplugging on the trail, but there are times that seeing a bar or two of service pop up in a remote area is a welcome surprise. Like many aspects of this mighty and temperamental trail, cell phone coverage on the PCT is unpredictable. Sometimes it shows up in places you least expect it, like Donohue Pass at 11,000 feet in the Ansel Adams Wilderness. On the other hand, it can be nonexistent in places where we take it for granted, like trailheads with big parking areas and nature centers.

Regardless of your carrier, you'll be disappointed with coverage along the PCT. If staying connected is vital for you, consider purchasing a second phone with another carrier or an unlocked phone with SIM cards for two carriers.

Finally, if you do use your phone on the trail, be sure to take it out of sight and earshot of others. Be courteous and don't intrude on anyone else's wilderness experience.

TRAIL ADVICE

Once you have your wilderness permit (if required) and a full pack, you are ready to start hiking. The following advice, most of it from the National Park Service and USFS, will help make your hike safer and more enjoyable.

The wilderness permit does not serve as a registration system for hikers. Leave your itinerary, route description, and expected time of return with a responsible person back home. Also leave instructions on what to do if you don't arrive or make contact as planned. You must be specific on what the contact is to do when the deadline arrives: "Call the sheriff of the county in which I am hiking; say that I am an overdue PCT hiker, and give them my description." Fill in all the details so your stand-in has no decisions to make. Be specific and make sure you connect as planned.

Stay on maintained trails unless you are good at using a compass and topographic maps. When off the trail, you can easily lose your sense of direction, especially in a viewless forest or in bad weather. If you become disoriented, don't panic. As soon as you think you may be off track, stop, assess your current direction, and then retrace your steps to the point where you went astray. Using a map, a compass, and this book, and keeping in mind what you have passed thus far, reorient yourself, and trust your judgment on which way to continue.

Note: About 10% of the PCT is on private land. Always obey signs and do not go off trail, camp, or follow side trails in these areas.

Solo hiking can be dangerous, particularly if you have large streams to ford. If you do set out alone, stick to frequently used trails so that you can get help if you become sick or injured.

Watch your step on trails. The mountains are no place to get a sprained ankle.

Take a wilderness first aid course. Accidents happen on the PCT, so make sure you're prepared to handle them. Your safety is your responsibility.

If you want to wear hiking boots, make sure they are well broken-in to avoid blisters. Wear two pairs of socks and carry moleskin just in case.

If you bring children along, be sure they have personal identification on them at all times. Tell them what to do if they get lost (they should stay put), and give them a whistle or other means of signaling for help. Don't leave them alone; there are mountain lions out there (see page 31).

Confusion about which trail to take at junctions frequently results in spread-out parties becoming separated. To avoid confusion and the possibility of someone getting lost, faster party members should wait for slower members at all trail junctions. If members of your party want to travel at different paces, then be sure enough of them have a marked map that shows the party's route and campsite for each night.

Be prepared for rain or snow any time of the year. Learn survival techniques, especially how to stay warm and dry in inclement weather.

Always use sun protection when hiking. Wear sunglasses and a hat, and always use a lip balm and sunscreen, both with an SPF of 30 or higher. Also note the expiration date on the tube or bottle.

Don't underestimate the power of moving water, particularly since streambeds tend to be quite slippery. One of the greatest dangers to backcountry travelers is crossing streams. Whitewater and areas above cascades and waterfalls are especially dangerous. Visit pcta.org/discover-the-trail/backcountry-basics/water/stream-crossing-safety for an in-depth discussion on how to safely navigate stream crossings.

Lightning is a hazard in the mountains. You can gauge how far away a lightning strike is by counting the seconds it takes for thunder to arrive after you see lightning flash. A 5-second delay means the strike was about a mile away. A 1-second delay means that it was about 1,000 feet away and you are too close for comfort—absolutely seek shelter. Do not continue upward into a thunderstorm. Get off ridges and peaks. Stay away from meadows and lakes, and avoid exposed lone objects such as large rocks, isolated trees, railings, cables, and sizable objects. Find shelter in forested areas among same-size trees. Your vehicle is a safe place to wait out a storm.

It's possible to hike portions of the PCT with your dog, but it requires a great deal of planning and preparation. Dogs are allowed on the PCT in some national and state parks but not others. Visit pcta .org/discover-the-trail/backcountry-basics/dogs for everything you need to consider when thinking about bringing your dog on your PCT adventure.

Water Caches

Water caches are containers of water left on or near the trail by an informal and unorganized community of volunteers. They are especially prominent along dry stretches of the Southern California portion of the PCT. Well-known water caches are noted in the sections of this book, **but they should never be counted on, under any circumstances.**

One of the intentions of long-distance hiking on trails such as the PCT is to promote self-reliance. Hikers should be prepared to carry enough water and not depend on water caches, as they can run dry, be tampered with, and sometimes contribute to large quantities of litter on the trail. The best way to monitor the water situation on the PCT is to regularly check the crowd-sourced PCT Water Report at pctwater.com.

LEAVE NO TRACE

With thousands of hikers using the PCT, there is a virtual string of people progressing down the trail, competing for drinking, camping, and bathing space—and elimination space. Welcome, Leave No Trace!

The Leave No Trace (LNT) philosophy became a movement helped along by professionals at the USFS and the National Outdoor Leadership School (NOLS). NOLS recorded

and reported on the impact of leading students into the same areas and the effect it was having on each ecosystem they visited, specifically those that were revisited annually. Learning what worked and what did not was based on these observations. It depends a lot on locale—coastal, desert, forest, mountain. Each ecosystem requires specific care.

There are only seven LNT principles, and they are all common sense. Most PCT hikers embrace them automatically.

The member-driven Leave No Trace Center for Outdoor Ethics teaches people how to enjoy the outdoors responsibly. These copyrighted principles have been reprinted with permission from the Leave No Trace Center for Outdoor Ethics: LNT.org.

1. Plan ahead and prepare. PCT hikers have no choice but to start early and plan ahead—to bring gear that can serve multiple purposes, to anticipate supply needs (food and fuel), and to handle the logistics of resupplying.

2. Travel and camp on durable surfaces. Just by our numbers, we stress the ecosystems we traverse. When hiking, stay on maintained trails, and don't cut across switchbacks, as this leads to trail erosion and wastes precious trail maintenance resources when volunteers must head out to repair damage.

Camp in existing sites, at least 200 feet away from water and the trail. Campsites too close to water sources cause water pollution. Also stay away from meadows, which are easily destroyed in one season by just a few inconsiderate acts. For an excellent sleep, try granite slabs. Never build new fire rings.

3. Dispose of waste properly. The old cliché is still true: if you can pack it in, you can pack it out. Litter and food scraps are not only unsightly but also an unnatural food source that attracts animals—bears and rodents in particular. Your food source is simply detrimental to their well-being. All trash, including cans, bottles, foil, tampons, disposable diapers, toilet paper, orange peels, and apple cores, must be packed out. Do not burn or bury trash or scatter organic waste. Carry plastic bags for trash.

When it comes to human waste in the wilderness, we all need to learn to handle it properly or we'll soon literally be on top of it. Giardia spreads when waste is not disposed of away from water sources (see page 35 for information on giardia). At least 200 feet from streams, lakes, and springs is perfect. Dig a hole in the soil down to the mineral layer (sand or rock) about 6–8 inches deep and large enough for your deposit. This part is a must-do before business. Have other materials at hand—leaves, smooth rocks, wet moss, cones, or smooth sticks. If you need toilet paper, have a couple of zip-top bags to carry it out in. Do not place a large rock over your waste. Think about this the next time before *you* move a rock to excavate beneath it. Simply cover the hole with the excavated soil.

The issue of human waste has become far more serious in the past few seasons. Campsites formerly noted for their desirability are now surrounded by a dozen paths, each leading to a stomped-out 10-foot-diameter area full of surface turds and tissue blooms. These are not only unsightly, smelly, and disgusting, but they are also an extreme health hazard. Before taking a long hike, know and practice how to safely treat human waste in the wilderness. It's your responsibility.

Chemicals found in both biodegradable and nonbiodegradable soaps and detergents pollute backcountry waters, and pollution by organic waste has caused bacteria to spread through many lakes and streams. Unfortunately, our own bodies, as carriers of bacteria, contribute to the problem. Reduce your impact by cleaning pots, washing clothes, and bathing yourself at least 100 feet away from any body of water. You can clean your pots quite well with a small piece of a scrubby sponge and some warm water. To eliminate the need for pot scrubbing, as well as the weight of pots, a stove, and fuel, you could eat cold meals; indeed, many trekkers have hiked the entire PCT this way.

4. Leave what you find. Along this trail, you are going to see wonderful sights. Leave each spot as you found it; do not add to or alter it. At your campsite, minimize your impact: don't clear away brush, level the ground, cut trenches, or build a fire ring. Don't destroy, deface, or carve up trees, shrubs, or any other natural or cultural features.

5. Minimize campfire impacts. Wildfires are caused by lightning strikes and human carelessness. The first cannot be prevented; the second is completely under your control. If you must build a fire, and it's legal and appropriate, use only deadwood lying on the ground, build it no larger than you actually need, and use an existing fire ring. Put it out at least half an hour before you are ready to leave, adding water to it and stirring the ashes. In the High Sierra, fires are usually banned at elevations above 9,000 feet. At a few popular backcountry lakes, camping and/or campfires are banned; these are mentioned in the text. Finally, fires are almost always banned in Southern California. And during dry summers, especially the second half of summer, campfires are often banned everywhere. Always check with the local land management agency to see if fires are allowed before you build one. For more information on wildfire safety, visit pcta.org /discover-the-trail/backcountry-basics/fire.

6. Respect wildlife. Water instabilities over the past decade have been a major stressor on wildlife in every biozone. Observing wildlife from a distance will allow you to see much more than if you approach. Wild creatures in general do not need your food. Don't hand it out, don't leave it behind, and don't surrender it. Protect it properly (see page 30), and enjoy eating it yourself.

7. Be considerate of other visitors. We each get to have our own wilderness experience, so don't, by sight or sound, deny others theirs. When you meet pack stock on the trail, speak quietly and remain in plain view. Allow them to pass by stepping off the trail on the downslope side; equestrians have the right-of-way. Close all gates. They prevent stock from wandering up and down the trail.

WEATHER

If you adequately prepare for inclement weather, your backpack trip won't be all that bad even if such weather occurs. What's more, while most of the discussion below is about avoiding rain and snow, and certainly that's the goal for most hikers, don't forget that the PCT is a world-class place to ski, snowshoe, mountaineer, and enjoy snowy solitude and beauty. During fall, winter, and spring, you truly have endless opportunities for winter recreation, with hundreds of access points.

The warmest temperatures are in mid-July through early August; they can vary from the 90s in southern Oregon to the 70s in the North Cascades. During this period, night temperatures for the entire two-state route are usually in the 40s but at times can be in the 50s or the 30s, and occasionally in the 20s.

In late June, with its long daylight hours, the maximum and minimum temperatures are almost as high as those in midsummer. In addition, you can expect to be plagued with mosquitoes through early August. A tent is a necessity; without one you won't get a mosquito-free sleep until later in the season when the nights are cooler. A tent not only helps you get a good night's sleep but may also prevent serious disease. Mosquitoes in Oregon and Washington have been identified as vectors in the transmission of West Nile virus and western equine encephalitis.

By late August, the days become considerably shorter and the temperatures lower. Evenings and nights in southern Oregon are comfortable, but those in northern Washington are nippy, if not freezing. Expect to see morning frost on your tent, and prepare for brisk days. Also, there's likely to be a water shortage, particularly in most of Oregon. An advantage of a hike at this time, however, is that both Oregon and Washington will have a magnificent variety of berries ready for picking. You will want to budget plenty of extra time for berry-grazing.

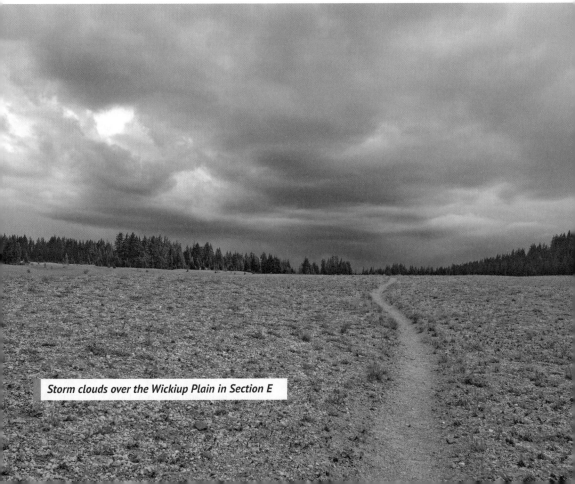

Storm clouds over the Wickiup Plain in Section E

Storms

Another consideration is storms. Storm frequency increases northward. In central Oregon, the period of good weather is only July–August, and even then occasional storms may be expected. If you visit southern Washington, be prepared for bad weather, even though you might get to hike a week or two at a time in beautiful midsummer weather. Expect bad or threatening weather in northern Washington. It is possible to hike two solid weeks in the North Cascades without receiving a drop of precipitation, but don't count on it—you might just as well receive a month of rain.

The cumulonimbus clouds that create thunderstorms build in the afternoon, and the storms themselves typically occur from midafternoon into early evening—that is, from about 2 or 3 p.m. until about 7 or 8 p.m. Therefore, if you have an exposed alpine pass to cross, try to do it before midafternoon. As mentioned in "Trail Advice" earlier in this chapter, if you see the clouds looming and hear distant thunder, be prepared to seek shelter. Exposed high lands are no place to be dodging lightning strikes.

Best Times to Hike

If you want to avoid snow-clad trails, incessant mosquitoes, and severe water shortages, hike the following segments at these recommended times (remembering, of course, that weather patterns vary considerably from year to year).

Seiad Valley, Siskiyou Mountains, southern Oregon: June–mid-September

Mount McLoughlin, Sky Lakes basin, Seven Lakes basin: Mid-July–late August

Crater Lake: July

Mount Thielsen, Windigo Pass, Diamond Peak: Mid-July–late August

Three Sisters: Late July–early August

Mount. Washington, Three Fingered Jack: Late June–mid-July

Mount Hood: Late July–mid-August

Columbia River Gorge, southern Washington: Mid-June–early September

Mount Adams, Goat Rocks, White Pass, Mount Rainier, Stampede Pass, Snoqualmie Pass, Stevens Pass: Mid-July–mid-August

Glacier Peak, North Cascades, E. C. Manning Provincial Park: Late July–early August

There are, of course, advantages and disadvantages to hiking in any season. In the North Cascades, for example, early June will present you with spectacular snow-clad alpine scenery—but also soft-snow walking and a slight avalanche hazard. Early July will present you with a riotous display of wildflowers—plus sucking mosquitoes and biting flies. Early August will present you with the best trail conditions—and lots of backpackers. Early September will present you with fall colors and ripe huckleberries—but also nippy nights and sudden snowstorms.

THRU-HIKING SEASON, SOUTH TO NORTH

Choosing an optimal hiking month is not an option for thru-hikers bound for the Canadian border. They must start at the Mexican border by mid-May, when there isn't too much snow at higher elevations. The hike through Antelope Valley (the western part of the Mojave Desert) can be grueling, usually too hot and always too dry. But a couple of weeks later, thru-hikers will be entering the High Sierra, which will be snowy. Not until early July, when hopefully they've reached I-80 at Donner Pass, will their problems be over—temporarily: snowstorms may await them in Washington in September.

Precipitation Considerations for Thru-Hikers

If you plan to thru-hike and can choose the year to do it, pick one in which the southern half of the Sierra and all lands south of it (Sections A–H, in *Pacific Crest Trail: Southern California*) are having a relatively dry year. (This requires some serious trust in *The Farmer's Almanac* and a huge dose of hiker optimism.) In theory, though springs will dry up earlier in Southern California, with a light Sierra snowpack, you can start a month sooner, in early April rather than in early May. However, by the time you reach Oregon, perhaps in early August, the snow problems may not be that bad and the snow will continue to melt as you advance north. Another bonus of hiking in such a year is that you can finish by early or mid-September, before the frontal storms start coming in thick and fast, besieging you with one snow dusting after another.

Perhaps the worst kind of year is one with heavy precipitation both in the central and southern Sierra Nevada and in Southern California. On the plus side, springs and seasonal streams will be flowing in Southern California. On the minus side, the snowpack can slow you down in Southern California's mountains, and especially in the Sierra. Hiking slower than average, you could run out of time, for Washington's North Cascades can be snowbound and that section can be indecipherable by the time you reach it.

In the Lake Tahoe and Desolation Wilderness vicinity, moisture from the Bay Area is funneled up the American and Yuba River canyons. The moisture rises and cools as it blows in from sea level to 10,000 feet. By about 3 p.m. on any day, thunderclouds may form over the crest and unleash a locally ferocious 25-minute rain- or hailstorm with all the accompanying lightning. Then, sunshine and ice-water puddles take over the trail. Scheduled storms tend to be behind you once you reach Sierra City.

Once hikers pass the Bridge of the Gods, the trail begins to move to the east side of the Cascades. Here, you can almost see the divide in the sky as clouds from the coast move in, hit the mountains, and as in the Sierra, halt and dump their load of water on the west side, leaving usually anxious PCT hikers quite dry.

For the most updated information on the water situation in Oregon and Washington, check the PCT Water Report (pctwater.com) or the website of the PCTA, pcta.org. It keeps track of trail conditions, including drinking-water availability, snow problems, and other issues pertinent to the PCT trekker.

Drought, Wildfires, and Flooding

Natural disasters and extreme weather conditions can cause all kinds of challenges and setbacks for thru-hikers. Preparation and awareness are essential and could save your life. Severe drought struck California between 2009 and 2016, spurring Governor Jerry Brown to declare a drought state of emergency for the entire region. This had a significant impact on the PCT and anyone who traversed it. Once-reliable natural water sources dried up, forcing hikers to carry even more water through long dry stretches. Wildfires burned longer and wider, some in areas still recovering from past fire damage. Stretches of trail were closed for months or even years to allow for recovery and trail repairs. An unprecedented string of wildfires in Oregon and Washington in late summer 2017 forced many hikers off the trail or resulted in hikes that were uncomfortably dominated by smoke and hazy views.

Conversely, the heavy rains and snowfall that hit California in the winter of 2016–17 led to dangerously high river levels; two thru-hikers drowned in separate incidents while crossing swollen rivers in the Sierra Nevada in July 2017. Others were forced to take so many detours or wait out brutal conditions that a new slogan emerged for the season: "2017—We tried."

The record rains and snowfall in the winter of 2016–17, as well as an exceptionally wet 2018–19 season, did help pull most of the state out of its emergency drought status, but experts say its aquifers, forests, and wildlife ecosystems have a long road to recovery and may be forever altered by their desiccated states.

Regardless of the drought status, the high volume of snowmelt has an impact on the depth and velocity of creeks and rivers. Plan your stream crossing for early morning when the snowmelt is at its lowest for the day. And don't be shy about asking to buddy up with another hiker or two if you are lightweight or inexperienced.

Hypothermia

Hypothermia is the rapid and progressive mental and physical collapse that accompanies chilling of the human body's inner core. The condition is caused by exposure to cold and is intensified by wetness, wind, and exhaustion. Therefore, it's always a good idea to carry raingear. An unexpected storm could otherwise soak you to the bone. Hypothermia almost always occurs at temperatures well above freezing. Anyone who becomes fatigued in wet and windy conditions is a potential victim. If you experience a bout of uncontrolled shivering, you should seriously consider yourself a candidate for hypothermia and take appropriate countermeasures.

The best defense against hypothermia is to avoid exposure. Stay dry. When clothing is wet, it can lose as much as 90% of its insulating value, draining heat from the body. Wool and synthetic fibers such as polypropylene and Polartec retain most of their insulating value when wet, unlike cotton, down, and some synthetics. Buy breathable garments with a durable water repellent (DWR), made by various manufacturers. Be aware of the wind. Even a slight breeze carries heat away from your body and forces cold air under, as well as through, clothing. Wind intensifies cold by evaporating moisture from the skin's surface. Put on raingear immediately, not after you are soaked. Add a layer of clothing under your raingear before shivering occurs. Wear a hat or ski cap, preferably made of wool or polypropylene, to protect and help retain body heat.

If your party fails to take these precautionary steps, a hiker with hypothermia may develop more advanced symptoms, which include slurred speech, drowsiness, amnesia, and frequent stumbling, followed by a decrease in shivering; hallucinations; and, finally, stupor, coma, and death. The victim may strongly deny he or she is in trouble. Believe the symptoms, not the patient. This is a serious condition to prepare for if you are planning on hiking solo.

It is far more dangerous to hike alone than in a group. You may not recognize the signs of hypothermia by yourself, and if you do, you may have a harder time restoring your body heat than if you had others to help you. In the mountains it is extremely important to keep your sleeping bag and a set of clothes dry. If they get wet and threatening weather prevails, try to get out of the mountains as quickly as possible. But don't abandon your pack to make a dash for the trailhead; this risks exposing yourself to the elements even more, and losing your shelter, food, and stove can be deadly. If the weather gets too bad, set up your tent in a sheltered area, keep warm and out of the elements, and stay put until the inclement weather abates. You'll be alive and have a great story to tell, and no one at work will care if you're a day late. You should not attempt to continue hiking in inclement weather.

HIGH-ALTITUDE PROBLEMS
Altitude Sickness

Altitude sickness may occur at elevations of about 8,000 feet or more. Symptoms include fatigue, weakness, headache, loss of appetite, nausea, vomiting, and shortness of breath on exertion. Everyone is affected differently; some are not affected at all. Symptoms are usually temporary and should not affect you for more than 48 hours. Sleep may be difficult for the first night and, if you are above 10,000 feet,

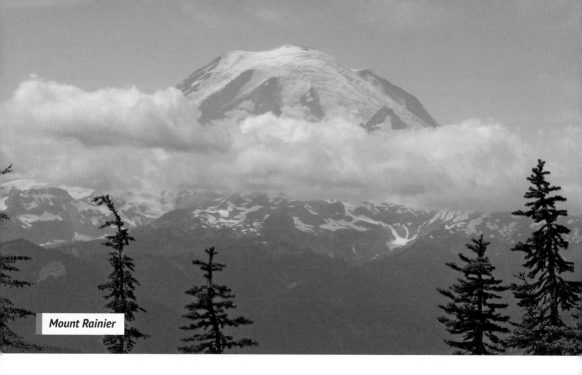

Mount Rainier

perhaps even for one or more additional nights. Regular periods of heavy breathing separated by periods of no breathing may awaken the sleeper with a sense of suffocation. Hyperventilation may also occur, causing light-headedness; dizziness; and tingling of the hands, feet, and mouth. Altitude sickness results from exposure to the oxygen-deficient atmosphere of high elevations. It is aggravated by fatigue and cold. Some people are more susceptible to it than others. As the body adjusts to the lower oxygen pressure, symptoms usually disappear. Resting and drinking extra liquids are recommended. If symptoms persist, descend to lower altitudes.

High-Altitude Pulmonary Edema

Though rare, this is a serious and potentially fatal condition. Cases have been reported at altitudes of 8,500 feet, but it usually occurs considerably higher. The basic problem, as with altitude sickness, is a reduction of oxygen, and early symptoms are often unrecognized or confused with altitude sickness. However, in the case of pulmonary edema, reduced oxygen initiates diversion

of blood from the body shell to the core, causing congestion of the lungs, brain, and other vital organs. Besides exhibiting symptoms similar to those of altitude sickness, the victim is restless, coughs, and eventually brings up frothy, blood-tinged sputum. The only treatment is immediate descent to at least 2,000 feet lower and, if available, administration of oxygen. You should secure medical help as soon as possible.

Blood in Urine

If you are at high elevations and exercising to the point of dehydration, you can, like serious long-distance runners, have reddish urine. You are not dying, but this is a good sign that you are overexerting yourself. Slow down.

Ultraviolet Radiation

You should always use sun protection when outdoors, but it is especially important above 9,000 feet, as the dangerous ultraviolet radiation at these elevations is very intense. Wear UV-absorbing or -reflecting sunglasses and a hat to protect your eyes. You can get quite a splitting headache if your eyes get too much radiation. Prolonged exposure to ultraviolet radiation increases your risk of skin cancer, so be liberal with sunscreen, and reapply frequently, on all your exposed skin.

TRAIL REGISTERS

Trail registers give hikers an idea of who did what, the relative degree of trail use, and annually and seasonally changing trail conditions and special concerns. By signing these registers, the backpacker over time develops a camaraderie with other trekkers. Though you may never catch up to those ahead of you, by trail's end you may feel that you've come to know them.

MAILING TIPS

If you will be on the trail long enough to bother with resupply points, you can use the table on the next page, which lists mostly post offices but also private businesses that accept packages. Expect to pay holding fees when mailing to private businesses, and be sure to check whether they accept UPS and FedEx only, USPS only, or all three. It's generally acceptable to mail a package to arrive about two weeks before you get there. If you mail it too early, your package may be returned to you.

Those who thru-hike the trail should consider buying *Yogi's Pacific Crest Trail Handbook* by Jackie McDonnell, as she gives up-to-date and complete post office hours, locations, and phone numbers. You should also visit pcta.org /discover-the-trail/thru-hiking-long-distance -hiking/resupply for additional sources of resupply locations. (Be aware that this kind of information has changed in the past and likely will in the future.) Finally, also check the introduction of each section for resupply information.

You can mail yourself almost any food, clothing, or equipment. Before you leave home, you should have a good idea of your consumption rate of food, clothing, and fuel for your stove. What you may not know is what you want to eat or what other items you may need in week two or three. So, when you decide what you want and need in the coming weeks, purchase those items at stores along the way and send

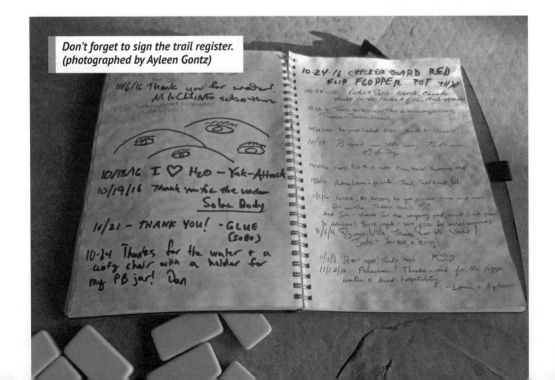

Don't forget to sign the trail register. (photographed by Ayleen Gontz)

packages forward for pickup. The buy-as-you-go approach supports local trail town economies, and the stores are nearly universally well prepared and stocked for hikers. However, if you have special dietary needs, you may want to ship your packages from home.

Address your package to:

[Your Legal Name]
PCT Hiker, ETA: MM/DD/YY
General Delivery
[Post Office, State Abbr. Zip Code]

Keep in mind that some post offices are seasonal. Hours of most are 9 a.m.–noon and 1–5 p.m. or longer. Some are open Saturday mornings. Plan your trip schedule accordingly to avoid waiting two or three days in town because an office was closed for the weekend (don't forget about the three-day weekends: Memorial Day, Fourth of July, Labor Day).

FEDERAL GOVERNMENT AGENCIES

The USFS has overall responsibility for managing the PCT. The large majority of the PCT lies on lands for which the USFS is the public steward.

The USFS partners with the Bureau of Land Management and National Park Service to manage and protect the trail. While all of these land-management agencies have similar regulations, each may have specific requirements. For example, some wilderness areas do not require a wilderness permit for entry, while others do. As stated earlier, the PCTA provides wilderness permits for trips of 500 miles or more on the PCT; however, hikers who plan to do less than 500 miles may need to apply

RESUPPLY POINTS ALONG OR NEAR THE ROUTE, SOUTH TO NORTH

OREGON
- Seiad Valley 96086
- Ashland, OR 97520
- Callahan's Mountain Lodge
  7100 Old US 99 S
  Ashland, OR 97520
- Fish Lake Resort
  OR 140, Mile Marker 30
  Eagle Point, OR 97524
- Mazama Village Camper Store
  USPS address:
  Mazama Village
  Crater Lake, OR 97604
  UPS/FedEx address:
  569 Mazama Village Dr.
  Crater Lake, OR 97604
- Diamond Lake, OR 97731
- Shelter Cove Resort & Marina
  27600 W. Odell Lake Road/OR 58
  Crescent Lake, OR 97733
- Elk Lake Resort
  60000 Century Dr.
  Bend, OR 97701
- Bend, OR 97703
- Sisters, OR 97759

- Big Lake Youth Camp
  26435 Big Lake Road
  Sisters, OR 97759
- Government Camp, OR 97028
- Timberline Lodge
  27500 E. Timberline Road
  Timberline Lodge, OR 97028
- Cascade Locks, OR 97014

WASHINGTON
- Stevenson, WA 98648
- Trout Lake, WA 98650
- Packwood, WA 98361
- Kracker Barrel Store
  48851 US 12
  Naches, WA 98937
- Summit Inn
  603 WA 906
  Snoqualmie Pass, WA 98068
- Skykomish, WA 98288
- Stevens Pass
  93001 NE Stevens Pass Hwy./US 2
  Skykomish, WA 98288
- Stehekin, WA 98852
- Goat's Beard Mountain Supplies
  44 Lost River Road
  Mazama, WA 98833

FEDERAL GOVERNMENT AGENCIES, SOUTH TO NORTH

- Klamath National Forest
  530-842-6131
  fs.usda.gov/klamath
  *Trinity Alps, Russian, and
  Marble Mountain Wildernesses*

- Cascade-Siskiyou National Monument*
  541-618-2200
  blm.gov/oregon-washington
  Soda Mountain Wilderness

- Crater Lake National Park*
  541-594-3000
  nps.gov/crla

- Rogue River–Siskiyou National Forest
  541-618-2200
  fs.usda.gov/rogue-siskiyou
  Sky Lakes Wilderness

- Fremont-Winema National Forest
  541-947-2151
  fs.usda.gov/fremont-winema
  Sky Lakes and Mount Thielsen Wildernesses

- Umpqua National Forest
  541-957-3200
  fs.usda.gov/umpqua
  Mount Thielsen Wilderness

- Deschutes National Forest
  541-383-5300
  fs.usda.gov/deschutes
  *Diamond Peak, Three Sisters,
  Mount Washington, and
  Mount Jefferson Wildernesses*

- Willamette National Forest
  541-225-6300
  fs.usda.gov/willamette
  *Diamond Peak, Three Sisters, Mount Washington,
  and Mount Jefferson Wildernesses*

- Mount Hood National Forest
  503-668-1700
  fs.usda.gov/mthood
  *Mount Jefferson, Mount Hood, and
  Mark O. Hatfield Wildernesses*

- Columbia River Gorge National Scenic Area
  541-308-1700
  fs.usda.gov/crgnsa

- Gifford Pinchot National Forest
  360-891-5000
  fs.usda.gov/giffordpinchot
  *Indian Heaven, Mount Adams, Goat Rocks, and
  William O. Douglas Wildernesses*

- Mount Rainier National Park*
  360-569-2211
  nps.gov/mora
  Mount Rainier Wilderness

- Okanogan-Wenatchee National Forest
  509-664-9200
  fs.usda.gov/okawen
  *Goat Rocks, William O. Douglas, Norse Peak,
  Alpine Lakes, Henry M. Jackson, Glacier Peak,
  and Pasayten Wildernesses*

- Mount Baker–Snoqualmie National Forest
  425-888-1421 and 360-677-2414
  fs.usda.gov/mbs
  *Norse Peak, Alpine Lakes, Henry M. Jackson, and
  Glacier Peak Wildernesses*

- North Cascades National Park*
  360-854-7200
  nps.gov/noca
  Stephen Mather Wilderness

- E. C. Manning Provincial Park*
  604-668-5953
  bcparks.ca/explore/parkpgs/ecmanning

*requires a wilderness permit for an overnight stay

directly to a federal government agency for a permit. You may also want to inquire about trailhead parking fees or check for temporary road or trail closures. (Also visit pcta.org /discover-the-trail/closures for information about closures on the trail.) The appropriate Bureau of Land Management, National Forest, and National Park offices are listed above.

If you need a wilderness permit, obtaining it online is often the most painless way to do so. In many wilderness areas, including those with quotas, permits are available through the National Recreation Reservation Service (NRRS) at recreation.gov. In most cases, reserved permits can be printed at home or picked up at a USFS ranger station within 14 days prior to date of entry. In some instances, hikers are required to pick up the permit in person. If in doubt, call the issuing authority for clarification. If you are seeking permits for single sections covering any wilderness, recreation.gov is the most efficient source for gaining your permits.

ORGANIZATIONS RELEVANT TO THE PACIFIC CREST TRAIL

The previously mentioned books should answer most of your questions about hiking or riding the PCT. But if questions linger, they may be answered by contacting one or more of the following organizations.

Pacific Crest Trail Association (PCTA)

The PCTA is part of the legacy (the PCT itself is the other part) of many advocates and volunteers, including Warren Rogers. As a young man, Rogers worked with Clinton C. Clarke, the father of the trail. Clarke put the trail on the map beginning in the 1930s, forming the Pacific Crest Trail System Conference and advocating for the idea with a reluctant USFS. World War II contributed to the slow demise of his beloved conference. He died in 1958.

Rogers eventually picked up the baton in 1971, forming the Pacific Crest Club to be a "worldwide fellowship of persons interested in the PCT," as his son, Don, put it. Then, in 1977, he founded the Pacific Crest Trail Conference, which addressed the needs of both the trail and its users. In 1987, when Rogers was no longer able to run these organizations, the club was merged with the conference, and for several years volunteer Larry Cash of Eugene, Oregon, was its chief officer. The conference campaigned against trailside clear-cutting, against mountain bikes, for additional water sources along the drier stretches, and for volunteer trail maintenance. In 1992 the organization

changed its name to the Pacific Crest Trail Association (1331 Garden Highway, Sacramento, CA 95833; 916-285-1846; pcta.org).

Over the years, the PCTA has become increasingly active in coordinating volunteer trail maintenance and leading efforts to promote safe and responsible use of the trail. The association has a formal partnership with the USFS, National Park Service, Bureau of Land Management, and California State Parks through a Memorandum of Understanding. In 2018 PCTA volunteers spent 118,524 hours maintaining the trail, promoting the PCTA, and helping to raise awareness. That same year, the organization raised more than $4 million in private donations.

What services does the PCTA provide the potential trekker? In addition to issuing long-distance permits and keeping members up-to-date on all things trail-related via its website and social media (its Twitter handle is @PCTAssociation), it publishes a monthly e-newsletter, "Trail Dirt," and a quarterly print magazine, *The Pacific Crest Trail Communicator*. While addressing general issues and timely matters, it provides informative and inspirational accounts by those who have hiked or ridden horses on much or all of the PCT. The association's website contains an active blog and more than 100 pages of content, including trip-planning aids, current trail and snowpack conditions, trip calculators, permit applications, and links to other useful sites.

While it's impossible to keep track of exactly how many people use the trail every year, the PCTA provides estimates on use via the number of annual long-distance permits it issues. The group maintains a 2,600-Miler List on its website and sends hikers who notify it of completion a medal or certificate. In 2018 the organization issued a record 7,313 permits to hikers and horseback riders, who came from all 50 states and 41 countries and territories.

Finally, the PCTA lobbies Congress to support trail maintenance and for adequate funding for the USFS and other federal land management agencies. Private donors provide the bulk of its funding, which supports volunteer programs, public engagement, and advocacy. The organization is also raising money to help acquire the nearly 10% of the PCT that remains on private land, working with willing sellers to ensure that future generations of users have a protected corridor. In 2019, in a historic leap toward achieving this goal, the PCTA announced that along Northern California's Trinity Divide in the Klamath and Shasta-Trinity National Forests, 17 miles of the PCT that was previously on private property, as well as 10,300 acres of land surrounding the trail, are now in public ownership and permanently protected. The organization also consults with and advises government agencies on future reroutes to make the trail safer, more practical, or more scenic.

American Long Distance Hikers Association–West

In 1993 Ray Jardine founded the Western States Chapter. After a couple of years, Ray left his organization, and a few of its members took it over and reorganized it. Its mission is to promote fellowship and communication among long-distance hikers and anyone who supports long-distance hiking. As the association's name implies, it is aimed at long-distance backpackers (that is, not day hikers and equestrians). It addresses relevant backpacking matters on long trails or treks, not only in the Western United States but also overseas, and members hail from around the country, not just from the West. If you're a long-distance hiker, there are at least two reasons to join the association: First, "The Distance Hiker's Gazette" contains good descriptions of various trails and routes, plus backpacking advice. Second, you can find camaraderie among distance hikers at the ALDHA-West Gathering, held each fall. To join the organization, visit aldhawest.org.

Equestrian Organizations

The vast majority of PCT users are hikers, but there is fair use from equestrians on certain stretches. Occasionally an equestrian party will attempt to do the whole trail. This is more difficult than hiking, as horses don't wear crampons and don't cross logs over deep, raging streams. Consequently, it's virtually impossible to do the whole trek in one long season without making serious diversions, such as skipping the High Sierra entirely or doing it later, after the snow has melted and streams are safe. Should you want to ride the entire trail without any diversions or leapfrogging, then do it over two or more summers, making sure you do the High Sierra between mid-July and mid-September (and Washington during August—before that, there is too much snow, and after that, too much chance of snowstorms). For help on planning your trip through California, contact the Backcountry Horsemen of California (bchcalifornia.org); for Oregon and Washington, start with the Back Country Horsemen of America (see below for more information). The PCTA also offers invaluable planning information on its website at pcta.org/discover-the-trail/equestrian-center.

BACK COUNTRY HORSEMEN OF AMERICA

Back Country Horsemen of America (BCHA) is open to both men and women, but it does not include all of the United States; it covers only 11 Western states plus several others of the contiguous 48 states. If you plan to ride in Oregon or Washington, you might start with this organization. It publishes a quarterly newsletter (available via its website, bcha.org). Plus, Back Country Horsemen of Montana publishes the *Back Country Horsemen's Guidebook* (see "Recommended Reading and Source Books: Backpacking, Packing, and Mountaineering," page 340).

ANIMAL AND PLANT CONCERNS

If you hike the entire PCT in Oregon and Washington, you'll see dozens of bird species. You'll also pass by dozens of mammal species but will see very few, except for deer, marmots, pikas, and squirrels. However, the animals are around; you'll hear quite a flurry of activity during the night. What follows is a brief synopsis of animal and plant problems you might face on the PCT.

Black Bears

With the possible exception of cougars, most animals will be scared of you and will not be a threat as long as you respect the animal's space. The wilderness of Oregon and Washington is the black bears' home; we can only visit. The threat they pose is that they are very intelligent and always searching for large quantities of food to build their nutrition stores.

Black bears, which can be a variety of colors and hues, are almost as far-ranging as cougars and are present along the entire PCT. Conflicts between bears and humans usually occur because bears want your food. And if a bear can nab your food, it will nab someone else's too. So, the bear becomes known as a nuisance bear. This is not the bear's fault. Human food needs to be properly stored by humans (more on that below).

Despite weighing up to 500 pounds, black bears can run up to 35 miles an hour. One day shy of Monument 78, we watched as a fully filled-out, lustrously black-coated adult bear moved itself quickly from the canyon creek up 450 vertical feet on the opposite mountainside.

Most bears actually fear people and will leave when they see you. You are more likely to see the back end of a bear than to meet one face-to-face. If a bear woofs, snaps its jaws, slaps the ground or brush, or bluff charges, you are too close. Back away! Don't take any pictures! Seriously, don't.

Take precautions to avoid this kind of bear–human interaction. Control your food, toiletries, and trash—anything with a smell that may be an attractant.

Locate your camp kitchen away from your sleeping area, and keep the area free of food spills. It's also best if your backpack doesn't smell of trout and your candy supply is stored away from your tent.

Don't leave food out or unattended—not even for a few minutes. Secure your food for the protection of yourself and the bear. Use a bear-proof canister to carry and store your food when backpacking. These work and can be rented at most USFS visitor centers.

If a bear is eating your food or shredding your pack in search of your snacks, don't throw rocks at its head or face, and don't attempt to retrieve your food items until the bear has left the area. You've lost. In the bear's mind, it is now his food. Let him have it, and you can walk away with a great story. If you try to reclaim the food from the bear, you won't.

In the unlikely event that you do encounter a black bear on the trail, don't run. Make eye contact without staring. Pick up small children to keep them from running. Back away slowly. Speak calmly but firmly to the bear to identify yourself as a human and not a prey animal; never scream.

If a bear approaches within about 75 feet, make yourself appear larger by spreading your arms, waving hiking sticks or branches, or holding your jacket open. Do not block the bear's escape route.

Attacks are rare, but if a bear is after you and not your food, throw rocks and make every attempt to frighten it away or fight it off aggressively with anything at hand (now is the time to use your bear spray). Don't bother to run; they're very fast.

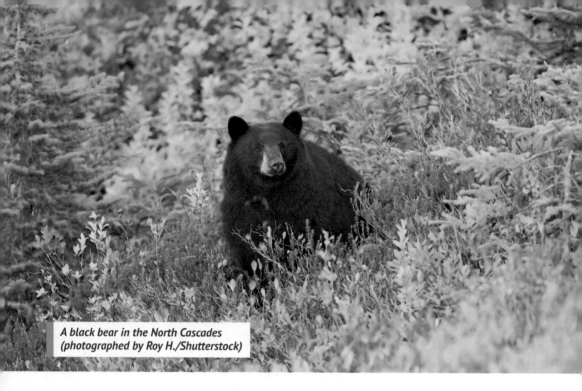

A black bear in the North Cascades (photographed by Roy H./Shutterstock)

Although black bears are carnivores by nature, they are mostly herbivores by habit; only about 10% of their diet is animal matter, and that is mostly insects. Humans are not part of their diet.

SAFEGUARDING YOUR FOOD

If you're thru-hiking, keep in mind that all of Yosemite and Lassen Volcanic National Parks and parts of Sequoia and Kings Canyon National Parks and Inyo, Sierra, and Humboldt-Toiyabe National Forests require hikers to carry bear-proof canisters. These are available for purchase at most outdoors outfitters and for rent at most main visitor centers and permit offices. They can be returned to the same location or mailed back to the USFS for a small fee (obtain a return label at the time of rental).

Food-storage boxes are also available for use by long-distance hikers on the PCT and John Muir Trail (JMT). A detailed list of their locations on parts of the JMT and PCT, along with other helpful info, can also be found at nps.gov/seki/planyourvisit/bear_box.htm and sierrawild.gov/bears/food-storage-map.

As a last resort, and only where bear canisters are not required, you may consider suspending your food in trees using the counterbalancing technique. (For step-by-step instructions on this method, consult nps.gov/seki/planyourvisit/bearhang.htm.) However, black bears are incredibly good tree climbers and very intelligent, so suspending your food in trees is generally not secure. In fact, it is so insecure that it is not really a deterrent, preventative, or protection as much as it is a mere delaying tactic. Although bear canisters are not required in Oregon and Washington national forests and parks, we strongly recommend storing your food in an approved canister. For more information on safeguarding your food, visit pcta.org/discover-the-trail/backcountry-basics/food/bear-canister-protecting-your-food.

BEAR TIPS

The USFS offers tips on how to avoid negative encounters with bears.

- Never give food to a bear.
- Carry and use a food-storage container designed to prevent access by bears.

- Be sure that your food, toiletries, and trash are stored and that your canister is closed properly at all times—bears are active 24 hours a day. Ensure that all your food, toiletries, and trash fit in the canister. To do this, remove all your food and toiletries from their original packaging to reduce bulk.

- Pack your canister before leaving the permit office to be sure that all items fit inside.

- If you do see a bear, do not approach it.

Cougars

These large cats, also called pumas or mountain lions (but they also live in lowlands), weigh up to about 200 pounds for males (about half that for females) and are about 7 feet long from nose to tail. The adults are tan-coated and have black-tipped ears and tail. Cubs are usually cuter and covered with dark-brown spots.

There seem to be two views about how threatening they are to humans. One is that they are merely curious, and that is why they track you. The other is that they are hungry, so they stalk you. Attacks on humans by cougars are rare, and most are nonfatal. However, a 2018 cougar attack, which occurred west of Washington's Snoqualmie Pass, was fatal, and wildlife specialists determined it was a case of a hungry animal stalking a cyclist who had acted like prey. Another fatal attack occurred that year in Oregon's Mount Hood National Forest.

Cougars are important to the natural community, and this is their home. They are seldom seen but have been known to attack humans without warning, so hikers need to be alert. Avoid hiking alone at dawn or dusk, and closely supervise children. Cougars are drawn to children and dogs because their size and motions mimic those of prey. If the trail tread is soft, look for their tracks: paw prints about 3 inches across, like those left by a large dog, but without claw marks, because cats walk with their claws retracted.

The following advice is from the National Park Service: Foremost, avoid hiking alone; there is safety in numbers. If you hike alone, you may be safer with a backpack than with a day pack because with the latter, more of your body, especially your neck, is exposed. Second, if you bring children, watch them closely; they are easy prey. Never approach a cougar. If you hear or see one, stay calm and don't scream. If you stumble upon an animal's corpse—whether fresh or rotting—depart the area immediately. This is probably a cougar's well-guarded meal.

If confronted by a cougar, do anything to make yourself appear larger: raise your outspread arms, wave hiking sticks or tree limbs, and gather other hikers next to you (pick up children). Act threatening, but allow the animal a path to escape. Absolutely avoid bending over or turning your back on mountain lions. Cougars will interpret these actions as those of their prey. Maintain eye contact and do not run. Prey such as deer run, so don't act like prey and excite its killing instinct. Stay calm, not fearful (this is not easy). Hold your ground, or back away slowly. To flee is to die. If the cougar behaves aggressively, wave your arms, shout, and throw sticks and/or stones at its body. Convince the cougar that you may be dangerous. If you are attacked, try to remain standing, as the animal will try to bite the neck or head. Use any instrument at hand to repel the cat. Always try to fight back. In 2007 an Auburn, California, woman successfully defended herself using a tree branch and ballpoint pen to fight off the cougar that was attacking her husband. The couple survived.

Rattlesnakes

Few animals are more unjustly maligned in legend and in life than the western rattlesnake, and no other animal, with the possible exception of the American black bear, causes more concern among walkers and riders along the PCT. Indeed, most thru-hikers will have several encounters with these common reptiles by the time they reach the High Sierra. Even so, PCT hikers are much more likely to be taken down by dehydration or giardia than by a rattlesnake.

Frequenting warmer climes generally below the red fir belt (although they have been seen much higher), rattlers are most often encountered basking on a warm rock, trail, or pavement, resting from their task of keeping the rodent population in check. Like other reptiles, rattlesnakes are unable to control their internal body temperature (they are cold-blooded), and therefore venture from their underground burrows only when conditions are suitable. Just as rattlers won't usually be seen in freezing weather, it is also no surprise that they are rarely seen in the heat of day, when ground temperatures may easily exceed 150°F—enough to cook a snake (or blister human feet, as many will learn). One will usually see rattlers toward evening, when the air is cool but the earth still holds enough heat to stir them from their lethargy for a night of hunting. They naturally frequent those areas where rodents feed—under brush, in rock piles, and beside streams.

It is their nocturnal hunting equipment that has inspired most of the legends and fears concerning rattlesnakes. In their wedge-shaped heads, rattlers have heat-sensitive pits, resembling nostrils, that can sense nearby changes in temperature as subtle as 1°F. Rattlers use these pits to locate prey at night, as they do not have well-developed night vision. More important perhaps is their sensitivity to vibrations, which can alert a rattler to footfalls more than 50 feet away. With such acute sensibilities, useful for detecting a meal or danger, a rattler will usually begin to hurry away long before a hiker spots it. Furthermore, if you do catch one of these reptiles unawares, these gentlemen among venomous snakes will usually warn you away with buzzing tail rattles if you get too close for comfort.

The easiest way to avoid a snakebite is to avoid snakes. More than 75% of rattler bites are inflicted on people who are handling a snake, and more than 80% of all bites are on the hand. The lessons: Don't catch snakes, and look before you put your hands under rocks or logs, or into tall grass. Snakes will usually graciously depart as you approach, if you make enough noise—a good reason to carry a walking stick.

If bitten, get help immediately. The only truly useful treatment for a rattlesnake bite is intravenous antivenin, which can be administered in most emergency departments. The sooner it is given, the better, even if you must

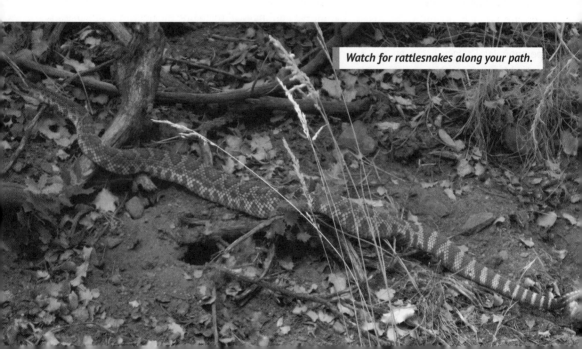

Watch for rattlesnakes along your path.

hike a distance for help. If you are solo, hike out immediately and call 911 as soon as you have service or hit the SOS on a satellite emergency notification device. If you are part of a group and are distant from possible medical attention, have the victim lie down, while another hiker goes for help. Keep the victim calm, and keep the puncture site below the heart. Because antiquated first-aid measures such as cold packs, tourniquets, and incision and suction devices are dangerous, they should never be used. There is no substitute for rapid evacuation to a hospital.

Mosquitoes

Mosquitoes occur near water from sea level up to around 11,000 feet—that is, near treeline. All mosquitoes can transmit various diseases, such as West Nile virus. If you're not bothered by the buzzing and biting, this should be reason enough to use some protection in the evening.

By early August, mosquito populations wane in the high mountains, as snow melts and meadows dry out (although they can still be abundant lower down, where water is available). Until then, you'll probably want to carry a tent with mosquito netting just to get a good night's sleep. This is especially true in June. From midmorning until late afternoon, when you are likely to be on the trail, wind usually keeps their numbers down. Of course, you can postpone your hike until August, but this is not an option for thru-hikers. Mosquitoes are pollinators, which explains why they are near their maximum numbers when wildflowers are so profuse. Without them, perhaps mountain wildflower gardens would be less glorious.

Ticks

Ticks, the slow-moving relatives of spiders, are another potential carrier of disease. They are usually found in lower elevations and seem most prevalent in late winter and spring. They neither jump nor fly but transfer from grass or brush to animals or you. You hardly see them and often do not feel their bite. This eight-legged creature can be as tiny as the dot of an *i* (larvae) or up to 0.25 inch (adult).

Bites by these blood-sucking arachnids cause two general problems for hikers and equestrians: 1) how to get them off and treat the wound, and 2) rare infections. Lyme disease has raised concern about infections from tick bites.

Ticks burrow their heads into the skin of the groin, armpits, hairline, or other body areas, especially where there is a constriction created by snug clothing, such as the waistband. The trick is to remove them, whole, without further injury. The most effective method is also the simplest—grasp the tick with tweezers as close to its attachment point as possible and pull gently upward and outward but firmly until it lets go. Try not to crush it, as doing so releases its fluid into the bite. After removing the tick, take precautions to prevent infection: Wash the wound with soap and water, apply a small amount of antibiotic ointment, and try to keep it clean. No further treatment is necessary.

Tick-borne infections are the feared hazard of tick bites and are sometimes difficult to diagnose, even by doctors, so prompt hospital attention is recommended for anyone who has symptoms that suggest such an infection.

Lyme disease is characterized by a migrating rash, fever, flulike symptoms, and worsening joint pain. It is easily treated with antibiotics in its early stages.

Spotted fever is marked by high fever; headache; and a red, spotty rash that becomes purple over time. This very serious illness should be promptly treated with antibiotics. It is quite rare throughout the Pacific West. Spotless forms of the fever are also occasionally contracted. Though difficult to diagnose, the victim's history of a prolonged tick bite will help steer the doctor toward the correct diagnosis.

Tick paralysis is a rarer condition of progressive severe weakness. It is usually completely reversed by removal of the tick. It rarely affects adults and is almost never seen outside of the Pacific Northwest.

Ticks need a few hours of attachment before they can transmit any disease they may harbor, so the quicker you remove them, the better. Check your clothing and skin carefully for ticks a couple of times daily, and especially after hiking through brush at low elevations. Wear long-sleeved clothing, with cuffs tucked under socks or into boots, and apply insect repellent liberally and often to skin and clothing.

Other Invertebrates

Flies can be a problem at lower elevations. Small black flies typically become numerous in warm weather—from about June through August. Flies are attracted to sweat from your face and body, but if you clean up, they generally cease to bother you. Occasionally, at low to mid elevations, you'll meet large, biting flies (usually deer flies), but they don't attack in numbers. Furthermore, when one is preoccupied with biting into your skin, it is easy to swat.

Another problem is the **yellow jacket,** a wasp that occasionally builds a ground nest under or beside a trail; if you trample on it, the yellow jackets will swarm you. You are very unlikely to meet them, though your chances increase if you ride a horse, for it tramples the ground far more than a hiker does. Their stings are multiple and painful, but not dangerous unless you happen to be allergic to bee stings. (More people in the United States die from bee stings than from rattlesnake bites.)

One of the best arguments for avoiding squirrels, which frequent popular campsites looking for food, is that they may be rabid or their **fleas** may carry the plague. Avoid fleas by avoiding rodents and their nests. Often rodents will opportunistically winter in a shelter that isn't visited until spring, when hikers will find the animals' nest, dust, and feces covering the surrounding floor. Hantavirus has been reported in Oregon and Washington, and it is caused, in every case in North America, by human contact with rodent excrement. Avoid areas where you find abandoned rodent nests.

Finally, there are **scorpions,** which are not strictly desert creatures. They are active at night and can give you a painful sting, although the species found along the PCT is not life-threatening.

Poison Oak

In some locations along the PCT, optimal conditions allow the waist-high shrub to assume the proportions of a small tree or a thick, climbing vine. Certainly, many PCT travelers would agree that, with the possible exception of flies or mosquitoes, poison oak is the most consistent nuisance along the trail. The allergic rash it causes in most people leads to several days of insane itching and irritation. It may, however, completely incapacitate a luckless few.

Poison oak dermatitis is best managed by avoidance, and avoidance is best accomplished by recognition of the plant, in all phases of its life cycle: In spring and summer, it puts forth shiny green leaves, each divided into three oval, lobed leaflets, which, even on the same plant, exhibit an unusual variety of sizes. Toward fall, the leaves and stems turn reddish, and the

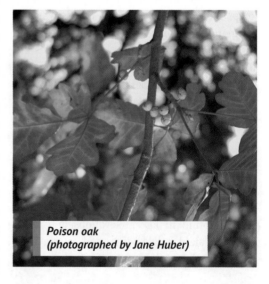

**Poison oak
(photographed by Jane Huber)**

small whitish flowers become smooth berries. In winter and early spring, when its leaves are gone, identification is most difficult: look for dusty-gray bark on stems, with smooth green, red-tipped new growth and possibly some white-green berries left over from the previous season.

Avoid touching any part of the plant in any season—all parts contain urushiol, an oil in the sap, that will, in a few days, cause an allergic reaction where it has penetrated the skin. If you do brush against the shrub, immediately wash the area with soap and water. Water helps to deactivate the toxin, and soap helps to extract the oil from skin. If you can't wash the area right away, try to avoid rubbing, which will spread the oil around. Better yet, avoid exposure entirely by wearing long-sleeved shirts and pants tucked into boot tops. But beware: Urushiol on clothing can be transferred to the skin even hours later. If you must wear shorts, try applying a commercial barrier cream, which helps keep the oil from reaching the skin. Above all, avoid smoke from burning poison oak, and never eat any of the plant—fatal internal reactions have occurred.

If you do develop the itchy, red, blistering, weeping rash of poison oak dermatitis, console yourself with the knowledge that it will be gone in a week or so. In the meantime, try not to scratch it—infection is the biggest hazard. Use calamine lotion, topical hydrocortisone cream, and oral Benadryl for itch relief. Severe allergic reactions, characterized by trouble breathing, dizziness, or swelling around the eyes or mouth, should be treated as soon as possible by a doctor.

Waterborne Microscopic Organisms

Many of the PCT's springs, streams, and lakes have clear water, but what you can't see might make you ill. The microscopic organisms are perhaps more threatening than any black bear you'll meet on the trail. One microscopic organism is *Giardia lamblia,* which causes giardiasis.

Although the condition can be incapacitating, it is not usually life-threatening. After ingestion by humans, giardia organisms normally attach themselves to the small intestine, and disease symptoms usually include diarrhea, increased foul-smelling gas, loss of appetite, abdominal cramps, and bloating. Weight loss may occur from nausea and loss of appetite. These discomforts may last up to six weeks. Most people are unaware that they have been infected and return home before the onset of symptoms. If not treated, the symptoms may disappear on their own, only to recur intermittently over a period of many months. Other diseases have similar symptoms, but if you drank untreated water, you should suspect giardiasis and so inform your doctor. If properly diagnosed, the disease is curable with prescribed medication.

There are several ways to treat found water to make it relatively safe to drink. The treatment most certain to destroy giardia is to bring the water to a boil (no need to boil for minutes; once it comes to a boil, the little assassins are gone). Chemical disinfectants such as tablets or drops may not be as reliable: although they work well against most waterborne bacteria and viruses that cause disease, they are not effective against a certain intestinal parasite, *cryptosporidium,* which can occur at water holes fouled by cattle. The most convenient safeguard is to use a portable water purifier. While relatively expensive and somewhat bulky, an ultraviolet-light water purifier or hollow-fiber technology in a straw or gravity filter gives you safe water in a minute or two—no chemical taste and no waiting for chemicals to act or for boiled water to cool.

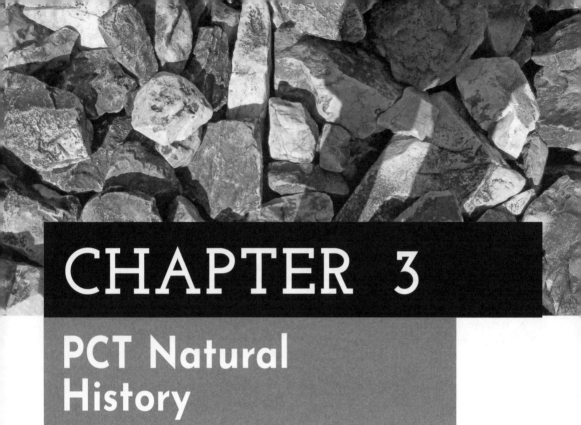

CHAPTER 3

PCT Natural History

GEOLOGY   *by Dan R. Lynch*

It is difficult to fully appreciate the Pacific Crest Trail's sights without a basic understanding of the earth, its rocks, and the forces strong enough to build mountains. Here, we will cover some of the fundamentals of geology and a brief history of how the Pacific Coast's mountain ranges came to be. Then, when you're resting after a difficult portion of your hike, you'll be able to look back on your route and admire it for the natural forces that produced such a picturesque landscape.

Rock Types Along the Pacific Crest Trail

The Pacific Crest Trail (PCT) follows the ridges and peaks of the Sierra Nevada and the Pacific Coast Ranges, but some of the regions connecting these mountains include low-lying deserts, valleys, and gorges. This diverse topography will lead you through an equally diverse assortment of rock types from all three categories of rocks—igneous, metamorphic, and sedimentary. These terms refer to how the rocks formed and are crucial to understanding geology.

Igneous Rocks

Many of the PCT's most rugged landscapes and highest peaks, including Mount Whitney and Mount Hood, are composed of igneous rocks. **Igneous rocks** are formed directly from the cooling

Above: Quartzite is common along the trail.

of fluid molten rock originating from deep within the earth, where temperatures can reach thousands of degrees. Molten rock still deeply buried is called **magma,** and if undisturbed, it will cool and harden very slowly to form **intrusive igneous rocks,** such as granite. But movement within our planet can force magma upward toward Earth's surface. During an **eruption,** when magma breaks through Earth's **crust,** or the outer, most rigid layer of the planet, magma becomes **lava** and can flow across the landscape, where it cools very quickly in the atmosphere. **Extrusive igneous rocks,** such as basalt, are the results of cooled, hardened lava. Aside from how quickly they cool, a primary difference between magma and lava is the amount of gas trapped within the molten rock. All molten rock contains various gases, and within the earth, magma's gases have nowhere to go. When magma erupts as lava, however, those trapped gases can rise and escape, creating bubbles in the resultant rock and, if the gases escape very quickly, even causing powerful explosions when erupting.

Igneous rocks are defined and distinguished from each other by their mineral compositions and structural variations, particularly their grain sizes. All rocks are composed of different mixtures of minerals; the mixtures in igneous rocks are determined by the varying properties of the magma or lava that formed them. **Minerals** can therefore be thought of as the building blocks of rocks; minerals are not rocks, but all rocks contain minerals. Minerals are solid materials composed of specific chemical compounds that crystallize, or harden in a particular repeating shape that reflects their molecular structure. This can be a fairly complex subject, but put more simply, a **crystal** is the natural shape a chemical takes on when it hardens. Table salt, for example, is a mineral called halite, which is composed of the chemical compound sodium

chloride and crystallizes in the shape of a cube (look at table salt through a magnifying glass to see for yourself). Quartz, the most common mineral, is a constituent of many rocks, as are minerals from the feldspar, mica, olivine, pyroxene, and amphibole groups, all of which form different crystal shapes.

As hot, thick, fluid magma or lava begins to cool, the minerals within it begin to crystallize. The longer the molten rock takes to cool, the larger the crystals are. In granite, for example, which cools for many years within the earth, the various minerals within it can crystallize to large, visible sizes. But in rhyolite—a rock with essentially the same mineral composition as granite but which instead cools rapidly on the earth's surface—the minerals have a much shorter time to crystallize, remaining small and nearly invisible without magnification. In both, each individual grain is a mineral crystal, no matter its size. This is called **grain size,** which helps identify rocks.

In the Cascade Range, you may encounter rocks that appear to be both coarse- and fine-grained. These rocks, which show large, angular grains suspended in a very fine-grained body of rock, are described as **porphyritic,** meaning that they have a mixture of textures. These rocks are the result of a body of magma that was beginning to cool within the earth, allowing some minerals to crystallize to visible sizes, but was then suddenly erupted, causing the rest of the rock to cool much more quickly around the large grains.

Intrusive igneous rocks form much of the backbone of the PCT; granite is particularly common along the trail, but others can also be found in the mountains. Extrusive igneous rocks are also very prevalent along your journey. While definitively identifying each type of rock is beyond the scope of this book, learning some of their key traits will help point you in the right direction.

PRIMARY IGNEOUS ROCKS ALONG THE PCT

Granite (*intrusive*)	Coarse-grained, hard; mottled coloration but predominantly white, gray, tan, or pink. It is composed primarily of quartz and feldspars, with some micas, amphiboles, and other minerals. As one of the most common igneous rocks, you will find it in many places; Yosemite and the rest of the Sierra Nevada Range are composed primarily of granite and granitelike rocks.	
Rhyolite (*extrusive*)	Fine-grained, hard; usually even coloration in shades of tan, gray, or pink, but may have faint bands. It has essentially the same composition as granite but cooled on the earth's surface and thus has very fine grains and some rounded gas bubbles. It is common throughout the Cascade Range; it is one of the rocks produced by volcanoes.	
Diorite (*intrusive*)	Coarse-grained; mottled coloration but predominantly white or gray. While visually similar to granite, it has far less quartz but more feldspars, amphiboles, and pyroxene minerals, making it less variable in color. It can be found throughout most of the PCT's ranges.	
Dacite (*extrusive*)	Typically porphyritic, with larger grains or crystals embedded in a much finer mass; predominantly light to dark gray. Similar to both andesite and rhyolite, dacite contains ample quartz and feldspars; as such, its lava is very thick and can contain large amounts of gas. This can result in explosive eruptions, such as in the famous 1980 eruption of Mount St. Helens. As such, it is common throughout the Cascade Range.	
Basalt (*extrusive*)	Fine-grained; very dark coloration, usually dark gray to black, but may also have brown surfaces. It has mostly the same composition as gabbro but cooled quickly on the earth's surface, particularly in large flows; it often contains rounded gas bubbles. The Columbia River Gorge is part of one of the largest basalt formations; basalt forms the valley's black walls.	
Andesite (*extrusive*)	Typically porphyritic with lighter colored larger grains embedded in a finer, darker mass. Andesite forms when oceanic crust melts and is mixed with continental magma; it is essentially a blend of basalt and rhyolite. Very common throughout the entire Cascade Range and forms much of the mountains and volcanoes there.	

A body of intrusive igneous rock still underground is called a **pluton;** rocks that formed deep underground are known as **plutonic rocks.** Sometimes magma is forced upward into cracks within older rocks, forming a near-vertical wall of rock within a different type of rock; this is called a **dike.** Bodies of extrusive igneous rocks are called **flows,** as their lava flowed away from its source. A **volcano** is a vent in the earth's crust from which lava erupts; the Cascade Range is well known for its large, cone-shaped volcanoes, known as **stratovolcanoes.** All these igneous bodies, as well as many more, are present along the PCT.

Sedimentary Rocks

All rocks, no matter how hard or high, eventually succumb to the effects of weather. Wind, rain, chemical exposure, and especially ice are all destructive forces that wear down and degrade rocks, reducing their once solid masses into mere grains of sand and silt. These particles, or **sediments,** end up being washed into rivers, lakes, and seas, where they settle into **beds,** or flat layers. But for the remains of many weathered rocks, these beds are just the first step in becoming a new type of rock.

Sedimentary rocks are those formed when sediments—particularly the remnants of older rocks, but also organic remains—are compacted and cemented to form a new rock body. As the weight of water and newer sediments press down on bedded sediments, the grains compress and lock together. In many cases, the addition of dissolved minerals, particularly calcite, can crystallize between grains of sediment and act as a glue to further adhere them. The resultant rocks are often flat, broad, and layered.

These rocks are identified by and often named for the type of sediment that comprises them. Sandstone, for example, is formed from compacted, solidified sand. Others, like shale, have more specific identifying traits, such as dense layering. But in general, whatever their composition, most sedimentary rocks (with the exception of chert) tend to be fairly soft and susceptible to weathering, their particles often only loosely adhered together. As a result, some sedimentary rocks may have harder and softer layers that weather at different rates, creating sculpted rock formations with dramatic layers, arches, and caves, such as the Vasquez Rocks along the trail north of Los Angeles.

Sedimentary rocks can offer us insight as to the climate and conditions at the time of their formation, including what kind of body of water in which the rock formed. The type of sediment is, of course, a key clue, but equally important is how those sediments are organized within the rock. For example, in shale, the size of the sediments is extremely fine—tiny particles of mud and clay—and such tiny, lightweight particles sink and settle very slowly. Therefore, for large beds to build up, the body of water—usually deep—must remain very calm for long periods of time. Layer after layer of sediments were undisturbed, which resulted in shale, a very fine-grained rock with many soft but well-preserved layers. When the same kinds of sediments settle in more turbulent waters, the fine layering does not occur, and the resultant rock—mudstone—is more of a mass with fewer features.

Not all sedimentary rocks are formed from rock and clay particles, however. Limestone, an extremely prevalent rock in the western United States, is formed entirely of ancient sea life. Coral reefs, both in ancient times as well as today, are home to corals, mollusks, and many other types of marine plants and animals that produce shells and skeletons made of calcium carbonate. As those organisms die and settle, the reefs build upon themselves through successive growth. The buried calcium carbonate skeletons begin to create a solid mass, and the sediments adhere together in the form of the mineral calcite. The result is limestone, a soft rock consisting primarily of calcite and frequently containing visible fossils. Similarly,

PRIMARY SEDIMENTARY ROCKS ALONG THE PCT

Sandstone	Composed of sand-size particles that settled in ancient lakes and seas. Usually gray or yellow to brown but can contain bands. The sand grains within sandstone are typically quartz held together by calcite and clays; grains can often be separated by hand. Common along the PCT in both desert and coastal areas.	
Shale	Composed of very fine mud-size particles that settled in calm, deep water. Fairly soft and often gray to tan or brown. Always with many fine layers that may be split apart with a knife into flat sheets; fossils may be found between layers. Very common along the PCT, especially in low-lying areas or closer to the Pacific Coast.	
Chert (*black chert is known as flint*)	Composed of extremely fine particles invisible to the eye. May be almost any color; usually gray to black, tan to brown, or reddish. Derived from seafloor sediments rich in diatoms, this silica-rich rock is extremely hard—a knife will not scratch it. When worn, especially in riverbeds, it can appear smooth and almost polished; freshly broken pieces will have very sharp edges. Common all along the PCT.	
Conglomerate	Composed of coarse pebbles embedded in a much finer grained mass; usually very mottled and variable coloration. Conglomerate formed in active bodies of water, particularly riverbeds, where larger rounded pebbles were buried in finer sediments, such as sand. When cemented and hardened, the result appears as though many river rocks were glued together. Most common in areas closer to the Pacific Coast.	

chert is a sedimentary rock that forms from the compaction of thick beds of silt rich in skeletons of diatoms, tiny aquatic organisms that make shells of silica, or quartz.

Many of the low-lying or desert regions of the PCT and surrounding areas are home to sedimentary rocks, but they can be prevalent in mountainous areas as well. As plutons and other igneous rock formations were forced upward due to movement within the earth, they were often forced up through sedimentary rocks. As a result, sedimentary rocks that formed long ago at the bottom of seas and lakes can now be found high on mountainsides or comprising foothills.

You'll see a few natural features throughout the PCT that are a result of weathering and are closely related to sedimentary rocks. **Talus slopes,** also known as scree, are the fragments and boulders that have fallen from mountains and cliffs and collected at their bases, forming steeply slanted hills comprised of loose rocks. **Alluvial fans** are fan-shaped accumulations of rocks, sand, and mud that originate from the mouth of a river or canyon. These are common where rivers meet flatter, broader planes and the flow slows and spreads outward, creating the fan shape. In desert areas, rivers that create alluvial fans are typically the result of flash floods, which later dry up to reveal the alluvial fan as a land feature.

Metamorphic Rocks

On the earth's surface, the weather is the primary force that changes rocks, but within the earth things are very different. Beginning less than 0.5 mile down into the earth's crust, the temperature begins to increase dramatically, and at greater depths it becomes hot enough to soften or melt rock. And the deeper within the earth you go, the greater the pressure becomes as well, as the weight of the world bears down from above. It is in these extreme conditions that rocks undergo their most dramatic changes, being softened and compressed and becoming

entirely new types of rocks in the process. The resulting rocks are called **metamorphic rocks** and are sometimes so completely changed by heat and pressure that it can seem impossible to tell what rock they originally were.

The movement that occurs within our planet can force rocks downward beneath the earth's crust. Although an extremely slow process (discussed in detail later), this movement is how rocks like limestone—consisting of ancient seafloor sediments from the earth's surface—can achieve such deep burial that they can be affected by the earth's interior heat. Igneous rocks, sedimentary rocks, and other metamorphic rocks can be **metamorphosed,** or changed, into metamorphic rock types. And depending on the varying amounts of heat and pressure, rocks can undergo varying amounts or different kinds of metamorphosis, all with potentially different resultant rocks.

PRIMARY METAMORPHIC ROCKS ALONG THE PCT

Slate (*foliated*)	Slate begins its life as shale; with heat and pressure, the layers of shale compact and harden, creating a more highly layered, harder, and brittle rock. Dark gray to black, slate is found sparingly along the Pacific Coast, usually in the more metamorphically active ranges, such as the Klamath Range.	
Schist (*foliated*)	Schist results from a fairly strong heating and compaction of many different kinds of rocks; the original rock determines the type of schist that results. Many schists are a result of metamorphosed sedimentary rocks and can show many fine layers, ample glittering micas, and pockets of hard gemstones, such as garnets. Schists are common throughout the PCT.	
Gneiss (*foliated*)	Gneiss (pronounced "nice") is the result of advanced metamorphism and can be derived from many types of rock. Gneisses tend to have broad layering and loosely organized bands of minerals, often with many glittering layers of micas. Gneisses are named for their parent rock; granitic gneiss, for example, began as granite and can appear to share many traits with granite. Gneisses are common throughout the PCT.	

Heat and pressure can plasticize, or soften, rocks, which can have a variety of effects: consolidation and hardening of the rock, reorganization of a rock's minerals into tightly packed layers (called **foliation;** any metamorphic rocks that exhibit layering are described as being foliated), or recrystallization of a rock's minerals into entirely new minerals, to name a few. Shale, for example, is a soft, layered sedimentary rock that, when metamorphosed, turns into slate, a harder and more densely layered rock that still somewhat resembles the original shale. Sturdier rocks, like granite, require more extreme conditions to metamorphose but can be changed as well.

Metamorphosis occurs on a gradient, and with increasing heat and pressure, a rock can continue changing. The shale-to-slate transformation, for example, is a low-grade metamorphism and can continue, with the slate eventually becoming phyllite, then schist, then gneiss—all increasingly harder, more foliated, more crystallized, higher-grade metamorphic rocks—if the heat and pressure continue to build. Along the way, the rock's minerals can recombine to form new minerals. Schist, for example, is an intermediate-grade metamorphic rock that can contain garnets, which are gems typically not present in the original rock.

There are many kinds of metamorphism, most of which are associated with movement in the earth's crust or the rising of hot plutons. As a result, metamorphic rocks are particularly common in mountainous areas—especially the Klamath Range—and in foothills that have often been pushed and transformed to make way for the growing mountains.

Along the trail, you'll likely encounter metamorphic rocks in the form of hard, dark, layered rocks that frequently appear to glitter with countless mineral flakes. Cliffs and other rock faces may also reveal metamorphic layers that bend or wrap around each other—these are called folds, and they illustrate the immense power that has affected these rocks.

Tectonic Plates

Many of the rocks you'll encounter along the PCT exist as a direct result of movements within our planet. Earth is not a solid, unchanging mass; it is dynamic and always evolving. This is due in large part to its layered structure. Earth has distinct zones of varying temperature and composition as they progress downward toward the planet's solid metal core. Earth's crust, the outermost layer upon which all life resides, is the top of the lithosphere, a rigid, rocky layer that is broken up into enormous segments called **tectonic plates.** These plates are like ill-fitting puzzle pieces; some plate boundaries rest on top of or beneath the edges of other plates. Generally, each continent and major ocean sits atop its own plate, and the boundaries or joints at which these plates meet are called **faults,** which can be the sites of major geological events.

Beneath the lithosphere is the asthenosphere, a molten layer upon which the tectonic plates sit. The asthenosphere consists of hot, soft rock and is in constant motion due to convection. Currents of rock rise, fall, and flow very slowly, taking the tectonic plates above them along for the ride. As the rigid tectonic plates of the lithosphere move, some collide, some spread apart, and others slide past each other. All these types of movements have played a role in the formation of the Pacific Coast region and the modern-day PCT.

Convergent Movement

This type of tectonic plate movement sees plates converging, or coming together, and is frequently associated with building mountains. Many times, mountains are a result of one plate being forced beneath another, causing the upper plate to rise and develop a mountain range. Along the Pacific Coast, however, the process was a little more complex, resulting not only in mountains but volcanoes as well. This process was particularly important in the development of the Cascade Range; this will be discussed in detail later.

Divergent Movement

This type of movement occurs when two tectonic plates spread apart, leaving a gap between them. This typically occurs on ocean floors where two oceanic plates are separating. Divergent movement is particularly prominent in the Atlantic Ocean but also occurs in the Pacific. When two oceanic plates separate, the space between them fills in with rising molten rock. This tectonic spreading can be a driving factor for convergent plate collisions on the other sides of the plates.

Transform Movement

Transform movement is the general term for when tectonic plates slide past each other, often grinding against each other in such a way as to cause earthquakes, as occurs along the San Andreas Fault in California. But smaller mountain ranges can also form when the two plates don't slide along each other cleanly. Angular pressure between the plates can push material upward between them; this is how Southern California's Transverse Ranges were formed.

Formation of the Pacific Crest Trail

With a basic understanding of rock types and tectonic plates, we can now begin to piece together the story of how the PCT's mountain ranges formed.

The PCT begins near Campo in Southern California, at the Mexico border, in the foothills of the Peninsular Ranges. The **Peninsular Ranges** are a series of mountain ranges that run north–south along the Baja Peninsula of Mexico and into Southern California; the Laguna, Santa Rosa, and San Jacinto Ranges are the Peninsular Ranges that PCT hikers will pass through. All the Peninsular Ranges formed around the same time as the Sierra Nevada Range and from similar geological events stemming from the movement of an ancient tectonic plate, called the Farallon Plate. Today, the Farallon Plate is mostly gone, almost completely subducted beneath North America, but around 200 million years ago, it was a major oceanic plate spreading eastward, toward the Pacific Coast, bringing islands along with it. As the islands docked with North America, collecting on the edges of the continent and building out the western coasts, the Farallon Plate began to dive below the North American Plate, heating up as it got deeper. As the plate melted, the resultant soft, hot rock began to rise toward the surface as plutons, or massive blobs of intrusive igneous rocks, particularly granite. In simplest terms, as the Farallon Plate continuously sank and melted, the hot rock produced rose and displaced the rock above it; as a result, the plutons were continuously pushed upward. As the Farallon Plate moved eastward, the overlying older rock moved westward and the younger granite plutons were exposed, composing the Peninsular Ranges as we know them today. The Peninsular Ranges' north-south-trending direction mainly follows the plate boundary, or fault, where the Farallon Plate was subducted, and where the Pacific Plate currently meets the North American Plate.

Just north of the Peninsular Ranges are the **Transverse Ranges,** named such because their east–west orientation is transverse to the north–south nature of the coast. The Transverse Ranges, which include the San Bernardino, San Gabriel, and Tehachapi Ranges, extend from the

Pacific Coast to the Mojave Desert and generally follow the San Andreas Fault. The San Andreas Fault is an extremely active fault system on the boundary of the Pacific and North American Plates in Southern California, notorious for the frequent and destructive earthquakes it causes. While technically a transform fault, the Pacific and North American Plates are not sliding past each other smoothly. Instead, they grind together as they pass, pressing into each other and generating incredible forces that not only shake the land but also push rocks upward. As the rocks were forced higher and higher, the Transverse Ranges were born.

California's most significant portion of the PCT runs along the **Sierra Nevada Range,** famous for dramatic sites like Yosemite National Park, Lake Tahoe, and Mount Whitney. This iconic mountain range also has a particularly interesting geological history. While the range's oldest rocks originate from the Cambrian period, around 541 million years ago, the soaring, snowy peaks we see today weren't present until around 70 million years ago.

Much like the Peninsular Ranges, the subduction of the ancient Farallon Plate caused the formation of intrusive plutons that rose and began to collect near the earth's surface in modern-day eastern California. As the multitude of plutonic rocks formed, they came to act as a singular massive body of rock known as the **Sierra Nevada Batholith** (a batholith is a large mass of intrusive rock, usually granite, that measures more than 100 square kilometers in size), which was not originally exposed on the earth's surface.

How it rose to form the Sierra Nevada Range is still actively debated; traditionally, it was thought to have been uplifted as a result of tectonic activity farther east. In a geologic region known as the Basin and Range Province (underlying much of Nevada, Arizona, and eastern California today), intense volcanic heat below the easternmost portion of the batholith is thought to have thinned it, making it lighter

weight than the western portion. This may have caused the batholith to tilt and rotate westward as the eastern end rose to become the peaks of the range. This theory, which stems from the tilted shape of the range, has been proposed for decades and is one that many may already be familiar with. Modern research, however, has suggested that perhaps there wasn't much uplift at all, but rather a collapse of the surrounding rock. As tectonic forces in the region lessened, surrounding areas may have subsided—especially the Basin and Range Province to the east—exposing the batholith and leaving it elevated. New research is still being conducted, but evidence for this theory is strong.

In either proposed method of formation, modern research suggests that the Sierra Nevada Range has towered over the eastern portion of the state for at least 70 million years. The range as we see it today has since been shaped by weathering, with notable help from past **glaciers** (thick masses of ice indicative of ice ages). The glaciers scoured through valleys and down the range's slopes, creating many of the lakes found there today.

As you pass from the Sierra Nevada Range to the **Klamath Range** in Northern California and southern Oregon, you also pass into dramatically different geology. As the Farallon Plate was subducted beneath the North American Plate, large islands and microcontinents (similar to New Zealand today) atop the Farallon Plate were pulled toward North America. As they collided with the West Coast, they accreted, or became part of the North American continent. The Klamath Mountains represent the accumulation of several of these accreted islands, forced upward as further plate collisions occurred. Later volcanic activity injected the Klamath Range with intrusive rocks from below, heating and heavily metamorphosing many of the range's bodies of rock, resulting in some of the stranger kinds of rocks along the PCT.

As you leave the Klamath Range and continue northward, you'll enter the longest section of the PCT: the **Cascade Range.** These iconic mountains, stretching from Northern California into Canada, are famous for their active volcanoes and rugged valleys formed during the subduction of the Juan de Fuca Plate beneath the North American Plate. The Juan de Fuca Plate, thought to be a remnant of the Farallon Plate, is a small plate off the coast of Oregon and Washington that is still actively subducting beneath North America. As it does, it descends eastward to where portions of it begin to melt, many miles from the plate boundary. As a result, when the rising magma formed by this melting is forced to the surface, it erupts inland. Due to the makeup of the magma, it produces lots of pulverized rock and ash when it erupts; subsequent eruptions can create a buildup of rock and ash around the vent, giving rise to a stratovolcano, or layered,

cone-shaped volcano. Throughout the past 37 million years or so, many Cascade volcanoes have erupted for a short time and then stopped when their magma supply moved to a new spot, where a new volcano began. Peak after peak began to rise and accumulate in this way, building much of the modern range. But this is just the most recent chapter in a long history of Pacific Coast eruptions along the Cascade Range. Much earlier, the adherence of a microcontinent that already contained a chain of volcanoes laid much of the groundwork for today's Cascades.

Along your way through the Cascades, you'll have to cross the **Columbia River** along the Washington–Oregon border, where you'll notice a marked change in geology. The black-walled river valley is part of the **Columbia Plateau,** a landform composed almost entirely of basalt

GEOLOGIC TIME SCALE

Throughout the book, we'll refer to various geological periods during which parts of the PCT were formed. This scale shows how these periods relate to each other and how many years ago they began.

ERA	PERIOD	BEGAN (in millions of years)
Cenozoic		
	Quaternary	2.58
	Neogene	23.03
	Paleogene	66.0
Mesozoic		
	Cretaceous	145.0
	Jurassic	201.3
	Triassic	251.9
Paleozoic		
	Permian	298.9
	Carboniferous	358.9
	Devonian	419.2
	Silurian	443.8
	Ordovician	485.4
	Cambrian	541.0

The Precambrian eon has not been included here. These dates are derived from the latest sources available in 2020, but, as in the past, they are bound to be slightly revised in the future. The oldest known rocks are about 4.3 billion years old; Earth's crust solidified about 4.6 billion years ago.

formed during a series of eruptions between 17 million to 6 million years ago. In one of the largest continuous lava formations in the world, the Columbia Plateau formed during a flood basalt, in which basalt lava flowed over huge, broad expanses, creating a relatively flat landscape. This unique section of your hike is in stark contrast to most of the PCT's geology, taking you to one of the lowest elevation portions of the entire route: the Bridge of the Gods, which you'll take to cross the river.

In many areas along the PCT, particularly the Sierra Nevada and Cascade Ranges, glaciers have played a large role in shaping the mountains as they appear today. Glaciers are massive formations of ice that appear at the poles and in high elevations during the glacial periods of ice ages. As they accumulate more ice, or as warming temperatures melt their ice, they grow or recede, flowing like a very slow river. But the immense weight of the ice can crush and break up rocks, the fragments of which become incorporated within the glaciers and add to its abrasive quality. As a result, mountain glaciers can carve large valleys.

The point at which a glacier begins to accumulate, high in the mountains, is called a **cirque,** and it is usually bowl-shaped. As glaciers melt, cirques often collect glacial meltwater, creating small but pristine mountain lakes called **tarns.** Tarns often have a natural dam, called a **moraine,** that keeps them filled— moraines are piles or ridges of rock created by glaciers as the pulverized rock within the ice is deposited. **Lateral moraines** form along the sides of a glacier, parallel to its flow direction, from gravel left behind as a glacier begins to melt. Conversely, **terminal or end moraines** form at the front of a glacier as gravel and sand are dumped when a glacier begins to melt and recede. Keep an eye out for these features as you progress along the trail.

From the shadow of Mount Whitney to the Columbia River banks, the PCT follows some of the most dramatic geology on the West Coast, and you'd be remiss to let it pass you by without taking notice of the millions of years of history just beneath your feet.

BIOLOGY

The California section of the PCT is noted for its great diversity of plants, animals, climates, and landscapes. The Oregon section of the PCT provides quite a contrast, having the most homogenous vegetation and landscape of this tristate route. The Washington section falls between these two extremes. Along the route covered by this volume, certain plants and animals appear time and time again. The most common entities appear to be:

Flower: lupine

Shrub: huckleberry

Tree: mountain hemlock, subalpine fir, western white pine

Invertebrate: mosquito

Fish: trout

Amphibian: western toad, tree frog (but all amphibians are faring poorly)

Reptile: garter snake

Bird: dark-eyed junco

Mammal: chipmunk, golden-mantled ground squirrel, deer

The average elevation of Oregon's section of the PCT is about 5,120 feet, whereas Washington's section is about 4,550 feet—lower in part because the weathering and erosional processes farther north are more intense (contrast Washington's 4,550 to California's 6,120 feet). Not only is the average trail elevation different between these two northwest states, so, too, is the typical terrain that the trail traverses. The Oregon section is flatter, drier, more volcanic, and less glaciated than Washington's section. In Oregon, a typical hike is through a mountain-hemlock forest while traversing rolling ridges and crossing lake-bound basins. In

Washington, a typical hike is through alternating forests of mountain hemlock and subalpine species while climbing over passes and dropping somewhat into glaciated canyons. Both states, of course, have many distinctive features worth investigating.

Flora

A backpacker who has just completed the California section of the PCT might conclude that southern Oregon's forests are more integrated than those of California. Passing through different environments of the Sierra Nevada, you may have noticed the segregation of tree species and concluded that as you ascend toward the range's crest, you pass through a sequence of forests: Douglas-fir, white fir, red fir, and mountain hemlock. Near the Oregon border, however, you discover that these four species and others reside together. Certainly, this aggregation would never be seen in the Sierra. The great diversity of environments found within that range has allowed each species to adapt to the environment most suitable for it.

In contrast, the southern Oregon environments, and therefore the plant communities, are not as sharply defined. Still, each plant species is found within a certain elevation range and over a certain geographic area.

If you've hiked through California's rugged Sierra Nevada, you'll find southern Oregon a much gentler, more uniform landscape. But despite its relatively subdued topography, it still supports a diverse assemblage of plants, and the discerning hiker soon learns what species to expect around the next bend. Ponderosa pines thrive in the drier southern Oregon forests, yet they are nonexistent in the dry pumice soils of the Crater Lake vicinity. Here, you'll find lodgepole pines, which, ironically, are water-loving trees. These are usually seen growing in boggy soils near lakes, creeks, and wet meadows, where they often edge out the mountain hemlocks, which are by far the most common tree

you'll see along the PCT in Oregon and Washington. The most suitable habitat for hemlocks appears to be shady north slopes, on which pure stands of tall, straight specimens grow. At lower elevations, mountain hemlocks give way to western hemlocks and Douglas-firs, and, as the environment becomes drier southward and eastward, these two species yield to ponderosa pines. The harder you look at a forest, even a small piece of it, the more you realize that this seemingly uniform stand of trees is, in fact, a complex assemblage of particular plants, animals, soils, rocks, and microclimates all influencing each other.

The trail description in this book commences at Seiad Valley, a man-made ranchland carved from a Douglas-fir forest. Near the end of the odyssey, along Agnes Creek and the Stehekin River, you also encounter a Douglas-fir forest. The two are hardly alike. The Douglas-fir forest of Northern California

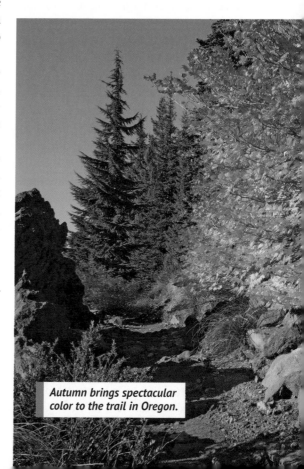

Autumn brings spectacular color to the trail in Oregon.

and southern Oregon contains, among other trees, incense cedar, ponderosa pine, white fir, Oregon oak, and madrone. Its counterpart in northern Washington contains, among others, western red cedar, western white pine, grand fir, vine maple, and Engelmann spruce.

The two forests vary considerably in the density of their vegetation. Not only does the rain-laden northern forest have a denser stand of taller conifers, but it also has a denser understory. Its huckleberries, thimbleberries, devil's club, and other moisture-loving shrubs are quite a contrast to the stiff, dry manzanita, ceanothus, and scrub oaks seen in the southern forest. Wildflowers in the northern forest are more abundant than their counterparts to the south. During rainstorms, they are too abundant, for their thick growth along the trail ensures that you'll be soaked by them from as high as your waist on down. Both forests have quite a number of species in common, but from central Oregon northward, the moisture-oriented species become prominent. Now you find bunchberry, dogwood, Oregon grape, Lewis monkeyflower, and other species growing on the dark, damp forest floor.

In contrast to trees, which are quite specific in their habitat selection, flowers can tolerate a broad range of environments. You'll find, for example, yarrow, a sunflower, at timberline on the slopes of Mount Hood and also on the Douglas-fir forest floor that borders the southern shore of the Columbia River. Both environments are moist, but the Mount Hood alpine meadows, at 6,000 feet above the bottom of the Columbia River Gorge, are a considerably harsher environment.

Some flowers prefer open meadows to shady forests; others prefer dry environments. Thistle, lupine, and phlox are found along the sunnier portions of the trail. Growing from crevices among rocks are the aptly named stonecrops, and on the pumice flats too dry for even the lodgepole pines to pioneer, the Newberry knotweed thrives.

In addition to adapting to specific climatic conditions, a plant may also adapt to a specific soil condition. Thus, you see on the otherwise-barren mica schist slopes of Condrey Mountain, near the southern Oregon border, acre after acre of pink, prostrate pussy-paws.

Lastly, a species may have a distribution governed by the presence of other species. Corn lilies thrive in wet meadows, but lodgepoles invade these lands and shade them out. Mountain hemlocks may soon follow and eventually achieve dominance over the lodgepoles. Then the careless camper comes along, lets the campfire escape, and the forest burns. Among the charred stumps of the desolate ruins rises the tall, blazing, magenta fireweed, and nature once again strives to transform this landscape back into a mature forest.

The Role of Fire

Fires were once thought to be detrimental to the overall well-being of the ecosystem, and early foresters attempted to prevent or subdue all fires. This policy led to the accumulation of thick litter, dense brush, and overmature trees—all prime fuel when a fire inevitably sparked. Human-caused fires can be prevented, but how does one prevent a lightning fire, so common in the Sierra?

The answer is that fires should not be prevented but only regulated. Left unchecked, natural fires burn stands of mixed conifers about once every 10 years. At this frequency, brush and litter do not accumulate enough to result in complete devastation; only the ground cover is burned, while the trees remain intact. Hence, through small burns, the forest is protected from flaming catastrophes.

Some pines are adapted to fire. Indeed, the relatively uncommon knobcone pine, growing in scattered localities particularly in the Klamath Mountains (Sections P, Q, and R of *Pacific Crest Trail: Northern California*), requires fire to survive: the short-lived tree must be consumed by fire for its seeds to be released. Seeds of the genus *Ceanothus* are also quick to germinate in burned-over ground, and some plants of this genus are among the primary foods of deer. Hence, periodic burns will help a deer population thrive, but without them, shrubs become too woody and unproductive for a deer herd. Similarly, gooseberries and other berry plants that sprout after fires help support several different bird populations.

Without fires, a plant community evolves toward a climax, or end stage of plant succession. A pure stand of any species, as mentioned earlier, invites epidemic attacks and is therefore unstable. But even climax vegetation does not last forever. Typically the climax vegetation is a dense forest, and eventually the trees mature, die, and topple over. Logs and litter accumulate to such a degree that when a fire starts, the abundant fuel causes a crown fire, not a ground fire, and the forest burns down. Over time, succession results in an even-age stand of trees, and the cycle repeats itself. In the past,

ecologists believed that stable climax vegetation was the rule, but we now know that unstable, changing vegetation is more common, even where man is not involved.

Fire also unlocks nutrients that are stored in living matter, topsoil, and rocks. Vital compounds are released in the form of ash when a fire burns plants and forest litter. Fires can also heat granitic rocks enough to cause them to break up and release their minerals. Even in a coniferous forest, the weathering of granitic rock is often due primarily to periodic fires. One post-fire inspection revealed that the fire was intense enough to cause thin sheets of granite to exfoliate, or sheet off, from granitic boulders.

Natural, periodic fires, then, are beneficial for a forest ecosystem and should be thought of as an integral process in the plant community. They have, after all, been around as long as terrestrial life has, and for millions of years have been common in western plant communities.

More than ever in our lifetime, we are faced with a forest emergency unlike one we've

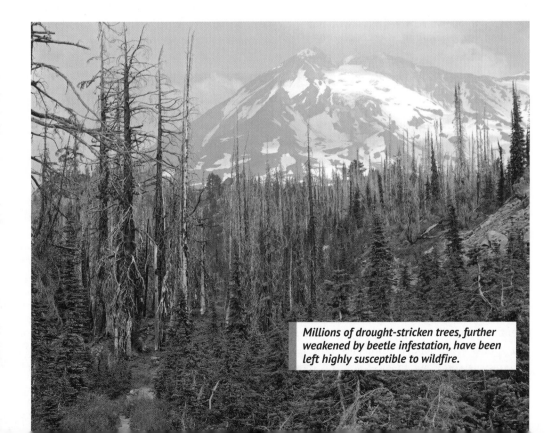

Millions of drought-stricken trees, further weakened by beetle infestation, have been left highly susceptible to wildfire.

ever seen. Since 2010, it is estimated that western forests have lost more than 100 million trees to drought, disease, pests, wind, and fire. Hikers will see this impact often on the trail, though it won't always be noted in the route description because change happens so rapidly. The borders of a forest can morph quickly into the devastation caused by pine beetles or into areas of blown-down trees. More important are the possible hazards presented to hikers, whether on the trail or in a camp; burned trees have weakened roots and therefore don't stand up well in high winds. Widow-makers are plentiful wherever you spot standing tree carcasses.

A few notes of caution:

- Take extra care with any open flame; have water on hand to completely extinguish the fire and its coals.
- Use existing fire rings, and never build a fire near dry leaves, forest duff, grasses, bushes, and branches.
- Be cautious in drainages around burn areas; flash floods are more common and destructive after a fire. Do not camp in drainages.
- Use a stove with a shut-off valve and a contained fuel source that cannot spill.
- Travel through burn areas quickly. Do not camp below hazard trees, especially on windy days.

Fauna

We have seen that plants adapt to a variety of conditions imposed by the environment and by other species. Animals, like plants, are also subject to a variety of conditions, but they have the added advantage of mobility. On a hot summer day, a beetle under a scant forest cover can escape the merciless sun by seeking protection under a loose stone or under a mat of dry needles.

Larger animals, of course, have greater mobility and therefore can better overcome the difficulties of the environment. Amphibians, reptiles, birds, and mammals may frequent the trail, but they scamper away when you approach. At popular campsites, however, the animals come out to meet you, or, more

exactly, to obtain your food. Of course, almost anywhere along the trail you may encounter the ubiquitous mosquito, always looking for a free meal. But in popular campsites, you'll meet robins, gray jays, Clark's nutcrackers, Townsend's and yellow-pine chipmunks, golden-mantled ground squirrels, and, at night, mice and black bears. You may be tempted to feed them, or they may try to help themselves, but please store your food properly to protect them from it; they will survive better on the real, organic food Mother Nature produces. Furthermore, an artificially large population supported by generous summer backpackers may in winter overgraze the vegetation. In the following paragraphs, we'll take a closer look at three species.

MULE DEER

Two subspecies of this large mammal can be found along much of the Oregon-Washington PCT. Mule deer, like other herbivores, do not eat every type of plant they encounter but tend to be quite specific in their search for food. Their primary browse is new growth on huckleberry, salal, blackberry, bitterbrush, and snowbrush, although they also eat certain grasses and forbs.

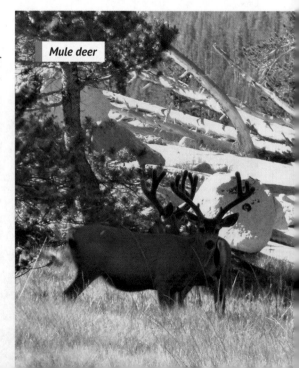

Mule deer

Together with other herbivores, parasites, and saprophytes (organisms feeding on decaying organic matter), they consume a small portion of the 100 billion tons of organic matter produced annually on the earth by plants.

Mule deer face a considerable population problem because some of their predators, such as wolves and grizzly bears, are either endangered or extinct in many parts of Oregon and Washington. In their places, coyotes and black bears have increased in numbers. Coyotes, however, feed principally on rabbits and rodents and only occasionally attack a fawn or a sick deer. Black bears occasionally kill fawns. The mountain lion, a true specialist in feeding habits, preys mainly on deer and may kill 50 of them in a year. This magnificent mammal, unfortunately, has been unjustly persecuted by people, and many deer that are saved from the big cat are lost to starvation and disease. Increasing human population compounds the problem. The expansion of settlements causes mountain lions to retreat farther, which leaves them farther from the suburban deer. Forests must be logged to feed this expansion of settlements, and then the logged-over areas sprout an assemblage of shrubs that are a feast for deer. The deer population responds to this new food supply by increasing in number. Then the shrubs mature or the forest grows back, and there is less food for the larger deer population, which is now faced with starvation. Forest fires produce the same feast-followed-by-famine effect.

GOLDEN-MANTLED GROUND SQUIRREL

There are two species of these ground squirrels: the Sierra Nevada golden-mantled ground squirrel, which ranges from the southern Sierra north to the Columbia River, and the Cascades golden-mantled ground squirrel, which ranges from the Columbia River north into British Columbia. On the eastern Cascade slopes of Washington, the Cascades golden-mantled ground squirrel lives in the same habitat as the yellow-pine chipmunk, but they have slightly different niches, or roles, to carry out in their pine-and-fir-forest environment. Both have the same food and the same burrowing habits, but the ground squirrel obtains nuts and seeds that have fallen to the forest floor, whereas the chipmunk obtains these morsels by extracting them from their source. The ground squirrel, like its distant cousin the marmot, puts on a thick layer of fat to provide it with enough energy to last through winter hibernation. The chipmunk, like the black bear, only partly hibernates. During the winter, it awakens periodically to feed on the nuts and seeds it has stored in its ground burrow.

WESTERN TOAD

Every Westerner is familiar with this drab, chunky amphibian. Along the Oregon–Washington PCT, you encounter its subspecies known as the boreal toad. This cold-blooded animal is amazingly adaptable, being found among rock crevices in dry, desolate lava flows as well as in subalpine wildflower gardens in the North Cascades. Its main environmental requirement appears to be the presence of at least one early-summer seasonal pond in which it can breed and lay eggs.

Although you may encounter dozens of boreal toads along a stretch of trail in one day (they occur in clusters), they prefer to actively hop or crawl about at night. Should you bed down near one of their breeding ponds, you may hear the weak chirps (they have no "croaking" vocal sacs) from dozens of males.

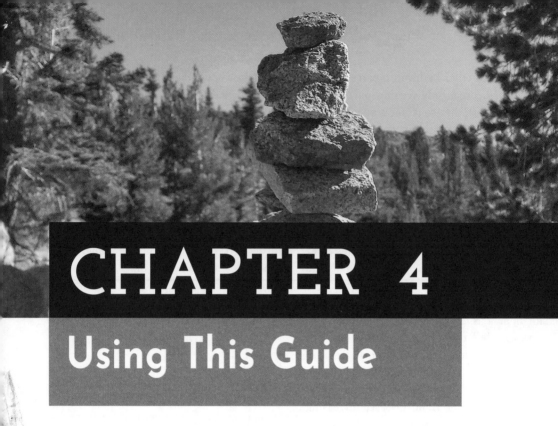

CHAPTER 4
Using This Guide

OUR ROUTE DESCRIPTION

*P*acific Crest Trail: Oregon & Washington is composed of the route description and area maps of the Pacific Crest Trail (PCT). In 12 section chapters, this guide covers the Oregon–Washington PCT as it heads north from CA 96 in northern California to BC 3 in British Columbia. Readers familiar with this guide's companion volume, P*acific Crest Trail: Northern California,* will note that its Section R is essentially the same as this one's Section A. The route description is divided into sections because most PCT hikers will be hiking only a part of the trail, not all of it. Each section starts at or near a highway and/or supply center (town, resort, park) and ends at another similar point. All of the sections are short enough to make comfortable backpacking trips ranging from about 4 to 12 days for the average backpacker. Each of these sections could be conveniently broken into two or more shorter sections to provide even shorter hikes.

At the beginning of each section is an introduction that mentions:

- The attractions and natural features of that section
- The declination setting for your compass
- The 7.5-minute topographic maps that cover that section, arranged south to north
- A mileage table of points on the route
- A campsite table with GPS coordinates and other pertinent information

- Weather and best times to go
- Supply points on or near the route
- Water availability or scarcity. If obtaining water is not an issue in certain sections, it will not be mentioned.
- Wilderness permits (if required)
- Special concerns (such as rattlesnakes, snow, and difficult-to-ford rivers and creeks)

Above: A buffed-out duck

Attractions and natural features will help you decide what part of the trail you want to hike.

The **declination setting** for your compass is important if you want to get a true reading. The declinations in this guide vary from 14°18'E near Seiad Valley to 15°24'E near the Canadian border. They were calculated in 2020 and are accurate within 30 minutes of arc, but note that declination changes over time. Visit ngdc.noaa.gov/geomag-web for the most current information before your hike.

If your compass does not correct for declination, you'll have to add the appropriate declination to get the true bearing. For example, if your compass indicates that a prominent hill lies along a bearing of 75° and the section you're hiking has a declination of 15°E, then you should add 15°, getting 90° (due east) as the true bearing of that hill. If you can identify that hill on a map, then you can find where you are on the PCT by adding 180°, getting 270° (due west) in this example. Note that this procedure is correct only for true-bearing (true field-sighting) compasses, which list degrees from 0° to 360° in a counterclockwise direction. Most hikers, however, use the generally less expensive reverse-bearing compasses, which are harder to use. (Indeed, a whole book has been written on using them for map-orienteering purposes.) Reverse-bearing, or backsight, compasses list degrees in a clockwise direction. With these compasses, you subtract. **No one should attempt a major section of the PCT without a thorough understanding of his or her compass and of map interpretation.**

Maps of the PCT can be ordered from REI at rei.com, where you can find various waterproof maps covering the PCT and the wilderness, parks, and forests it crosses. At the USGS Store (store.usgs.gov), you can order waterproof strip maps featuring the PCT. And National Geographic sells its waterproof topographic maps, which were created in partnership with Halfmile and the Pacific Crest Trail Association, online at natgeomaps.com.

The **Points on the Trail table** for each section lists the location, mileage, elevation, and GPS coordinates in degrees, minutes, and seconds (DMS) of major points in that section. If you average 22 miles a day—the on-route rate you'll need to do to complete the tristate PCT in four months—you can determine where to camp and estimate when you'll arrive at certain supply points. Specific information on camping is listed in a **Campsites and Bivy Sites table.**

On page xi, we've included a mileage table for the entire PCT. Any two adjacent points represent the start and end of a section. (We have also listed mileages for the 8 sections covered in *Pacific Crest Trail: Southern California* and the 10 sections covered in *Pacific Crest Trail: Northern California*.) The table also lists how long each section is, so you can pick one of appropriate length, turn to that section's introduction, and see if it sounds appealing. Of course, you need not start at the beginning of any section, as roads cross the PCT in most sections.

Supply points on or near the route are mentioned, as is what you might expect to find at each. You will realize, for example, that you can't get new clothes at Mazama Village but can in Ashland. Many supply points are just a post office and/or small store with minimal food supplies. By *minimal* we mean a few odds and ends that typically cater to passing motorists, for example, beer and potato chips (which nevertheless are devoured by many a trail-weary trekker).

Water is self-explanatory, as are **weather** and **permits.**

Finally, each section's introduction may mention **special concerns** you could encounter along the route, such as hordes of mosquitoes, snow avalanches, and early-season fords. If you are thru-hiking all of the PCT, you will be going through some of its sections at very inopportune times and will face many of these problems. Backpackers hiking a short stretch can pick the best time to hike it, thereby minimizing their problems.

When you start reading the text of a section, you will notice that a pair of numbers follows the more important trail points. For example, Section D (page 126) begins at OR 138 (1,847.8–5,923'), which means that this point is at mile 1,847.8 and an elevation of 5,923 feet. By noting these figures, you can determine the distance you'll need to hike from point A to point B, and you can get a good idea of how much elevation change is involved.

The route description tells something about the country you are walking through—the geology, the biology (plants and animals), the geography, and sometimes a bit of history. Longer highlights of interest are noted.

In the descriptions, an **alternate route** is a trail segment that the author thinks is worth considering given certain circumstances. Along this guide's alternate routes, there are occasional second mileage figures, which represent the distance along the alternate route to that point. A **side trip,** unlike an alternate route, returns to the main trail.

Note: If alternate routes and side trips vary considerably from the PCT, especially in wilderness areas that require their own backcountry permits, your PCT long-distance permit may not comply with local regulations.

FOLLOWING THE TRAIL

The route of the PCT is mostly along trail tread, but occasionally it is along a stretch of road. Except where the trail tread may momentarily die out, there is no cross-country trekking, although early-season hikers may go miles on snow, when accurate route finding becomes imperative. Quite naturally, you want to stay on the route. For that purpose, we recommend relying on the route description and maps in this book. To be sure, there are various markers along the route—PCT emblems and signs, metal diamonds and discs nailed to tree trunks, plastic ribbons tied to branches, blazes, and ducks. (A blaze is a place on a tree trunk where bark has been removed in the shape of a lowercase letter *i*. Typically a blaze is about 4–6 inches long. A duck is a stack of two or three rocks placed on a large boulder, log, sand, or gravel. It may be more elaborate, such as a pile of several small rocks whose placement is obviously unnatural.)

Our route descriptions depend on these markers as little as possible because they are so ephemeral. Furthermore, the blazes or ducks you follow, not having any words or numbers, may or may not mark the trail you want to be on.

One way to find a junction is to count mileage from the previous junction. If you know the length of your stride, that will help. We have used yards for short distances because 1 yard approximates the length of one long stride. Alternatively, you can develop a sense of your ground speed. Then, if it is 2 miles to the next junction and your speed is 3 miles an hour, you should be there in 2/3 hour, or 40 minutes. Be suspicious if you reach an unmarked junction sooner or later than you expect. We sometimes go to great lengths to describe the terrain so that you can be alerted to upcoming junctions. Without these clues, you could easily miss the junction in early season, when snow still obscures many parts of the trail.

THE MAPS

Each section contains topographic maps complete with shaded relief, contour elevation, and both UTM and latitude/longitude grids. All individual section maps are at a scale of 1:63,360, or 1 inch equals 1 mile, and include a north indicator. Refer to the legend at right for the different stylings between the PCT and other trails, as well as the many symbols featured throughout the maps.

Map Legend

PCT featured section	———————	Cabin rental	♠	Peak/summit	▲▲
PCT continued section	– – – – – – –	Campground	▲	Picnic area	⊼
Alternate route	———————	Campsite	◮	Picnic shelter	⟁
Side trail	• • • • • • • • •	Fee station	$	Pit toilet	⌂
Freeway	▭▭▭▭▭	Food service	❙❙	Post office	⊠
Major road	⊏▭▭▭▭▭⊐	Footbridge	✕	Ranger station	⌂
Minor road	⊂▭▭▭▭▭⊃	Gate	•–•–	Restroom	♟♟
Unpaved road	≡≡≡≡≡≡≡	General point of interest	●	Scenic view	⋈
Railroad	⊢⊣⊢⊣⊢⊣	Information kiosk	⑦	Shelter	⊏
Power line	•—•—•—•—	Laundromat	⎅	Shower access	⚒
Water body	▬	Lodging	⊨	Spring	○
River/creek/stream	~~~~	Lookout/fire tower	♙	Store	⬤
Boundary	—•—••—•—	Mile marker	211	Trailhead	⚐
National/state forest	▭	One-way (road)	◀	Tunnel	⊃
National/state park	▬	Overlook	▲	Waterfall	//
Wilderness area	▭	Parking area	🅿	Water source	⛉
Wildlife area	▬				
American Indian reservation	▬				
Military area	▬				

Contour lines   UTM grid   Latitude/Longitude grid

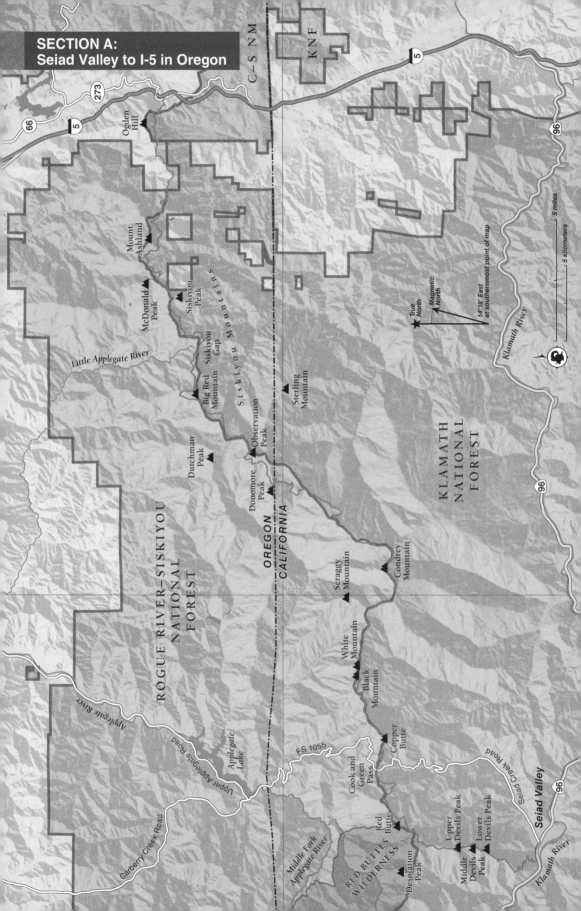

KNF

C–S NM

273

66

5

5

96

Ogden Hill

Mount Ashland

McDonald Peak

Siskiyou Peak

S i s k i y o u   M o u n t a i n s

Little Applegate River

Big Red Mountain

Siskiyou Gap

Observation Peak

Dutchman Peak

Sterling Mountain

Donomore Peak

OREGON
CALIFORNIA

5 miles

5 kilometers

True North

Magnetic North

14°18' East at southernmost point of map

Klamath River

ROGUE RIVER–SISKIYOU NATIONAL FOREST

K L A M A T H   N A T I O N A L   F O R E S T

Applegate River

Scraggy Mountain

Condrey Mountain

White Mountain

Black Mountain

Upper Applegate Road

Applegate Lake

FS 1055

Cook and Green Pass

Copper Butte

Seiad Creek Road

96

Seiad Valley

Upper Devils Peak

Lower Devils Peak

Middle Devils Peak

Red Butte

RED BUTTES WILDERNESS

Desolation Peak

Middle Fork Applegate River

Carberry Creek Road

Klamath River

W123

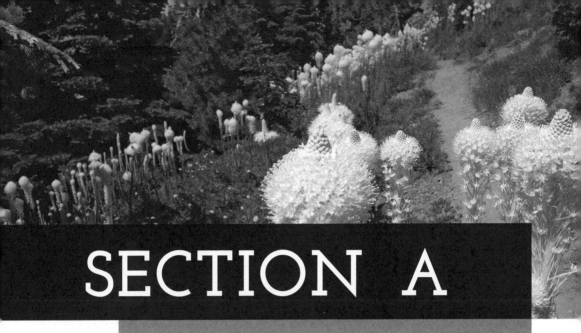

SECTION A

Seiad Valley to I-5 in Oregon

IN THIS SECTION YOU MAKE A LONG TRAVERSE east to get over to the Cascade Range. The long trek west from Burney Falls to Marble Mountain was not only beautiful but also quite necessary because a route going north from Burney Falls past Mount Shasta would be a dry, hot one indeed. Before the Pacific Crest Trail (PCT) route took on its current position, this sun-drenched corridor was the one most hikers followed to the former Oregon Skyline Trail—Oregon's section of the PCT.

Section A's route stays remarkably high for most of its length, dropping significantly only at each end. Although high, it has been only mildly glaciated, and because glaciers haven't scoured away the soil, thick forests abound. These, unfortunately, are rampant with logging roads. From Reeves Ranch east, you are always paralleling one road or another. Views, however, are pleasing enough, and surprisingly few logging operations are visible

Above: When bear grass, a member of the lily family, blooms, it creates an unexpected display on steep, open slopes such as these near Wrangle Gap.

from the trail. Before early July these roads are an advantage, for significant stretches of trail are still snowbound. The roads, being more open, are quite easy to follow, though they still have enough snow patches to stop motor vehicles. As you progress east on trail or road, you walk across increasingly younger rocks, first late-Paleozoic/early-Mesozoic metamorphic rocks, then mid-Mesozoic granitic rocks of the Mount Ashland area, and finally mid- to late-Cenozoic volcanic rocks of the I-5 area.

DECLINATION 14°18'E

USGS MAPS

Seiad Valley, CA	*Dutchman Peak, OR–CA*
Kangaroo Mountain, CA	*Siskiyou Peak, OR–CA*
Dutch Creek, CA	*Mount Ashland, OR*
Condrey Mountain, CA	*Siskiyou Pass, OR*

POINTS ON THE TRAIL, SOUTH TO NORTH

	Mile	Elevation in feet	Latitude/Longitude
CA 96 at Seiad Valley	1,655.9	1,373	N41° 50' 31.6050" W123° 11' 46.2365"
Lower Devils Peak saddle	1,662.0	5,004	N41° 52' 38.4404" W123° 12' 10.8769"
Cook and Green Pass	1,670.8	4,736	N41° 56' 30.2671" W123° 08' 42.5427"
Tin Cup Trail junction	1,675.9	6,062	N41° 57' 13.3974" W123° 04' 43.7775"
Alex Hole Spring	1,683.2	6,588	N41° 55' 57.1204" W122° 58' 08.1853"
Mud Spring spur road	1,685.3	6,732	N41° 57' 21.9898" W122° 57' 15.8434"
Bearground Spring	1,687.6	5,980	N41° 58' 01.1165" W122° 55' 52.1374"
Wards Fork Gap	1,689.1	5,287	N41° 59' 02.3006" W122° 55' 02.6162"
California–Oregon border	1,691.7	6,068	N42° 00' 12.9299" W122° 54' 32.6165"
Sheep Camp Spring	1,696.1	6,866	N42° 01' 58.1213" W122° 52' 24.4280"
Wrangle Gap	1,698.3	6,499	N42° 03' 01.3896" W122° 50' 46.1155"
Long John saddle	1,703.6	5,892	N42° 03' 16.5404" W122° 47' 44.7886"
FS 2080	1,711.9	6,054	N42° 04' 19.4700" W122° 41' 28.5500"
Old US 99 and Mount Ashland Ski Road	1,718.7	4,207	N42° 03' 53.0761" W122° 36' 09.7241"

CAMPSITES AND BIVY SITES

Mile	Elevation in feet	Latitude/ Longitude	Number of tents	Feature	Notes
1,660.5	3,778	N41° 51' 56.6234" W123° 12' 40.8055"	2	Vista	Small shaded saddle
1,679.3	6,201	N41° 56' 49.7202" W123° 01' 19.3522"	4	Vista	Shaded bivy on crest saddle

CAMPSITES AND BIVY SITES (continued)

Mile	Elevation in feet	Latitude/ Longitude	Number of tents	Feature	Notes
1,685.3	6,662	N41° 57' 28.4202" W122° 57' 20.9522"	>3	Mud Spring nearby	
1,685.3	6,662	N41° 57' 28.4202" W122° 57' 20.9522"	>3	Mud Spring nearby	
1,687.7	5,987	N41° 58' 08.8324" W122° 55' 50.4781"	2	Springs nearby	Decent sites in an area of several springs
1,698.3	6,400	N42° 03' 00.9286" W122° 51' 21.3113"	5	Wrangle Campground	Vault toilet, fire pit, picnic table
1,702.6	5,975	N42° 02' 47.7020" W122° 47' 55.3646"	>2		Shaded bivy sites, fire ring
1,708.2	6,604	N42° 04' 53.5948" W122° 44' 21.8705"	2	Grouse Gap Shelter	Vault toilet, picnic table, fireplace; views to Mount Shasta
1,710.0	6,513	N42° 04' 30.3900" W122° 42' 53.1300"	>4	Mount Ashland Campground	Campground straddles both sides of FS 20; vault toilet; water nearby
1,718.7 (alt.)	3,967	N42° 04' 25.9300" W122° 36' 09.4300"	>4	Callahan's Mountain Lodge	1.3 miles off-trail; restrooms, showers, laundry, restaurant

WEATHER TO GO

This section's PCT can be snowbound at higher elevations before early July. However, you could start in mid- or late June and bypass snowbound portions of the trail in some places using nearby roads that parallel it. Serious snowstorms can occur by late September or early October.

SUPPLIES

No supplies are available once you leave Seiad Valley. Along this crest route, virtually all roads south will get you down to CA 96, which has a smattering of hamlets, and virtually all roads north will ultimately channel you down to the Ashland–Medford area. However, we don't think you should descend either direction because you would then be way off-route. Even in an emergency situation, you're likely to get help from people driving along the near-crest roads long before you could reach any settlement. If you're thru-hiking, you'll want to end Section A in Ashland, and routes to it are described in this trail chapter. You won't find any more sizable towns within easy reach of the PCT—other than Sisters—until you reach the Oregon–Washington border area, more than 400 miles beyond this section's end. If you need new or specific gear, Bend is a bit of a hitch, but there is a large REI there. If you think you'll need a new pack, water filter, or hiking shoes, certainly stop in Ashland.

PERMITS

Using a stove or campfire in California forests requires a current California campfire permit. Visit readyforwildfire.org/permits/campfire-permit for more information.

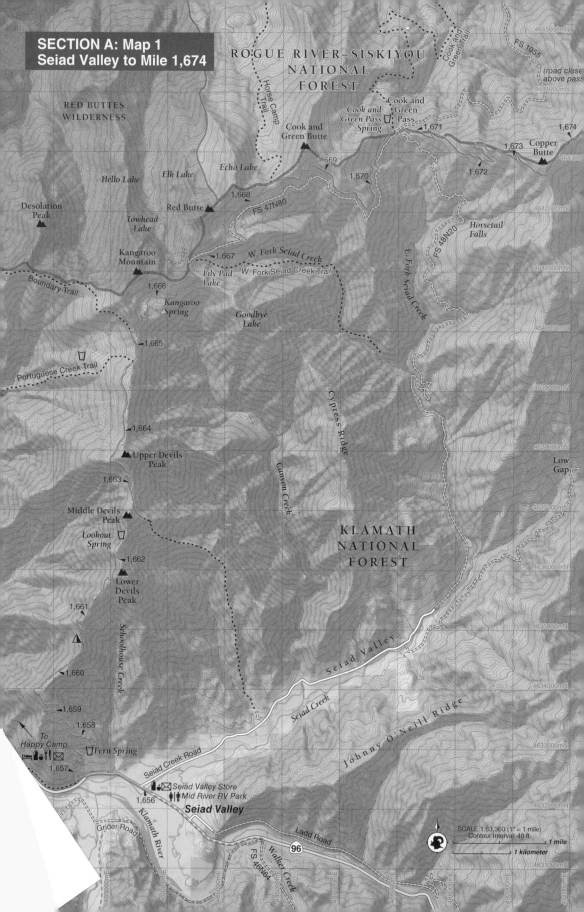

ROGUE RIVER–SISKIYOU
NATIONAL
FOREST

RED BUTTES
WILDERNESS

Horse Camp Trail

Cook and Green Trail

FS 1055

(road closed
above pass)

Cook and Green Butte

Cook and Green Pass Spring

Cook and Green Pass

1,671

1,673

Copper Butte

1,674

1,669

1,670

1,672

Hello Lake

Elk Lake

Echo Lake

1,668

Desolation Peak

Towhead Lake

Red Butte

FS 47N80

Horsetail Falls

Kangaroo Mountain

1,667

W. Fork Seiad Creek

FS 48N20

E. Fork Seiad Creek

Boundary Trail

1,666

Lily Pad Lake

W. Fork Seiad Creek Trail

Kangaroo Spring

Goodbye Lake

1,665

Cypress Ridge

Portuguese Creek Trail

Low Gap

1,664

Canyon Creek

Upper Devils Peak

KLAMATH
NATIONAL
FOREST

1,663

Middle Devils Peak

Lookout Spring

1,662

Lower Devils Peak

1,661

Schoolhouse Creek

Seiad Valley

1,660

Seiad Creek

1,659

Johnny O'Neill Ridge

1,658

To Happy Camp

Fern Spring

1,657

Seiad Creek Road

Seiad Valley Store

Mid River RV Park

1,656

Seiad Valley

Grider Road

Klamath River

Ladd Road

96

Walker Creek

FS 46N64

SCALE 1:63,360 (1" = 1 mile)
Contour Interval: 40 ft.

1 mile

1 kilometer

SEIAD VALLEY TO I-5 IN OREGON
>>>THE ROUTE

Begin this section at the Seiad Valley Store and post office (1,655.9–1,373') in California. Walking west along the highway, you immediately cross Seiad Creek Road, which heads northeast up to Horsetail Falls and beyond to Cook and Green Pass. Not much farther, you reach Schoolhouse Creek. Follow the road as it curves west, and reach a trailhead (1,656.7–1,372'). As it is an exhausting 4,400-foot ascent to the Kangaroo Mountain meadows, it's prudent to begin in the cool shade of the morning.

Under a cover of madrone, Douglas-fir, incense cedar, and Oregon oak, your trail curves west and climbs moderately to reach a junction (1,656.9–1,556') with a trail that parallels CA 96 west 1.4 miles before ending close to a stream-gaging cable that spans the mighty Klamath River.

From the junction with the CA 96 trail, where you cross under some minor power lines, your trail heads right (north) into a shaded ravine harboring poison oak.

WATER ACCESS

You soon reach Fern Spring (1,657.6–1,935'), a small seep trickling from a pipe into a concrete cistern. You may find a trail register here.

Your well-engineered trail switchbacks up shady, though fly-infested, south-facing slopes, then follows a ridge system northeast up toward Lower Devils Peak.

FIRE Along this stretch you'll see trees that were scorched in two widespread fires, both started by lightning, in the summers of 1987 and 2012. The damage here was minor and rather beneficial compared with that north of Lower Devils Peak. The Portuguese Creek terrain west of the PCT and the Kangaroo Roadless Area were significantly affected.

Where the ridge fuses with the peak's flank, you climb some short switchbacks, then traverse north across west-facing slopes to a junction (1,661.8–4,882').

WATER ACCESS

From here a 40-yard-long trail goes over to Lookout Spring. This trickling spring is usually reliable, though one has to marvel at how any water flows at all, considering the spring is so close to the Devils Peak crest.

From the junction you climb about 300 yards in a final push up to the Lower Devils Peak saddle, on the Devils Peak crest (1,662.0–5,004').

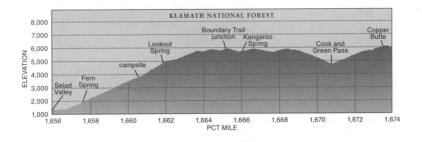

SIDE TRIP From the saddle you can follow a faint, rocky trail 0.25 mile east over to the remains of Lower Devils Peak Lookout, which was dismantled in 1976. The views from it are fine, but the many views ahead rival those from the lookout site. The lower room of the lookout still remains, albeit roofless.

From the crest saddle you start across the first of several major burns you'll traverse before Lily Pad Lake.

PLANTS Note the charred remains of knobcone pine here. These pines depend on major fires, the heat of which opens their cones to release their seeds. The short-lived trees die in the process, but new pines soon sprout. Without periodic fires, the population would die out.

On the east ridge of Middle Devils Peak, you meet an unmaintained trail (1,662.6–5,133') that starts down the ridge to the right (southeast).

PLANTS As you cross the northeast-facing slopes of Middle Devils Peak, you pass the first of several small groves of Brewer spruce, a rare species. Note the trees' drooping "Douglas-fir" branches, their oversize "hemlock" cones, and their scaly "lodgepole" bark.

North of the peak you reach a saddle, and from here, as well as from short switchbacks above it, you have views of snowcapped Mount Shasta (14,180') to the east and the Marble Mountain Wilderness to the south. Beyond the switchbacks you reach the western arm of Upper Devils Peak (1,663.6–5,782').

Your trail now traverses north, and along it you pass the charred remains of a forest before reaching a small grove of weeping spruce. Just past it you descend briefly to a saddle, which

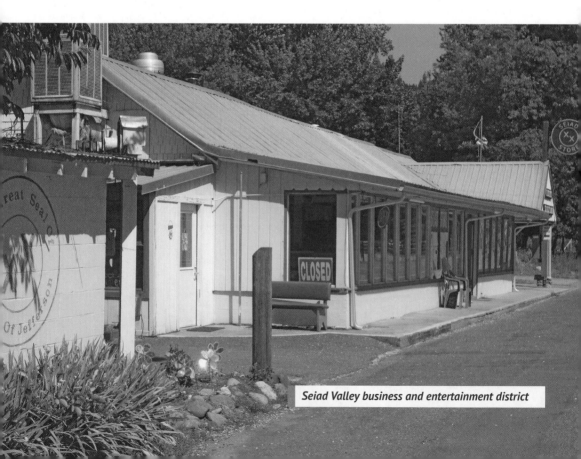

Seiad Valley business and entertainment district

has a junction with faint Portuguese Creek Trail (1,664.8–5,797').

WATER ACCESS

If you need water, you can drop west about 300 vertical feet along this trail to the seasonal headwaters of Portuguese Creek and then follow the creek down another 300–600 feet to find flowing water.

The PCT next climbs north and quickly reaches a junction with the Boundary Trail (1,665.2–5,894'). You'll likely have noted by now a high, often snowy peak along the western skyline, 7,309-foot Preston Peak.

Now you head 100 yards southeast to a minor saddle on nearby Devils Peak crest, which also happens to be the south ridge of rusty Kangaroo Mountain. The mountain's glaciated, broad-floored basin greets you as you start a short, switchbacking descent, and along it you may see two tiny ponds.

GEOLOGY Heading north from the switchbacks, you discover a creek that disappears into a sinkhole dissolved from a layer of light-gray marble that contrasts strongly with the orange, ancient, ultramafic intrusives of this area. These rocks are likely the northern extension of the rock types you see along the PCT in the Marble Mountain Wilderness, on the distant southern skyline.

Heading east, you reach a spring (1,666.0–5,715') in spongy ground. From this spring—the easternmost of the Kangaroo Springs—the trail soon reaches a southeast slope and traverses it. Soon you reach Kangaroo Mountain's east ridge and leave burned, trailside vegetation behind, although you'll see burned slopes

on lands south of you all the way to Cook and Green Pass.

From the east ridge you can gaze down at Lily Pad Lake. Your trail stays high above this lake and arcs northwest over to a narrow ridge, which is a small part of the Red Buttes Wilderness boundary. Along this ridge you may find a trail register, and just past it is a junction with a spur trail (1,666.7–5,904'). This goes 115 yards north along the boundary ridge to a jeep road. Westward, within the wilderness, the jeep road is closed, but eastward it is still open and is definitely used. The PCT parallels it at a distance down to Cook and Green Pass.

With that goal in mind, you go just 200 yards northeast on the PCT before intersecting an old trail that starts from the jeep road just above you and drops to Lily Pad Lake. Now you descend gently east to a ridge that provides views down into the lake's glaciated canyon. From the ridge you circle a shallower, mildly glaciated canyon and cross the jeep road (1,667.7–5,674'), which has been staying just above you.

Just several yards before this crossing, a spur trail leads about 20 yards downslope to a nearby spring, which hopefully will be flowing when you arrive here, but don't count on it. The PCT has kept below the road to avoid an old chromite mine, which lies just southwest of the road crossing. Next you travel through a stand of trees, then climb past more brush to a junction on a crest saddle (1,668.3–5,877').

SIDE TRIP From here Horse Camp Trail 958 generally descends north toward nearby Echo Lake.

Leaving the saddle and the last outcrop of marble you'll encounter on your northbound trek, you make a long, mostly brushy descent, first east and then north, down to Cook and Green Pass (1,670.8–4,736').

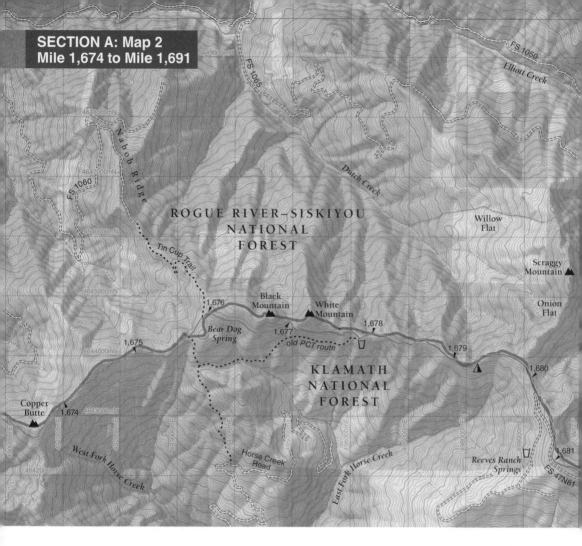

FS 1050

Elliott Creek

FS 1065

Nabob Ridge

FS 1060

Dutch Creek

ROGUE RIVER–SISKIYOU
NATIONAL
FOREST

Willow
Flat

Tin Cup Trail

Scraggy
Mountain ▲

Black
Mountain ▲

White
▲ Mountain

Onion
Flat

1,676

1,678

Bear Dog
Spring

1,677

old PCT route

🚻

1,679

1,675

KLAMATH
NATIONAL
FOREST

1,680

△

Copper
Butte
▲

1,674

West Fork Horse Creek

Horse Creek
Road

East Fork Horse Creek

Reeves Ranch
Springs 🚻

1,681

FS 47N81

WATER ACCESS

Get water by going along a trail that leads northwest from the pass. You'll reach a spring in 150 yards; if it's dry, continue another 225 yards to a creeklet.

Here, along the crest border between Klamath National Forest to the south and Rogue River–Siskiyou National Forest to the north, a major U.S. Forest Service road crosses the pass and then descends 12.1 miles to the Seiad Valley Store, at the start of this section. The PCT route is about 2 miles longer.

Northbound from Cook and Green Pass, the road has been permanently closed.

From this pass you follow an obvious trail east up the ridge toward Copper Butte.

PLANTS On it you pass scattered knobcone pine in a vegetative cover that includes manzanita, western serviceberry, tobacco brush, and Sadler's oak.

GEOLOGY Like tombstones, slabs of greenish-gray, foliated mica schist stand erect along the trail and, in the proper light, reflect the sun's rays as glacially polished rocks do.

Your trail makes a long switchback up to the crest, passing a clear-cut in the process. There are other clear-cuts to the south, on slopes east of Seiad Creek, and this patchwork

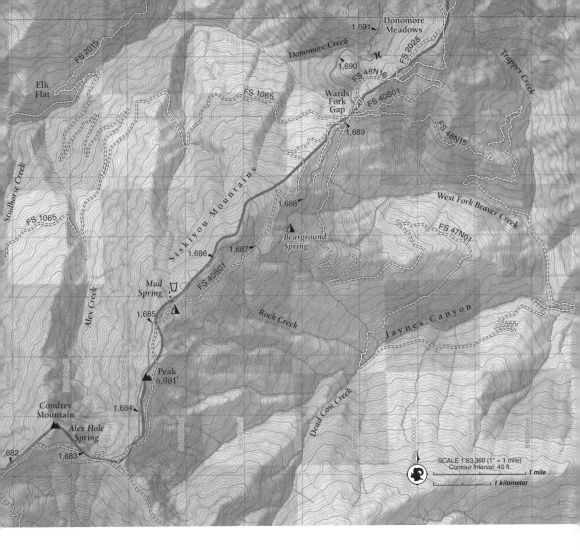

landscape of forest and clearing contrasts with the burned slopes, which are mostly west of the creek.

PLANTS Once back on the crest, the PCT enters a stand of white fir, red fir, mountain hemlock, Douglas-fir, ponderosa pine, and knobcone pine—a combination you'd never see in the Sierra Nevada, where these trees are altitudinally zoned to a much

greater extent. On the north slopes just below the crest, you'll also find weeping spruce.

Make a slight ascent to the south ridge of Copper Butte, on which you meet an abandoned trail (1,673.5–6,040') that once descended south to Low Gap, Salt Gulch, and Seiad Valley. Your course now becomes a northeast one and you keep close to the crest, crossing several forested crest saddles before arriving at an open one

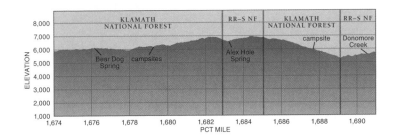

(1,675.7–6,056'), from which a pack trail begins a brushy descent south to Horse Creek Road 46N50. This road descends southeast many miles to the hamlet of Horse Creek on CA 96.

Continue northeast to another saddle (1,675.9–6,062'). Here you'll find Tin Cup Trail 961, which descends north-northwest 1.7 miles to FS 1060.

Leaving the saddle, you start a contour east and from brushy slopes can identify the spring area, across the meadow south of you, by noting a large log near the forest's edge. By Bear Dog Spring, immediately below the trail, your brushy contour becomes a forested one of Douglas-fir, Jeffrey pine, and incense cedar. Beyond a deep crest saddle, you soon start along the south slope of White Mountain. You cross somewhat-open slopes again, reach its spur ridge, and then arc east across the upper limits of a meadowy hollow. At its east end is a junction (1,677.9–5,933') with the old PCT.

WATER ACCESS

This trail will lead you to a seasonal seep near the hollow's west edge. Late-season hikers will have to descend the hollow a short distance to get their water.

Just beyond this junction, you reach another saddle, and from it you climb east to a higher crest. You stay close to it on a path that glitters with mica flakes before you eventually curve southeast and descend an open slope. Next you parallel a road across a long saddle, then almost touch the hairpin turn of FS 47N81 (1,680.2–6,234').

WATER ACCESS

You can take the lower road branch right (south) 0.8 mile to Reeves Ranch Springs, located below the road. The northernmost spring is seasonal, but the two others appear to be perennial. Dense groves of alder give away the springs' location but also make reaching them an effort.

The PCT parallels the east side of the road's upper branch, climbing first south, then east, and eventually traversing the south slopes of Condrey Mountain before descending 0.75 mile to a saddle (1,683.2–6,588').

From here a spur road leaves FS 47N81 to descend west-southwest, and another spur road descends north 0.25 mile to delightful, willow-lined Alex Hole Spring. Here, where your far-reaching view north is framed by cliffs of mica schist, your only neighbors may be deer, chipmunks, and mountain bluebirds.

On the PCT, you start to parallel ascending FS 47N81, then veer north away from it to climb the main Siskiyou crest. You almost top Peak 6,981 before descending into a mountain-hemlock forest. Long-lasting snow patches can make the next mile to the Mud Spring spur road difficult to follow; if so, you can take the crest road, just east of you, to the same destination. If you encounter snow along here, you are certain to encounter more snow to the east. Just yards away from FS 40S01, the PCT crosses the Mud Spring spur road (1,685.3–6,732').

WATER ACCESS

CAMPING You can continue left (northwest) 0.2 mile down this road to its end, where there are refreshing clear-water springs. Hikers rely on these fragile springs, so only gather water here. Hikers looking for campsites may prefer to camp about 100 feet from the PCT near the start of the spur road leading down to the springs.

Past the spur road you have an open, near-crest traverse that passes a prominent rock midway along your approach to less imposing, misnamed Big Rock (1,686.1–6,674'). You descend northeast across its open, gravelly east slope of glistening mica, briefly enter a patch of fir, leave it, and head south back into forest as you descend to a crossing of FS 40S01 (1,687.0–6,271'). Your trail now enters an old logging area as it first continues south, then turns northeast and descends to cross a dirt road (1,687.6–5,980') that lies immediately north of Bearground Spring.

CAMPING This is an area of several springs, each fragile and susceptible to contamination. In this vicinity, you should be able to find a decent place to sleep on a durable surface—such as snow, rock, or mineral soil—in an established site at least 200 feet (about 75 paces) away from water sources.

From the Bearground Spring road, you start among shady Shasta red fir and make a steady descent northeast, crossing an abandoned logging road midway to a saddle. Nearing this saddle, you cross narrow FS 40S01 at its hairpin turn, immediately recross the road, and in a couple of minutes reach a six-way road junction on the saddle, Wards Fork Gap (1,689.1–5,287'). Southbound FS 47N01 traverses over to FS 47N44, and from that junction both descend to Beaver Creek. Along the creek, FS 48N01 descends to CA 96, reaching it just 0.7 mile northeast of Klamath River, a small community with a store and post office. FS 48N15, descending east from the saddle, will also get you to Beaver Creek. FS 1065 traverses left (west) from the saddle but later drops to FS 1050, which descends west to Hutton Campground and the nearby Applegate Lake area.

Between north-climbing FS 48N16 and east-climbing FS 40S01, the PCT starts to climb northeast from Wards Fork Gap. This short

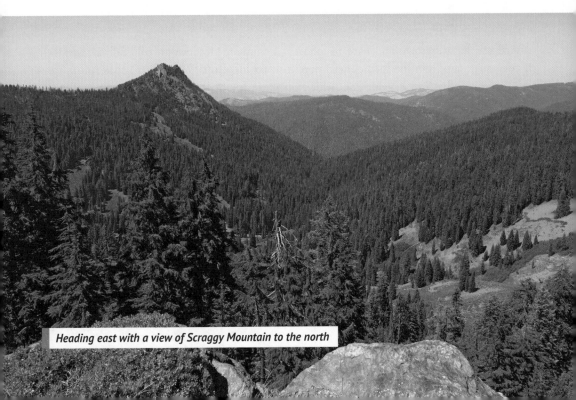

Heading east with a view of Scraggy Mountain to the north

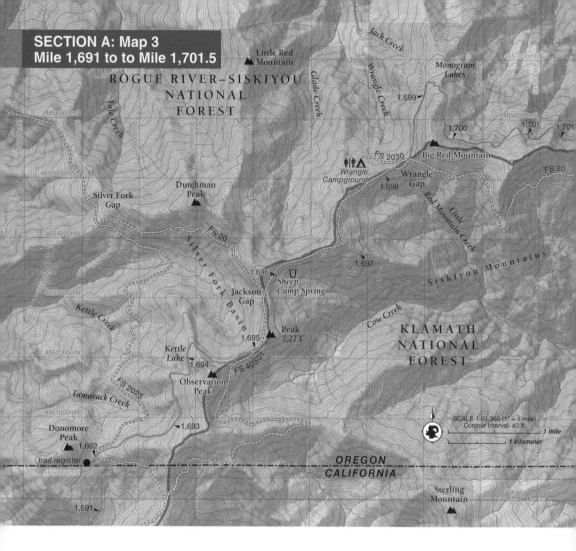

ROGUE RIVER–SISKIYOU
NATIONAL
FOREST

Little Red
Mountain

Jack Creek

Wrangle Creek

Glade Creek

Monogram
Lakes

1,699

1,700   1,701   1,701

Tate Creek

Silver Fork
Gap

Dutchman
Peak

FS 2030

Wrangle
Campground

Big Red Mountain

FS 20

Wrangle
Gap

1,698

FS 20

Little Red Mountain Creek

Silver Fork Basin

1,697

1,696

Sheep
Camp Spring

Jackson
Gap

Siskiyou Mountains

Kettle Creek

Peak
7,273'

Cow Creek

KLAMATH
NATIONAL
FOREST

1,695

Kettle
Lake

1,694

FS 40S01

FS 2025

Tamarack Creek

Observation
Peak

1,693

Donomore
Peak

1,692

trail register

OREGON
CALIFORNIA

SCALE 1:63,360 (1" = 1 mile)
Contour Interval: 40 ft.
1 mile
1 kilometer

Sterling
Mountain

1,691

stretch can be overgrown and hard to follow. If you can't, then from the saddle, head north briefly up FS 48N16 to a bend, from which a logging spur continues north. You'll see the PCT just above it, paralleling it first north then west. Walk south up FS 48N16 midway to its second bend, and you should be able to find the northbound PCT without much trouble.

On it you make a short climb north before embarking on a long traverse that circles clockwise around a knoll to Donomore Creek. You parallel the creek east to within 100 yards of the Donomore Meadows road and then cross the crystal-clear water (1,690.5–5,585') as it bubbles beneath a short, wooden bridge. You then wind north up an amorphous ridge that may be crisscrossed with cow paths. Long, sloping

Donomore Meadows are colorfully arrayed with corn lily, leopard lily, bear grass, pussy-paw, cow parsnip, meadow penstemon, paintbrush, lupine, and maybe more. This beautiful hillside has been protected forever and placed back into public ownership through the efforts of people like you who organized under the umbrella of the Pacific Crest Trail Association.

In 0.5 mile you cross the Donomore Meadows road at a point about 80 yards east of a cabin,

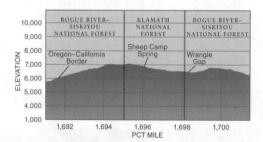

then parallel a jeep road, immediately below you, which follows the meadow's edge north. At the meadow's upper end, your trail curves east above it, then switchbacks west for a short, partly steep ascent northwest into Oregon (1,691.7–6,068'). Here, on shaded trail at a nondescript uphill switchback, northbound hikers can finally boast of navigating the entirety of California, from Mexico to Oregon, by walking on trail more than twice the straight-line distance. Here, find a trail register and a fractured sign with mileages to various borders. One more switchback north brings you up to a logging-road saddle (1,692.0–6,190').

Now you cross wide FS 2025, then climb east up a clear-cut crest and leave it to make a long, curving traverse north to the west ridge (1,693.6–6,731') of twin-topped Observation Peak. Kettle Lake, below you, immediately comes into view as you start an uphill traverse east. You climb east to Kettle Creek, then climb north high above Kettle Lake before rounding the large northwest ridge of Observation Peak. A southeast traverse through stands of mountain hemlock—snowbound until mid-July—gets

you to Observation Gap (1,694.7–7,048'), a shallow saddle from which you have your first vista including Mount McLoughlin through Jackson Gap. From the saddle you go 0.3 mile on your crest trail, cross FS 40S01, travel around the east slopes of Peak 7,273, and then parallel the crest north to just below Jackson Gap (1,695.8–6,975'). You'll certainly notice landscape terracing in the Jackson Gap area, done to prevent erosion on the burned-over slopes. Crossing this gap about 100 feet above you is broad FS 20, which you'll parallel all the way to the end of this section. Before mid-July, snowdrifts will probably force you to take this road rather than the PCT.

WATER ACCESS

Leaving the cover of hemlock and fir, you arc clockwise across the upper slopes of an open bowl, soon reaching a spur road (1,696.1–6,866') to Sheep Camp Spring, located 10 yards south along it.

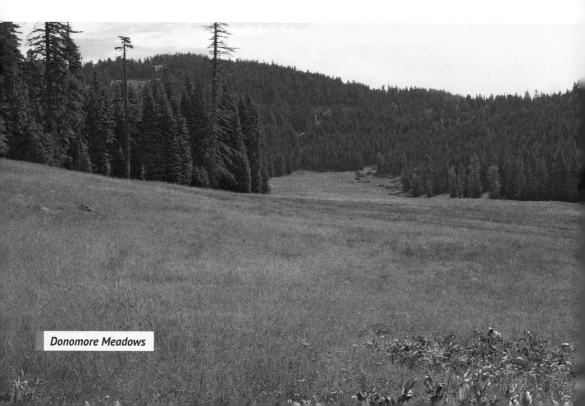

Donomore Meadows

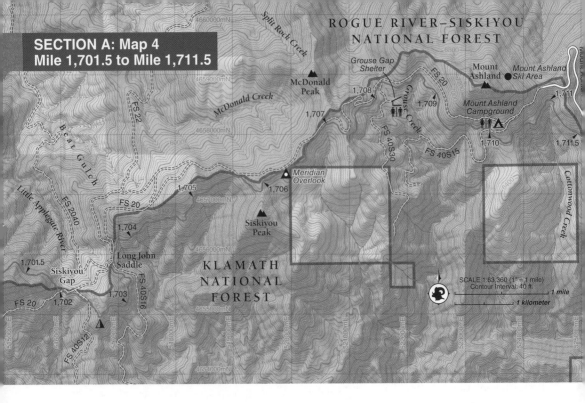

ROGUE RIVER–SISKIYOU
NATIONAL FOREST

Departing east from the spur road, you gradually descend, with unobstructed views, to a spur ridge, then arc northeast to Wrangle Gap (1,698.3–6,499'), reaching it 0.25 mile after you cross to the north side of FS 20.

CAMPING From Wrangle Gap, a spur road descends steeply west to Wrangle Campground. This little-used recreation site, nestled among Shasta red fir, has a large stone shelter complete with fireplace, two stoves, and tables. You'll have to get water from a nearby spring or lower down, from Wrangle Creek. The spring is at the upper end of a small bowl. To reach it from the shelter, head 210° for 150 yards. Using developed sites such as this reduces impacts elsewhere on the trail.

From Wrangle Gap the PCT makes a long climb north to the end of Big Red Mountain ridge and starts to wind southeast up it. The route gives you sweeping panoramas of southern Oregon and its pointed landmark, Mount McLoughlin—an Ice Age volcano. After crossing the ridge you contour south then east, leaving Big Red Mountain's slopes for a winding,

moderate descent to the west end of Siskiyou Gap (1,702.0–5,904'), where you cross FS 20.

TRAIL INFO The next 0.25 mile of trail lies on private land, and the U.S. Forest Service had to build a trail twice as long as a direct route would have been to Long John Saddle beginning at the crossing of FS 40S12.

Your trail first parallels FS 20 briefly over to its junction with FS 40S12, then parallels that road briefly over to a ridge crossing. Then it makes a long swing around a hill, offering you some Mount Shasta views, before finally reaching a five-way road junction (1,703.6–5,892') on forested Long John Saddle.

FS 20 traverses north across the level saddle, and a minor logging road descends northeast. Between the two, the PCT starts

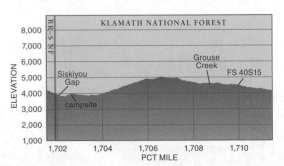

to parallel FS 20 north, then climbs northeast through an old logging area. After a mile of progress, you come to a spur ridge and exchange this scarred landscape for a shady forest climb north. From a ravine, your gradient eases to give you a pleasant stroll northeast to an open crest saddle. On it, your tread almost disappears as it parallels FS 20 for a few yards; then it becomes prominent again and climbs 0.5 mile to a saddle just north of Siskiyou Peak.

VIEWS From this saddle you'll see chunky Pilot Rock on the eastern skyline. If you're thru-hiking the PCT, you should pass by it in a few days.

Your trail now winds northeast toward a saddle on the main crest, crossing a spur road (1,706.2–6,888') that is just 25 yards below its departure from crest-hugging FS 20. The saddle is signed as Meridian Overlook, as it is a viewpoint close to the Willamette Meridian.

You parallel FS 20 northeast, sometimes below it and sometimes above it, to another saddle (1,707.4–6,981'), which is south of the main crest. Here the road bends north to descend, but you first go south briefly before switchbacking to descend northeast to reach FS 40S30 (1,708.2–6,604') at its junction with FS 20 on expansive Grouse Gap.

CAMPING This road takes you 0.2 mile south to a fork, from which you branch left on FS 40S30A for a minute's walk to Grouse Gap Shelter. You can usually get water from the creeklet just northeast of and below the shelter; however, late-season trekkers will likely have to backtrack on FS 40S30A to FS 40S30 and take that road 0.3 mile southwest to an obvious gully with a spring-fed creeklet.

The fenced-in shelter provides protection from the elements and offers dramatic sunrise views of Mount Shasta.

From Grouse Gap the PCT parallels FS 20 and passes several seeping springs before gradually dropping away from it down to a crossing of FS 40S15 (1,710.0–6,513'), which climbs 0.5 mile

northeast to this crest road. From their junction, FS 20 contours 0.5 mile northeast to the Mount Ashland Ski Area; eastward, the road is paved.

CAMPING An alternative to camping at Grouse Gap Shelter is to camp at Mount Ashland Campground, which straddles both sides of FS 20. To reach it, leave the PCT and follow FS 40S15 about 250 yards up to its bend left, from which you'll see an abandoned logging road that climbs upslope to the campground. The piped water isn't always flowing; when it's not, get water from a little stream just above the campground's upper (north) sites.

From FS 40S15 the PCT contours southeast to the bend and then traverses northeast to an open bowl below the ski area. From there it travels southeast to a saddle, where you cross FS 20 (1,711.6–6,175'), now known as Mount Ashland Ski Road. Continuing down-ridge (southeast), follow the PCT down to FS 2080 (1,711.9–6,054').

RESUPPLY ACCESS

Follow FS 2080 north down to Bull Gap (5,508'), where you meet FS 200, which climbs southwest to the Mount Ashland Ski Area. Continuing north, take FS 200, which in 3.5 miles rejoins FS 2080, down to Glenview Drive in Ashland. Descend this road north, then descend Fork Street. You quickly reach Pioneer Street and follow it two blocks to Lithia Way. The Ashland Post Office is one block southeast on it, at the corner of First Street. To get back to the PCT, head southwest one block to East Main, and walk southeast. East Main becomes two-way Siskiyou

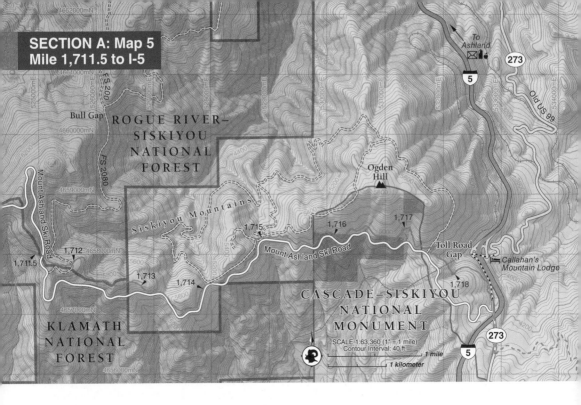

Boulevard, and from here you can continue southeast to OR 66 (Ashland Street). Take this east past the Ashland Shopping Center to I-5. Because hitchhiking on freeways is legal in Oregon, you can hitchhike 9 miles to the Mount Ashland Ski Area exit.

Alternatively, continue on OR 66, and then go south up OR 273 to the Mount Ashland Ski Area exit, about a 12-mile route. This route is described in the opposite direction at the end of this chapter.

If you decide against the resupply route, continue east down the forested trail. The PCT stays on or north of the crest, but after 0.7 mile it crosses to its south side and in 0.25 mile crosses a jeep road that climbs northeast back to the nearby crest.

The PCT continues its eastern descent on private land now, first past grass and bracken ferns and then mostly past brush. Soon the trail switchbacks and quickly reaches the shady grounds of the former Mount Ashland Inn.

A minute's walk below the inn site, you cross a saddle and then parallel Mount Ashland Ski Road for a generally brushy 0.7-mile traverse over to another saddle (1,714.1–5,140'). Next you make a similar traverse, this one to a saddle with four roads radiating from it (1,715.0–5,037'). Eastbound, the PCT is confined between an old crest road and Mount Ashland Ski Road for the first 0.3 mile and then parallels the latter as both descend east around ridges and across ravines. Three closely spaced

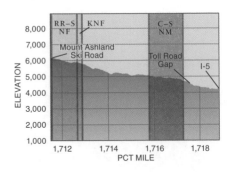

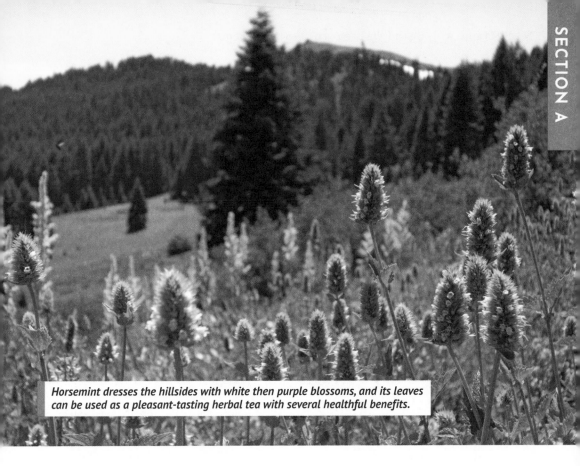

Horsemint dresses the hillsides with white then purple blossoms, and its leaves can be used as a pleasant-tasting herbal tea with several healthful benefits.

streams near the end of this descent provide spring-fed water before they coalesce to flow into the East Fork Cottonwood Creek.

Because you are on private land, you aren't allowed to deviate from the trail's tread and aren't allowed to camp. About 0.4 mile past your last spring-fed stream, you cross a road (1,717.5–4,566') that descends steeply southwest to nearby Mount Ashland Ski Road, which here turns southeast to cross a broad saddle. Then, after a 0.1-mile steep descent of your own, you cross a road that climbs gently west to a union with the first road at paved Mount Ashland Ski Road. Both dirt roads are private (off-limits), as is a third road that you parallel east, then momentarily turn south to cross in another 0.1 mile. Now you parallel this road, staying just above it, dip in and out of a streambed with a sometimes-flowing freshet, then soon curve away from the road as you glimpse busy, nearby I-5. Your path ends at an abandoned segment of Old US 99, which you take 140 yards around a hollow to a fork. Here you go left and descend an old, closed road 150 yards to trail's end on Old US 99. This trailhead is 250 yards north of where your section ends, at the junction of Mount Ashland Ski Road at Old US 99 (1,718.7–4,207'), and that junction in turn is immediately north of where I-5 crosses over the highway.

GEOLOGY The Mesozoic granitic rocks you've traversed along the eastern crest of the Siskiyou Mountains are now overlaid by thick, Cenozoic, basaltic andesite flows, and the Shasta red fir and mountain hemlock give way to Douglas-fir and orange-barked madrone.

RESUPPLY ACCESS #1

If you've hiked the PCT through much or all of California, you may want to celebrate your entry into Oregon by visiting Callahan's Restaurant. Go 1.2 miles north on Old US 99 to OR 273, and on it cross under I-5 at its Mount Ashland exit. The restaurant is just east of it. This ever-popular place, expensive by backpacker standards, is one of the better dining options along or near the entire PCT. The "bottomless" hiker dinner includes all the spaghetti you can eat, just as the "bottomless" hiker breakfast includes all the pancakes you want. Laundry, camping, showers, and meals can all be had in the hiker package for just 66 bucks (excluding tips). Check online (callahanslodge.com) for its complete offerings for thru-hikers, including huge discounts on its luxurious rooms.

To resupply for another stretch of the PCT in southern Oregon, you can hitchhike 9 miles down I-5 to the OR 66 interchange and take the highway west into downtown Ashland.

RESUPPLY ACCESS #2

An old, temporary PCT route offers you another way down to Ashland.

From Callahan's (0.9 mile from the end of Mount Ashland Ski Road), you can go 6.2 miles down tree-lined OR 273 to a junction with OR 66. Just east of it is the shallow upper end of Emigrant Lake, a popular fishing area; the deeper parts are relegated to water skiers, boaters, and swimmers. Northwest, OR 66 leads you 1.8 miles to the main entrance of the Emigrant Lake Recreation Area. Here a paved road heads southeast 0.4 mile up to a lateral dam, then curves north 0.6 mile to a public campground. Continuing 2.8 miles northwest on OR 66, you meet Dead Indian Memorial Road before it turns west and climbs to cross I-5 at the outskirts of Ashland. Some backpackers prefer to celebrate in Ashland rather than at Callahan's, as there is quite a selection of good to excellent cafés and restaurants. In addition, Ashland's Oregon Shakespeare Festival runs most of the year. Just north of the festival's grounds is the Ashland Hostel (150 N. Main St.; theashlandhostel.com), which welcomes hikers and even has a PCT register.

Lush vistas, such as this one from near Sheep Camp Spring, are often seen throughout Oregon.

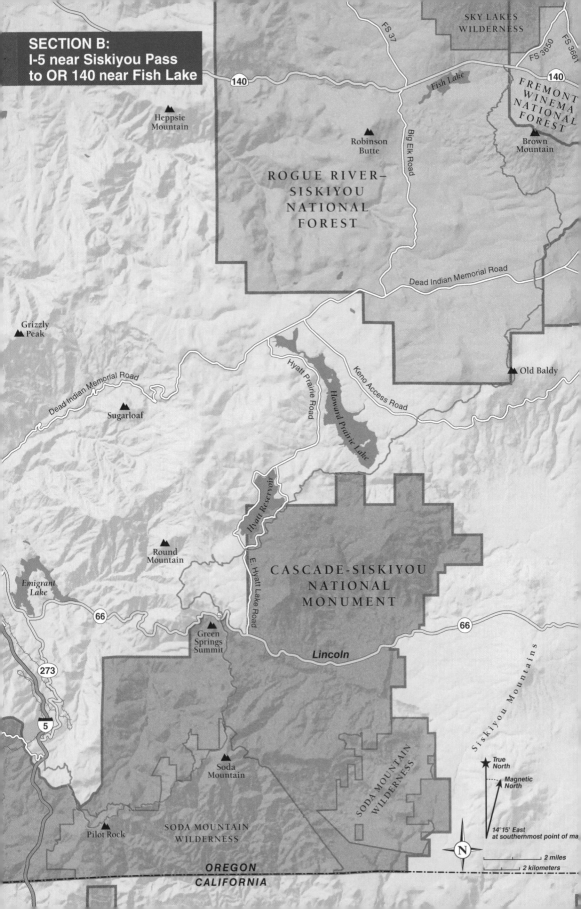

SECTION B:
I-5 near Siskiyou Pass
to OR 140 near Fish Lake

SKY LAKES
WILDERNESS

FS 37

FS 3650

FS 3661

140

Fish Lake

FREMONT
WINEMA
NATIONAL
FOREST

140

Heppsie
Mountain

Robinson
Butte

Big Elk Road

Brown
Mountain

ROGUE RIVER–
SISKIYOU
NATIONAL
FOREST

Dead Indian Memorial Road

Grizzly
Peak

Hyatt Prairie Road

Keno Access Road

Old Baldy

Dead Indian Memorial Road

Sugarloaf

Howard Prairie Lake

Hyatt Reservoir

Round
Mountain

E. Hyatt Lake Road

CASCADE-SISKIYOU
NATIONAL
MONUMENT

Emigrant
Lake

66

66

273

Green
Springs
Summit

Lincoln

5

Siskiyou Mountains

Soda
Mountain

★ True
North

Magnetic
North

SODA MOUNTAIN
WILDERNESS

Pilot Rock

SODA MOUNTAIN
WILDERNESS

14° 15' East
at southernmost point of ma

N

2 miles

2 kilometers

OREGON
CALIFORNIA

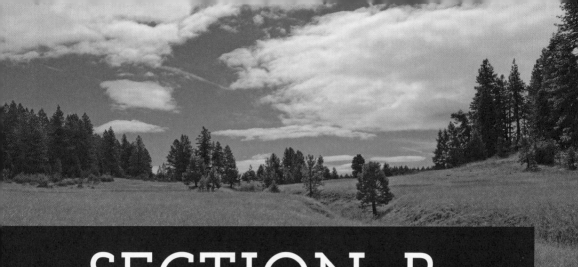

SECTION B

I-5 near Siskiyou Pass to OR 140 near Fish Lake

SECTIONS A AND C are among the highest stretches of the Pacific Crest Trail (PCT) in either Oregon or Washington. Between them, Section B, in contrast, is one of the lowest sections in either state—and certainly the driest. It abounds with logged lands that the PCT frequently passes through or skirts around, and the trail often runs closely parallel to logging or jeep roads. There is also a notable lack of drinking water. But despite these detractions, Section B has benefited from the Pacific Crest Trail Association's relationship-building with the Bureau of Land Management, some minor PCT relocations, and the designation of Cascade-Siskiyou National Monument and Soda Mountain Wilderness, which have greatly improved the PCT experience. Parts of this section—Hobart Bluff and Green Springs Mountain—have become quite popular with the local Rogue Valley population.

DECLINATION 14°15′E

Above: Traversing west of Hyatt Meadows

USGS MAPS

Siskiyou Pass, OR	Mount McLoughlin, OR
Little Chinquapin Mountain, OR	Emigrant Lake, OR
Soda Mountain, OR	Lake of the Woods South, OR (alternate route)
Brown Mountain, OR	Lake of the Woods North, OR (alternate route)
Hyatt Reservoir, OR	

POINTS ON THE TRAIL, SOUTH TO NORTH

	Mile	Elevation in feet	Latitude/Longitude
Old US 99 and Mount Ashland Ski Road	1,718.7	4,207	N42° 03' 53.0761" W122° 36' 09.7241"
I-5 near Mount Ashland Ski Road	1,718.9	4,271	N42° 03' 49.9640" W122° 36' 09.3417"
Pilot Rock Trail junction	1,723.5	5,155	N42° 01' 52.5507" W122° 34' 02.3093"
Spring	1,728.1	5,330	N42° 03' 12.8748" W122° 30' 27.7178"
Hobart Bluff spur trail junction	1,732.3	5,284	N42° 05' 42.3789" W122° 28' 23.4922"
OR 66 at Green Springs Summit	1,735.6	4,558	N42° 07' 48.3050" W122° 28' 57.8615"
Little Hyatt Reservoir	1,741.1	4,618	N42° 09' 31.3606" W122° 29' 08.4397"
Hyatt Prairie Road	1,742.7	5,105	N42° 09' 51.9100" W122° 27' 54.4500"
Eve Springs Road	1,749.3	4,617	N42° 12' 2.5600" W122° 23' 14.0500"
Keno Access Road	1,752.4	4,748	N42° 13' 35.9860" W122° 21' 01.8369"
Dead Indian Memorial Road	1,761.6	5,383	N42° 17' 35.6258" W122° 16' 16.9201"
Brown Mountain Trail junction	1,765.5	5,234	N42° 20' 11.7216" W122° 15' 40.8504"
High Lakes Bike Trail junction	1,773.2	4,952	N42° 23' 37.8240" W122° 17' 24.2520"
OR 140 near Fish Lake	1,773.4	4,970	N42° 23' 45.1043" W122° 17' 29.2840"

CAMPSITES AND BIVY SITES

Mile	Elevation in feet	Latitude/ Longitude	Number of tents	Feature	Notes
1,725.1	5,020	N42° 02' 28.8665" W122° 32' 55.2950"	>2		
1,739.9	4,680	N42° 09' 23.0436" W122° 30' 10.8638"	2	Nearby spring	Drive-in spot on left in shade
1,741.1	4,615	N42° 09' 28.9434" W122° 29' 11.6839"	2	Little Hyatt Reservoir	Keene Creek; shaded
1,742.7	5,052	N42° 10' 01.4772" W122° 27' 49.7268"	56	Hyatt Lake Campground	0.2 mile off-trail; reservations required; toilets, showers, table, grill, horse stalls
1,744.7	5,019	N42° 10' 59.7180" W122° 26' 55.8600"	12	Wildcat Campground	0.3 mile off-trail; vault toilets, water, picnic table, fire ring
1,749.3 (alt.)	4,600	N42° 12' 56.1276" W122° 23' 59.2584"	41	Willow Point County Campground	Vault toilets, picnic table, fire ring
1,750.4	4,560	N42° 12' 36.1152" W122° 22' 26.6736"	30	Klum Landing County Campground	0.3 mile off-trail; toilets, water, showers, picnic table, fire ring
1,763.3	5,305	N42° 18' 48.6538" W122° 15' 52.6313"	5	South Brown Mountain Shelter	Woodstove, potable water
1,765.5 (alt.)	4,983	N42° 23' 04.9999" W122° 12' 45.0000"	40	Aspen Point Campground	Flush toilets, drinking water, picnic table, fire ring
1,773.2 (alt.)	4,600	N42° 23' 39.1717" W122° 19' 05.6176"	20	Fish Lake Campground	PCT campsite available; flush toilets, drinking water

WEATHER TO GO

If you intend to hike this section, try to do it in late June, when snow problems can be minimal yet seasonal creeks are still flowing.

SUPPLIES

If you need major supplies, get them in Ashland before you start hiking this section. Directions to this city are given at the end of the previous section. Because this section is short, the need for supplies will be minimal, and minimal supplies are all you'll find at Hyatt Lake, Howard Prairie Lake, Lake of the Woods, and Fish Lake Resorts. All but Hyatt Lake are somewhat out of your way, especially Lake of the Woods. Three resorts accept packages from UPS but not from the US Postal Service. These are: Hyatt Lake Resort, 7979 Hyatt Prairie Road, Ashland, OR 97520; Fish Lake Resort, OR 140, Mile Marker 30, Medford, OR 97501; and Lake of the Woods Resort, 950 Harriman Route, Klamath Falls, OR 97601.

WATER

In this section you'll have to hike up to 23 miles between on-route water sources, though several sources lie just off the trail.

I-5 NEAR SISKIYOU PASS TO OR 140 NEAR FISH LAKE

>>>THE ROUTE

Section B's starting point is at the junction of Mount Ashland Ski Road and Old US 99 (1,718.7–4,207'), immediately north of I-5. To reach it by car, start in Ashland at the OR 66 exit and drive 9 miles south on I-5 to the Mount Ashland exit. If you're driving north, note that this exit is 16.5 miles past the CA 96 exit in Northern California. From the exit proceed 0.6 mile south on Old US 99 to the junction with Mount Ashland Ski Road.

From this junction, start hiking south up the highway, crossing under noisy I-5 (1,718.9–4,271') 200 feet south. You hike straight for 0.3 mile and then start to curve east–northeast. In 500 feet, you should see the resumption of PCT tread (1,719.3–4,357')—marked with a PCT emblem on a trailside post—that crosses a gully

running down the highway's east side. If you reach a road branching east, you've gone about 120 yards too far.

On the PCT, you cross the gully and, in 350 feet, cross a jeep road. Head east across private land about 0.75 mile, and then your winding path angles north but quickly switchbacks. On a southward track, climb moderately toward a ridge. Then wind gently 0.3 mile south up to a crest and, after a moment's walk down a spur ridge, reach a Y junction (1,721.4–4,897') 100 yards southwest of a roadside gravel quarry. One of the roads descends to a broad saddle, and you do the same, keeping east of the road as the trail, now an abandoned jeep road, winds 0.2 mile down to a major intersection (1,721.7–4,834'). Here, a pipe gate guards nothing, and

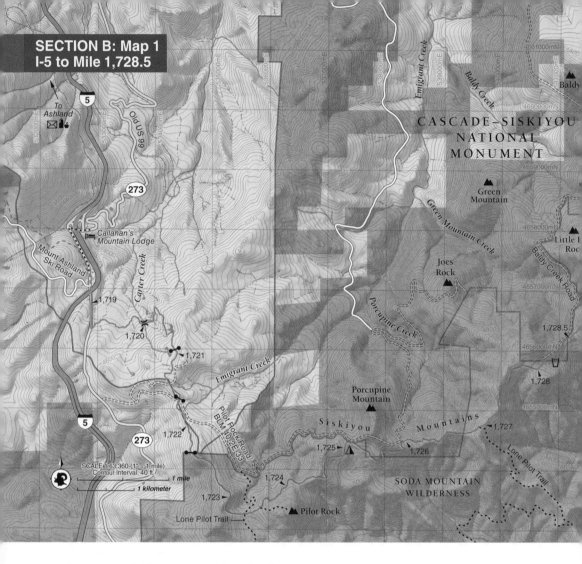

To Ashland

CASCADE–SISKIYOU
NATIONAL
MONUMENT

Baldy

Green
Mountain

Little I
Roc

Joes
Rock

Callahan's
Mountain Lodge

Mount Ashland
Ski Road

1,719

1,720

1,721

Emigrant Creek

Porcupine
Mountain

1,728.5

1,728

Siskiyou Mountains

1,727

1,725

1,726

SODA MOUNTAIN
WILDERNESS

Lone Pilot Trail

1,724

1,723

Lone Pilot Trail

Pilot Rock

Pilot Rock Road
BLM 40-2E-33

SCALE 1:63,360 (1" = 1 mile)
Contour Interval: 40 ft.

1 mile

1 kilometer

---

roads go every which way, two of them leading south along the west side of a crest.

Still on private land, the PCT begins beside the western southbound road. In 0.2 mile, however, it almost touches the wider, eastern one and then climbs 0.3 mile through a cool forest of Douglas-fir and white fir. As the trail enters the Soda Mountain Wilderness and emerges onto southwest-facing slopes, the forest thins rapidly, junipers appear, and temperatures rise. Hike southeast across a long, open crest; past its low point and a pipe gate, the trail, mixing with old jeep tracks, can become rather vague. Your faint trail passes through a cluster of trees, bearing toward steep-sided Pilot Rock. In a few minutes you cross a secondary crest, bend south, and head east to what was once a minor

road (1,723.4–5,112'), which you cross and then parallel as it reaches a prominent intersection atop a broad saddle.

The Pilot Rock Trail (1,723.5–5,155') heads right (east) from this saddle, soon climbing steeply toward the base of Pilot Rock.

SIDE TRIP If you have time, you might first make an excursion to the

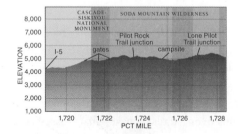

summit of Pilot Rock. Take the well-built side trail from the PCT to the rock's base, from which you'll see an obvious chute up to the top. This route is relatively safe, and no rope is required. However, acrophobes or careless climbers could get into trouble.

The PCT makes an obscure start along the former road's south edge and after 275 yards crosses it for a northeast climb to a nearby volcanic point. Your route goes east briefly along an abandoned road and then descends northeast 180 yards to a trailside outcrop with a summit that provides fair views across the northern landscape. Continuing your northeast descent, you round a ridge in 0.25 mile and momentarily reach a crest. Parallel this northeast a few minutes before turning east across it. Immediately, a dramatic volcanic landscape unfolds before you, with a huge, blocky pinnacle in the foreground plus towering Pilot Rock and snow-capped Mount Shasta to the south.

Beyond the pinnacle, the trail quickly angles north and then makes a pleasant, winding descent through a Douglas-fir forest to a crest saddle (1,725.1–5,020'). An old road from the southeast climbs to this saddle, crosses it, and swings west, joining Pilot Rock Road, which climbs east from OR 273.

From the crest saddle, the trail first descends southeast where it crosses in and out of the Soda Mountain Wilderness (1,725.4–4,937'), as it remains in the Cascade-Siskiyou National Monument, and then curves northeast to a ravine. The PCT is now routed on an abandoned, overgrown roadbed, which you follow east a few minutes and then climb north to a crest (1,726.3–5,019'). A short segment of trail leads east across north-facing slopes to a road, up which you walk about 50 yards to a minor crest saddle and the trail's resumption, on your left (1,726.5–5,060'). This trail segment goes just 110 yards before you cross the jeep road and parallel it east. Your path again crosses

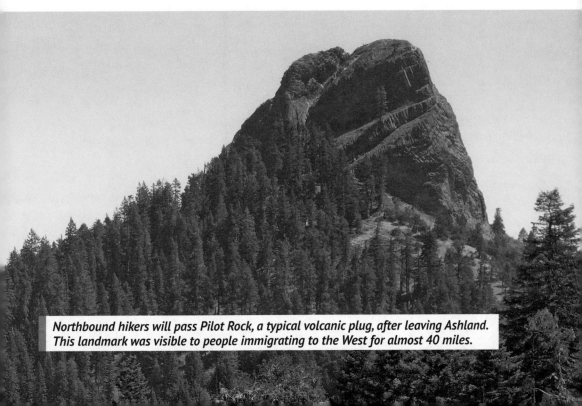

Northbound hikers will pass Pilot Rock, a typical volcanic plug, after leaving Ashland. This landmark was visible to people immigrating to the West for almost 40 miles.

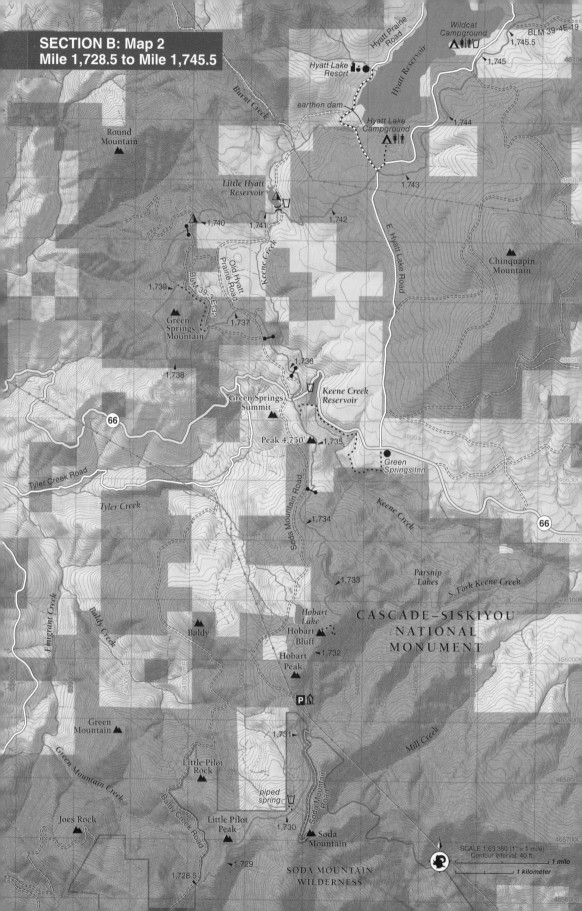

Round
Mountain

Burnt Creek

Hyatt Prairie Road

Wildcat
Campground

BLM 39-4E-19

1,745.5

1,745

Hyatt Lake
Resort

Hyatt Reservoir

earthen dam

Hyatt Lake
Campground

1,744

1,743

Little Hyatt
Reservoir

E. Hyatt Lake Road

1,742

1,740

1,741

Chinquapin
Mountain

Old Hyatt Prairie Road

Keene Creek

1,739

BLM 39-3E-32

1,737

Green
Springs
Mountain

1,738

1,736

66

Green Springs
Summit

Keene Creek
Reservoir

Peak 4,750'

1,735

Green
Springs Inn

Tyler Creek Road

Keene Creek

66

Tyler Creek

1,734

Soda Mountain Road

Parsnip
Lakes

1,733

S. Fork Keene Creek

CASCADE–SISKIYOU
NATIONAL
MONUMENT

Emigrant Creek

Baldy Creek

Baldy

Hobart
Lake

Hobart
Bluff

1,732

Hobart
Peak

P

Green
Mountain

1,731

Mill Creek

Green Mountain Creek

Little Pilot
Rock

Baldy Creek Road

piped
spring

Soda Mountain Road

Joes Rock

Little Pilot
Peak

1,730

Soda
Mountain

1,729

SODA MOUNTAIN
WILDERNESS

1,728.5

SCALE 1:63,360 (1" = 1 mile)
Contour Interval: 40 ft.

1 mile

1 kilometer

into the Soda Mountain Wilderness (1,726.7–5,221'), and twice more you cross this former jeep road, the second time where the Lone Pilot Trail (1,726.9–5,307') starts a descent southeast.

The trail now parallels the jeep road northeast, and after 0.25 mile it provides almost continuous views of Mount Shasta for 0.5 mile. Pilot Rock, your former guiding beacon, is now hidden.

WATER ACCESS

Beyond the views, the trail enters forest and descends gently east, crossing a broad saddle just before turning northeast to enter an open area with a refreshing spring (1,728.1–5,330'). With nearly 18 miles since the last on-trail spring, the water situation ahead happily starts out much better. This spring is your first reliable water in many miles, but you should purify any that you collect here.

Still following the old jeep road, the PCT descends northeast to a saddle (1,728.5–5,140'). From it Baldy Creek Road descends north, while another road once descended east, a third contoured northeast, and just above it your former jeep road climbed northeast. The PCT parallels the old jeep road's northwest side, twice crosses it, skirts past the south slope of unassuming Little Pilot Peak, and then dips to the north side of a saddle (1,729.3–5,551').

WATER ACCESS

Continue northeast 0.25 mile, then bend east, passing between two open slopes. Past the second slope, the trail curves northeast, and you quickly see a pond and an adjacent spring 80 yards down (northwest) from the trail (1,730.1–5,475'). Before leaving here, tank up, for your next reliable trailside water will be at Little Hyatt Reservoir, a dry 11 miles away. As always, treat the water before drinking it.

Continuing the trek, you meet an old trail in 0.2 mile that climbs 300 yards to a saddle junction with Soda Mountain Road. The jeep road that has been accompanying you since Pilot Rock ends at this road about 0.3 mile south of the saddle. The PCT stays below the saddle, traversing open slopes that give you views west to Mount Ashland and all the countryside below. Beyond the views, the trail drops to a shaded saddle, traverses north along a crest, and then drops past power lines to a crossing of gravel Soda Mountain Road (1,731.4–5,291') at a parking area with a pit toilet.

Just east of an open saddle, you start north-northeast through a meadow with vegetation that sometimes obscures the trail, but in 100 yards you reenter forest cover for a shady traverse around Hobart Peak to a long saddle.

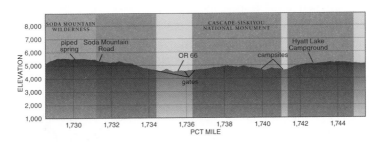

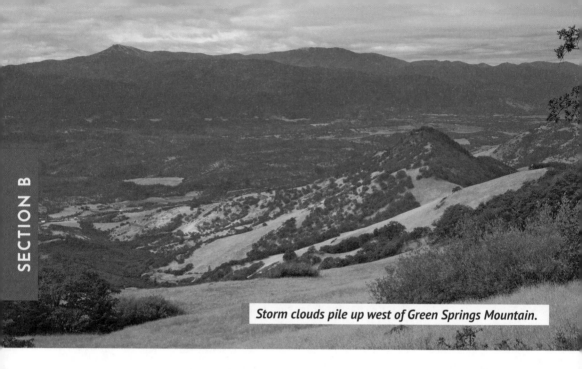

Storm clouds pile up west of Green Springs Mountain.

You soon meet the Hobart Bluff spur trail (1,732.3–5,284').

SIDE TRIP This trail climbs left (west) 0.3 mile to the juniper-capped summit. From it you'll see distant Mount Shasta to the south-southeast, Soda Mountain to the near south, Pilot Rock behind Hobart Peak to the southwest, Mount Ashland to the west, the spacious Rogue Valley to the northwest, and pyramidal Mount McLoughlin, which you'll see up close at the start of Section C, to the north-northeast.

From the Hobart Bluff spur trail, the PCT travels through a woodland of Oregon oak before emerging on more-open slopes and then curving northwest down into forest cover. The private land in the area is well marked with signs that implore you to stay on the trail. Forest temporarily gives way to a dry-grassland slope; then after another pipe gate, the PCT descends north-northeast, giving you a last view of the Ashland environs. You climb again and almost top Peak 4,750 and then descend north-northwest, spying Keene Creek Reservoir on your right (east) before crossing OR 66 at Green Springs Summit (1,735.6–4,558').

WATER ACCESS

You can reach the tempting reservoir by hiking 0.25 mile northeast along OR 66 and then dropping to the nearby shore.

Immediately east of north-climbing Old Hyatt Prairie Road, the PCT climbs gently northeast from Green Springs Summit and then rolls northwest across private land. The trail eases through a fresh pipe gate 0.4 mile past the highway, then slips through another gate 0.6 mile from the previous one, before passing under a small power line and crossing a one-lane road about 90 yards past that (1,736.8–4,700').

Just 0.2 mile past the road crossing, you cross Old Hyatt Prairie Road (1,737.0–4,705') and then climb south-southwest to a crossing of BLM 39-3E-32 (1,737.4–4,812') and the beginning of the Green Springs Mountain Loop Connector Trail. Thanks to a realignment of the trail corridor, the PCT takes this vista-rich route clockwise around Green Springs Mountain.

Head 15 yards southwest across the road, then turn southeast and go 65 more yards before once again settling on a southwest track on the Loop Connector. While the new tread is more than twice the distance of the old, the southwest vistas eclipse the eastside views. The new route meets the old at a small saddle where it turns to descend gently northwest on open slopes with views west. The trail soon turns northeast through a shady fir forest.

The PCT slips through a pipe gate and drops 300 yards to BLM 39-3E-32 (1,739.8–4,735'), which you cross near a bend. You descend briefly northeast to jeep tracks beside the Ashland lateral canal, now a dry gully. It once diverted water from Keene Creek west down to Ashland and then to the Rogue River, but today Keene Creek flows as it used to, ultimately down to the Klamath River.

WATER ACCESS

The PCT climbs east to a ridge, drops into a gully, crosses a second ridge, and in a second gully meets a trail (1,741.1–4,618') that climbs north 0.1 mile to Little Hyatt Reservoir.

CAMPING Under ponderosa pines along the reservoir's east shore, you can fish or just stretch out and relax. Swimming is best near the dam, from which you can jump into the tranquil water. It is a great place for a layover day, for it lacks the noise and congestion found at larger Hyatt and Howard Prairie Lakes. At Little Hyatt Reservoir you can camp in the de facto campground above the east shore.

From the reservoir, head east down to the nearby outlet, cross it, and then follow it momentarily up to the reservoir's dam and adjacent Old Hyatt Prairie Road (1,741.2–4,623').

Moving along, you resume the PCT 25 yards south of where it ended at Old Hyatt Prairie Road. The trail first climbs southeast, then climbs generally northeast past old roads and an informational kiosk to a three-way road fork (1,742.7–5,105') at which the northbound Hyatt Prairie Road branches northwest and East Hyatt Lake Road heads east and south.

RESUPPLY ACCESS

CAMPING From this fork, you can head northwest to follow steps over a fence and then follow a trail north 0.25 mile to a campsite that is 80 yards west-southwest of Hyatt Lake Campground's shower rooms. The campsite was specifically established for PCT hikers and has a picnic table and trash can. From the road fork, walk 170 yards northeast down to the entrance road, descend another 170 yards to a sign-in booth/fee station, pay for a shower, and then take the camp's west-climbing road over to the nearby shower rooms. If you don't camp at Little Hyatt Reservoir, you'll almost certainly want to do so at Hyatt Lake Campground. From the campground's north end, a shoreline trail heads west over to the lake's nearby dam, and from its far side, you can walk over to Hyatt Lake Resort, which has a café and a limited supply of groceries, plus showers and a laundry room. By this route, the resort is a 0.75-mile side trip from the road fork.

The campground entrance trail is found 170 yards northeast of the road fork along East Hyatt Lake Road. The PCT crosses East Hyatt Lake Road and curves east around the south side of the recreation area's administration building.

The PCT climbs east to a usually dry ravine and then heads northeast, crossing ravines and rounding ridges. The tread stays above usually visible East Hyatt Lake Road and snag-tarnished Hyatt Reservoir. Cross a southeast-climbing spur road (1,744.7–5,121'), down which you could walk 160 yards northwest to the main, paved road and then follow it 220 yards west to the entrance road of the Wildcat Campground. Next you wind over to east-climbing Wildcat Glades Road 39-4E-19.3 (1,745.6–5,086'). Heading east on the PCT, you soon cross an older road (1,746.1–5,198') to Wildcat Glades and immediately reach a seeping creek that drains the nearby glades.

Along the seeping creek's north bank, the trail starts upstream but quickly veers north and passes two sets of jeep tracks as it climbs a ridge. After a switchback, the trail swings to the east side of a secondary summit and then in 200 yards approaches the main one (1,746.8–5,510'). The scramble up to it (5,610') gives you a disappointing view. Now halfway through Oregon's Section B, you descend northeast along a crest, almost touch a saddle, and then turn east for a long descent. Midway along it, a jeep road climbs south across your trail to a nearby saddle. Just past this road is a fair view of Mount McLoughlin and Howard Prairie Lake. The descent ends when you cross Eve Springs Road (1,749.3–4,617'), which climbs southwest to a nearby rock quarry.

RESUPPLY ACCESS

CAMPING At this crossing, you are only a few yards south of Howard Prairie Dam Road. You can take it 1.6 miles northwest to a spur road that descends 0.25 mile to Howard Prairie Lake and the Willow Point County Campground. Just off this spur road, you'll also find a ranger station. From the spur-road junction, you can hike 0.7 mile west up to a paved road, follow it north 1 mile, and then branch right 0.4 mile down to bustling Howard Prairie Lake Resort, which logically caters more to boating enthusiasts than to backpackers. However, you can purchase meals and limited supplies there. Howard Prairie Lake, though shallower than Hyatt Lake, is considerably better in appearance because all the trees were removed before its basin was flooded.

From the quarry-road crossing, the PCT parallels Howard Prairie Dam Road east to a quick junction (1,749.4–4,626') with a road that descends an easy 0.5 mile to Soda Creek before climbing 0.75 mile to Wildcat Glades Road. Water obtained from Soda Creek is certainly better than that in Grizzly Creek, your next on-route source. Beyond the Soda Creek road, the PCT crosses a broad, open saddle. At its far end (1,749.5–4,621'), where a secondary road starts a climb east, the PCT starts a climb northeast and quickly leaves Howard Prairie Dam Road.

On the ascent, you get a couple of views down the length of Howard Prairie Lake, but these disappear before the trail's high point, the views being blocked by Douglas-firs, grand firs, sugar pines, and incense cedars. The easy ascent is mirrored by an equally easy drop to a crossing of a little-used road (1,750.4–4,705').

CAMPING You can follow this road 0.2 mile southwest down to Howard Prairie Dam Road and then turn northwest and go 100 yards to reach the Klum Landing County Campground with water faucets and picnic tables. Like the Little Hyatt Reservoir de facto campground, this campground is a good place to spend a layover day. Relax, fish, or perhaps swim out to Howard Prairie Lake's interesting island.

WATER ACCESS

Klum Landing County Campground is certainly desirable, even if it is 0.3 mile off route. You are now 9.3 miles past your last on-route water, near Little Hyatt Reservoir, and your next reliable on-route water, Christis Spring, is 34.5 miles away. Fortunately, a couple of near-trail sources occur in the next 5 miles.

Past the little-used road, the PCT drops northeast to a well-maintained road (1,750.7–4,635') that goes southeast to the start of the little-used road. Southbound hikers may want to take this well-maintained road to Howard Prairie Dam Road and then to Klum Landing County Campground. The PCT now heads north through a meadow whose seasonally tall grasses and herbs can hide the tread.

WATER ACCESS

Quickly, however, the trail enters forest cover, the tread becomes obvious, and you wind down to a canal, cross it and its maintenance

road, and in 90 yards drop to a long bridge over Grizzly Creek (1,751.2–4,459').

Working toward the next near-trail water source, you climb east, cross a forgotten road in 160 yards, and then continue up to a crossing of paved Moon Prairie Road (1,751.6–4,587'). The trail now turns northeast and climbs gently to a crossing of paved Keno Access Road (1,752.4–4,748'), a major trans-Cascade route for logging trucks bound for Klamath Falls. The PCT continues northeast 0.2 mile and climbs to an old road—now just a 25-foot-wide deforested strip—whose traffic was preempted by the newer logging road. From it, you round the northwest corner of a clear-cut, pass a minor spur road, and then curve east to a bend in Brush Mountain Road (1,753.1–4,987'). Southbound hikers: Please note that the last few yards of trail can be hidden by mulleins, thistles, and other "weeds" that characteristically spring up in logging areas; therefore, just plow west from the bend.

You initially climb southeast from the bend but gradually curve northeast up through a shady forest of Douglas-fir and grand fir, cross a broad ravine, climb to an adjacent ridge, and just beyond it reach a gravel logging road (1,754.7–5,501'). This descends 0.3 mile to Big Draw Road, which is also your immediate objective. Resume a moderate climb northeast, and soon approach that road, beside which the PCT bends north. In about 100 yards, look for a trail junction (1,755.2–5,708') leading about 100 yards right (east) to a piped spring.

WATER ACCESS

You should seriously consider walking 25 yards east over to the road and down it 75 yards

continued on page 90

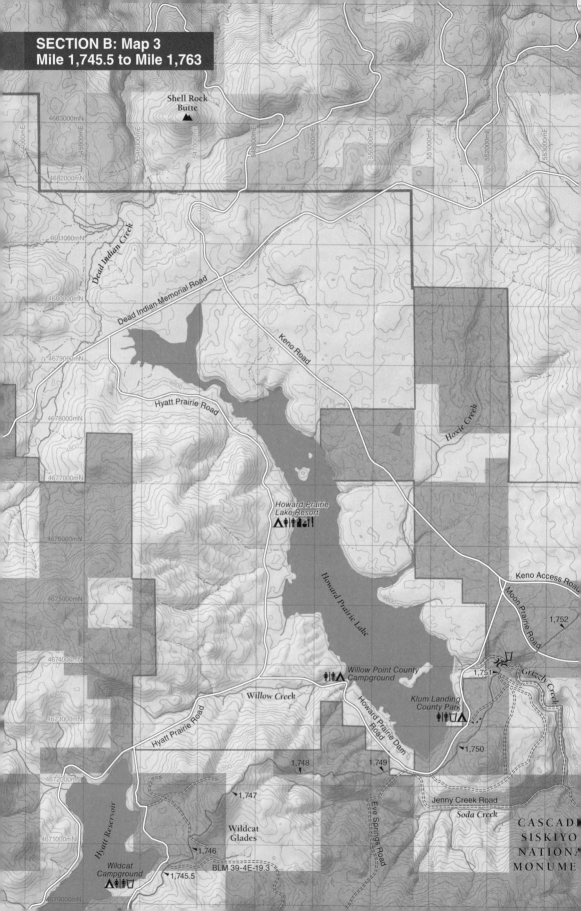

Shell Rock Butte

Dead Indian Creek

Dead Indian Memorial Road

Keno Road

Hyatt Prairie Road

Hoxie Creek

Howard Prairie Lake Resort

Howard Prairie Lake

Keno Access Road

Moon Prairie Road

1,752

1,751

Willow Point County Campground

Klum Landing County Park

Grizzly Creek

Willow Creek

Hyatt Prairie Road

Howard Prairie Dam Road

1,750

1,748

1,749

Eve Springs Road

Jenny Creek Road

Soda Creek

1,747

Hyatt Reservoir

Wildcat Glades

BLM 39-4E-19.3

1,746

Wildcat Campground

1,745.5

CASCADE SISKIYOU NATIONAL MONUME

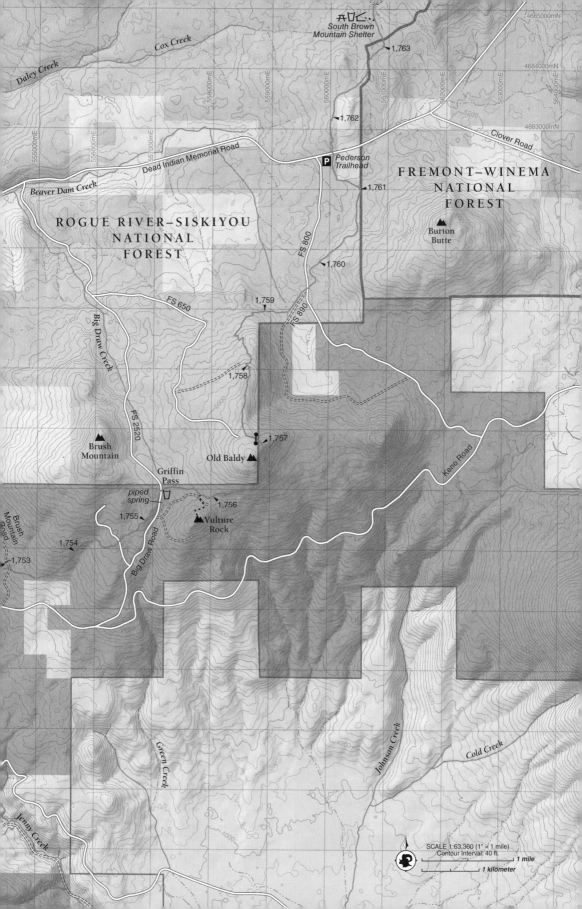

continued from page 87

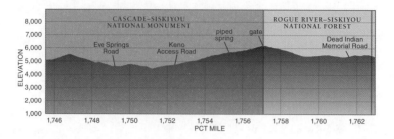

Where the PCT turns north, it parallels Big Draw Road up to the road crossing (1,755.4–5,715'), which is 250 yards short of ill-defined to an eastbound spur road. This spur road immediately reaches a piped spring, providing the hiker with fresh water—a good, reliable source until the off-route Fish Lake Resort, a long 20.2 miles ahead. Since most long-distance backpackers average 15–20 miles a day, they should plan to gather water here.

Griffin Pass. A signed side trail immediately south of the road crossing leads hikers to a gate allowing access to the Big Springs area. A boardwalk trail leads hikers to the aforementioned piped spring that typically flows in early summer. Still on Bureau of Land Management land, you parallel the Rogue River–Siskiyou National Forest boundary east, immediately crossing the seasonal Big Springs creeklet. In 0.3 mile, the trail bends southeast for a brief climb to a broad, shady saddle; then it angles northeast for a brief, moderate climb to Old Baldy's clear-cut slopes. The eastside ascent around this conical landmark is an easy one, and the peak's brushy terrain allows plenty of views south across miles of forest to majestic Mount Shasta.

PLANTS Chinquapin, tobacco brush, and greenleaf manzanita yield to noble fir as the curving trail climbs to a northeast spur ridge, from which you traverse 140 yards northwest to the Rogue River–Siskiyou National Forest boundary (1,757.1–6,162').

SIDE TRIP You can scramble south to Old Baldy's nearby summit (6,339') for 360-degree views. Abandoned by fire lookouts, it is now under the watchful eyes of turkey vultures. From it you can see Mount Shasta (bearing 176°), Yreka (185°), Soda Mountain (217°), Pilot Rock (223°), Hyatt Reservoir and Mount Ashland (242°), and Mount McLoughlin (354°). With

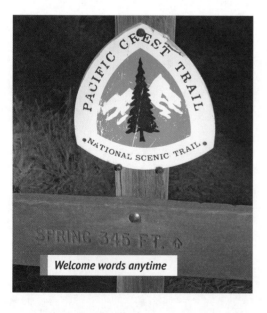

Welcome words anytime

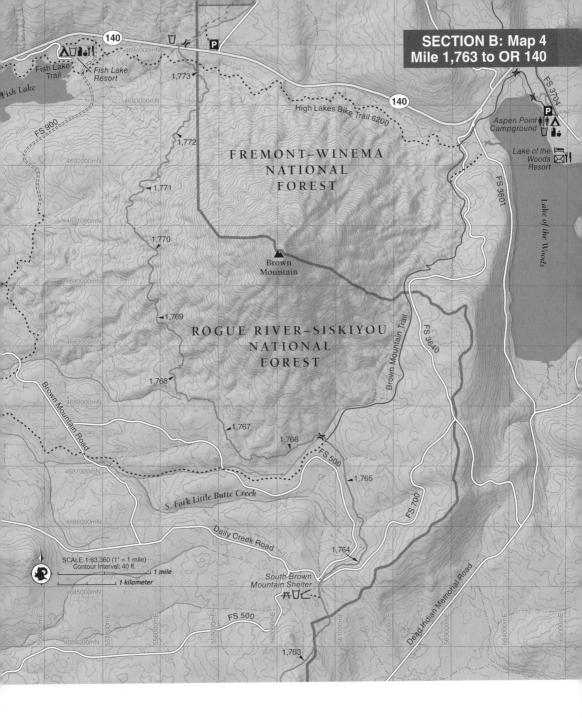

FREMONT–WINEMA
NATIONAL
FOREST

ROGUE RIVER–SISKIYOU
NATIONAL
FOREST

Fish Lake Trail

Fish Lake Resort

Fish Lake

FS 900

High Lakes Bike Trail 6200

Aspen Point Campground

Lake of the Woods Resort

FS 3704

FS 3601

Lake of the Woods

Brown Mountain

Brown Mountain Trail

FS 3640

Brown Mountain Road

S. Fork Little Butte Creek

Daily Creek Road

FS 500

FS 700

FS 500

South Brown Mountain Shelter

Dead Indian Memorial Road

SCALE 1:63,360 (1" = 1 mile)
Contour Interval: 40 ft.

1 mile

1 kilometer

these landmarks identified, a careful observer should be able to trace the PCT route over miles of country.

Now within U.S. Forest Service land, as you will be almost continuously to the Washington border, you start northwest and quickly bend

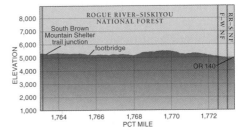

ROGUE RIVER–SISKIYOU
NATIONAL FOREST

RR–S NF
F–W NF

South Brown Mountain Shelter trail junction

footbridge

OR 140

ELEVATION

8,000
7,000
6,000
5,000
4,000
3,000
2,000
1,000

1,764   1,766   1,768   1,770   1,772
PCT MILE

north to descend a pleasant, forested ridge. The PCT touches on a saddle and then switchbacks down the northwest slopes of the ridge, swings east almost to Forest Service Road 890, turns north, and quickly crosses a closed road. Parallel FS 890, soon cross FS 800 (1,759.6–5,398'), and then wind north to a trailhead parking area by a crossing of Dead Indian Memorial Road (1,761.6–5,383'). The parking area is about 300 yards east of the road's junction with FS 800.

Northbound, the PCT climbs away from Dead Indian Memorial Road, cuts northeast across a broad ridgecrest, and then descends through an old logging area to a broad saddle crossed by an abandoned road, a route now used in winter by snowmobilers. About 0.3 mile north of it, you reach an important junction (1,763.3–5,305').

WATER ACCESS

CAMPING The spur trail left (west) goes a mere 180 yards to the 12-foot-square South Brown Mountain Shelter. More important is an obvious well, situated about 10 yards from the shelter.

Onward, the PCT winds north briefly down to a crossing of unpaved FS 700 (1,763.5–5,268') and loops around the headwaters of South Fork Little Butte Creek.

From FS 700, the PCT first contours northeast and then north, paralleling FS 500, which you sometimes see below as you cross an old logging area. Some ravines you cross may contain water, particularly if you are hiking through in the mosquito-plagued month of June. Finally, the trail drops to cross the Brown Mountain Trail (1,765.5–5,234') and a branch of South Fork Little Butte Creek. If you are covering hundreds of miles of PCT rather than just Section B, you may want to follow the Brown Mountain Trail over to Lake of the Woods Resort.

ALTERNATE ROUTE AND RESUPPLY ACCESS

On the Brown Mountain Trail, initially head east, and in 0.25 mile begin descending 4.3 miles until it meets FS 3640. Just after joining the road, you will zigzag north, northeast, and northwest and then head right (east) and continue 600 feet to a crossing of FS 3601. Continue past the northeast corner of Lake of the Woods, nearly touching it while passing beneath a U.S. Forest Service facility. Another 0.3 mile northeast and the trail begins a clockwise turn on wider trail, crossing a couple of large bridges on the way south along the east side of the lake.

CAMPING Hungry PCT trekkers curve south to pass the Fremont-Winema National Forest picnic and camping areas along the shore and head southeast a mile to reach the Lake of the Woods Resort restaurant and general store. Here you can restock with enough supplies to last you until Crater Lake Post Office, 51.3 miles away by this alternate route. The resort also serves good meals, and its store has a small post office where you can pick up goodies you've mailed to yourself. In summer this lake is crowded with water-skiers, swimmers, campers, and anglers. You'll find the lake's waters are stocked with kokanee, rainbow and eastern brook trout, and brown bullhead.

To continue your alternate route, turn back northwest on the wide campground trail or head over to the main paved road and then northwest to OR 140. The trail doesn't access the highway as easily as the maps indicate. It's a reachable but messy 300 feet from trail to highway.

But, on the trail, 0.1 mile after the first bridge going north is a lateral trail that goes over to the resort entrance road. From there you turn left and in moments reach OR 140. You then hike 0.2 mile west to a pole-line road. Hike into this messy turnout and start north, but in 5 yards branch right from it, making a hairpin turn onto a minor road. Follow it 100 yards to the start of Rye Spur Trail 3771. This alternate route to an OR 140 trailhead is about 2 miles shorter than the PCT route. You will reach OR 140 at the end of Section B about 4.5 miles east of the PCT's highway crossing. However, rather than head west to it, climb north to meet it in popular Sky Lakes Wilderness. By climbing north, you pass more than a dozen lakes worth camping at, plus about two dozen trailside ponds— quite a contrast with the virtually waterless PCT segment to which this is an alternate.

A continuation of this alternate route, which is also shorter than the continued PCT route, is described in the early part of Section C (page 101).

From the Brown Mountain Trail junction, the PCT follows the seasonal creek west until the stream angles south; then the trail goes west 0.5 mile before turning northwest and dropping 20 feet to a hollow. A 60-foot gain northwest from it takes you to a minor ridge (1,767.0–5,240').

The trail continues its long, irregular arc around the lower slopes of Brown Mountain. Although the trail on the map superficially appears to be an easy hike, careful study reveals that it has plenty of ups and downs— some of them steep—as you'll find out. As you traverse the northwest slopes of Brown Mountain, views of Mount McLoughlin—a dormant volcano—appear and disappear. Nearing OR 140, you reach a junction with the High Lakes Bike Trail 6200 (1,773.2–4,952').

RESUPPLY ACCESS

Unless you are ending your hike at OR 140, you'll want to visit the Fish Lake environs both for water and for supplies. A layover day wouldn't hurt. Trail 6200 winds 0.3 mile west down to a seasonal pond, soon crosses the equally seasonal Cascade Canal, rambles across varied slopes, and then treads a stringer separating a youthful upper lava flow from an equally youthful lower one. Next it descends more or less alongside the lower flow and intersects FS 900 just before that road starts a traverse across the flow.

CAMPING   Now 1.5 miles from the PCT, you wind 100 yards west to a junction just before Fish Lake. Here a spur trail branches left, going 55 yards to a PCT campsite perched above the lakeshore. However, you might want to head 300 yards north then west over to Fish Lake Resort's campground. Note the trail's end, for it may not be too obvious, and you'll want to find it later when you return to the PCT.

But first, head over to the resort's office and café, located just above the boat dock. Food and supplies cater to the beer-drinking fishing crowd, though a beer (or two) will probably sound very tempting after your long, dry haul. Pick up your parcel if you've mailed one to the resort. You can get a hot meal and a shower (or take a swim) and then perhaps do some laundry before returning to the PCT campsite.

After your stay at Fish Lake, return via Trail 6200 to the PCT. In 85 yards along the PCT, you cross an old, abandoned highway bed and soon reach broad, straight OR 140 (1,773.4–4,970').

WATER ACCESS

Cascade Canal flows underneath OR 140 about 40 yards west of your crossing. You'll meet the canal just beyond the highway. Don't expect any water flowing in it after midsummer. The first near-trail water will be at Christis Spring, just off the PCT and 11.5 miles from the highway.

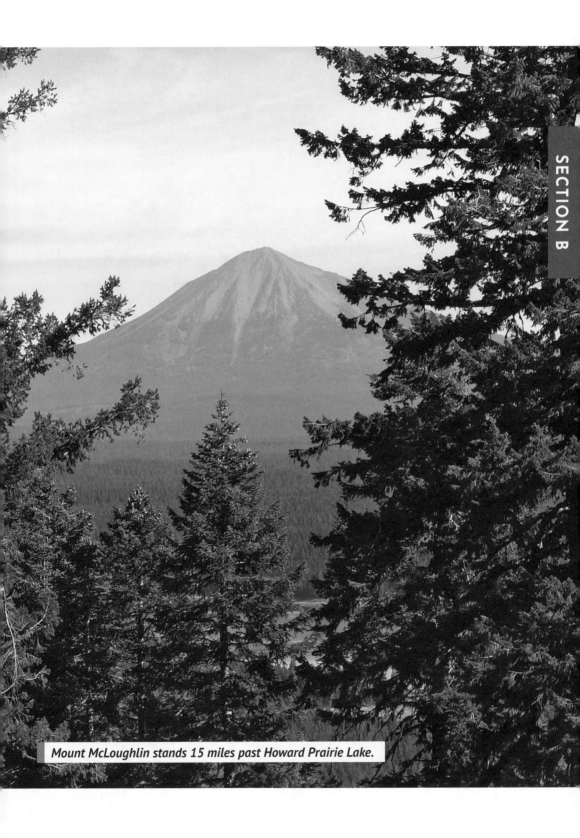

Mount McLoughlin stands 15 miles past Howard Prairie Lake.

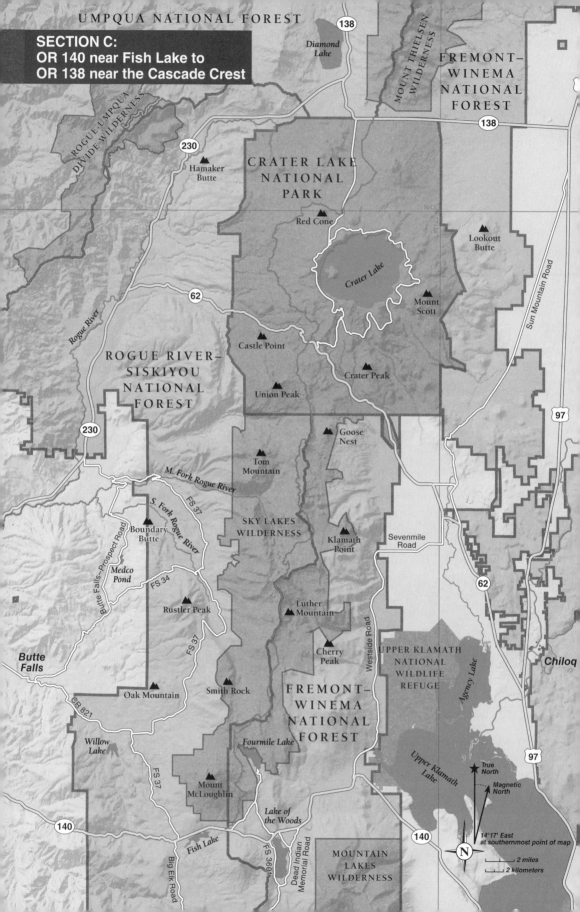

SECTION C:
OR 140 near Fish Lake to
OR 138 near the Cascade Crest

FREMONT–
WINEMA
NATIONAL
FOREST

ROGUE–UMPQUA
DIVIDE WILDERNESS

138

Diamond
Lake

MOUNT THIELSEN
WILDERNESS

138

230

Hamaker
Butte

CRATER LAKE
NATIONAL
PARK

Red Cone

Lookout
Butte

N43

Crater Lake

Mount
Scott

62

Castle Point

Crater Peak

Rogue River

ROGUE RIVER–
SISKIYOU
NATIONAL
FOREST

Union Peak

230

Goose
Nest

M. Fork Rogue River

Tom
Mountain

FS 37

S. Fork Rogue River

SKY LAKES
WILDERNESS

Klamath
Point

Sevenmile
Road

Boundary
Butte

Medco
Pond

Butte Falls–Prospect Road

FS 34

Rustler Peak

Luther
Mountain

UPPER KLAMATH
NATIONAL
WILDLIFE
REFUGE

FS 37

Cherry
Peak

Westside Road

97

62

Butte
Falls

OR 821

Oak Mountain

Smith Rock

FREMONT–
WINEMA
NATIONAL
FOREST

Agency Lake

Chiloq

Willow
Lake

Fourmile Lake

FS 37

Upper Klamath
Lake

True
North

Mount
McLoughlin

Lake of
the Woods

Magnetic
North

140

Fish Lake

FS 3601

Dead Indian Memorial Road

MOUNTAIN
LAKES
WILDERNESS

140

97

14°17' East
at southernmost point of map

N

2 miles

2 kilometers

Big Elk Road

Sun Mountain Road

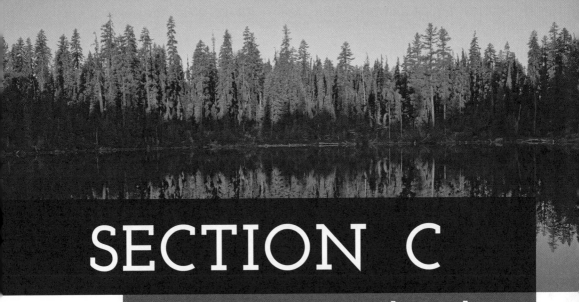

SECTION C

OR 140 near Fish Lake to OR 138 near the Cascade Crest

BOTH SECTIONS A AND B have a paucity of lakes and a surplus of roads, but in Section C the scenery changes, and at last you feel you are in a mountain wilderness. The bulk of Section C is composed of two attractive areas: Sky Lakes Wilderness and inspiring Crater Lake National Park. The number of lakes in the wilderness rivals that in any other mountain area along the Pacific Crest Trail (PCT), while the beauty and depth of Crater Lake make it a worldwide attraction.

Unfortunately, the original PCT route avoided Crater Lake entirely, taking a low route along the lower slopes of the former volcano Mount Mazama. So in our first edition (1974), we recommended an alternate route, mostly along paved Rim Drive, that traveled along Crater Lake's west rim. In the 1990s the National Park Service linked existing use trails with new tread to produce an alternate, hiker-only PCT rim route. Equestrians, however, still must take the low route. These alternate routes and others in Sky Lakes Wilderness are described along with the official PCT route.

Above: Lake Notasha in dawn's stillness

DECLINATION 14°17'E

USGS MAPS

Mount McLoughlin, OR	Pelican Butte, OR
Union Peak, OR	Pumice Desert West, OR
Lake of the Woods North, OR	Devils Peak, OR
Crater Lake West, OR	Pumice Desert East, OR

POINTS ON THE TRAIL, SOUTH TO NORTH

	Mile	Elevation in feet	Latitude/Longitude
OR 140 near Fish Lake	1,773.4	4,970	N42° 23' 45.1043" W122° 17' 29.2840"
Mount McLoughlin Trail junction, westbound	1,777.7	6,251	N42° 26' 00.1242" W122° 16' 09.3770"
Red Lake Trail junction (cross the alternate route)	1,786.8	6,035	N42° 30' 50.1223" W122° 13' 49.4046"
Sky Lakes Trail junction	1,790.4	6,158	N42° 33' 43.2000" W122° 13' 08.4000"
Snow Lakes Trail junction (end of alternate route)	1,796.0	6,693	N42° 37' 08.1181" W122° 12' 52.7805"
Middle Fork Basin Trail junction to Ranger Spring	1,804.3	5,763	N42° 41' 07.2882" W122° 10' 17.3742"
Jack Spring spur trail junction	1,808.9	6,205	N42° 44' 12.7984" W122° 11' 44.4483"
Stuart Falls Trail junction, south end	1,810.5	6,061	N42° 45' 24.9024" W122° 11' 48.2337"
Stuart Falls Trail junction, north end	1,816.0	6,311	N42° 48' 58.6602" W122° 10' 52.4387"
OR 62	1,820.9	6,177	N42° 52' 16.8406" W122° 10' 48.3659"
Dutton Creek Trail junction	1,823.0	6,093	N42° 53' 29.1812" W122° 10' 10.6921"
Lightning Spring Trail junction	1,827.4	5,869	N42° 55' 34.8066" W122° 13' 05.2751"
Bald Crater Loop Trail junction	1,835.9	6,129	N43° 00' 04.3200" W122° 11' 22.5600"
North Entrance Road junction	1,839.2	6,496	N42° 59' 44.6951" W122° 08' 08.8608"
OR 138 near the Cascade crest	1,847.8	5,923	N43° 05' 20.0308" W122° 05' 30.5370"

CAMPSITES AND BIVY SITES

Mile	Elevation in feet	Latitude/ Longitude	Number of tents	Feature	Notes
1,765.5 (alt.)	5,793	N42° 27' 21.0209" W122° 15' 0.7202"	29	Fourmile Lake Campground	Vault toilets, water, picnic table, fire ring, horse corrals; 9 equestrian sites
1,765.5 (alt.)	5,856	N42° 28' 28.9340" W122° 14' 09.5295"	>4	Badger Lake	Fire pit
1,765.5 (alt.)	6,036	N42° 29' 51.2448" W122° 13' 34.7927"	2	Long Lake	Fire pit
1,776.3	5,779	N42° 25' 25.0209" W122° 16' 20.9873"	2		Dry camp among trees
1,777.8	6,287	N42° 26' 04.3274" W122° 16' 12.6546"	2		Dry camp among trees
1,784.8	6,297	N42° 30' 13.4415" W122° 15' 20.7289"	2	Spring nearby	

CAMPSITES AND BIVY SITES (continued)

Mile	Elevation in feet	Latitude/ Longitude	Number of tents	Feature	Notes
1,786.8 (alt.)	5,903	N42° 31' 21.0591" W122° 14' 09.8876"	>4	Island Lake	Fire ring
1,786.8 (alt.)	5,807	N42° 32' 19.2776" W122° 14' 28.0294"	>4	Red Lake	Fire ring
1,789.4	6,052	N42° 32' 52.4173" W122° 13' 45.1842"	3		Flat spot near trail in trees; fire ring
1,790.4	6,156	N42° 33' 30.6393" W122° 13' 06.6045"	2		Flat spot near trail in trees
1,790.4 (alt.)	6,076	N42° 33' 51.5801" W122° 12' 42.5281"	3	Deer Lake	Fire ring
1,790.4 (alt.)	6,026	N42° 34' 04.6356" W122° 12' 03.6346"	2	Lake Notasha	
1,790.4 (alt.)	6,016	N42° 34' 23.0832" W122° 12' 13.0054"	3	Isherwood Lake	
1,790.4 (alt.)	5,981	N42° 35' 51.6436" W122° 11' 52.6578"	>4	Trapper Lake	
1,790.4 (alt.)	6,021	N42° 35' 56.5207" W122° 12' 08.6124"	2	Margurette Lake	
1,792.0	6,526	N42° 34' 41.6736" W122° 13' 35.4163"	2		Flat spot near trail in trees
1,792.7	6,600	N42° 35' 03.9825" W122° 13' 40.7562"	3		Flat spot near trail in trees
1,793.7	6,580	N42° 35' 33.2651" W122° 13' 13.0587"	2		Flat spot near trail in trees
1,799.4	6,744	N42° 38' 57.6468" W122° 12' 26.5015"	3	Stream nearby	Fire ring
1,805.8	6,151	N42° 42' 12.2467" W122° 10' 51.9391"	>4		Flat spot near trail
1,808.9	6,225	N42° 44' 13.5061" W122° 11' 43.6475"	4	Jack Spring nearby	
1,810.5 (alt.)	5,466	N42° 47' 55.5451" W122° 12' 48.7888"	2	Stuart Falls Camp	Red Blanket Creek
1,820.9 (alt.)	6,000	N42° 52' 03.6552" W122° 09' 55.6272"	214	Mazama Campground	Flush toilets, water, showers, laundry, picnic table, fire ring, bear-proof food-storage locker, general store
1,823.0	6,058	N42° 53' 29.1812" W122° 10' 10.6921"	2	Dutton Creek Camp	May be closed due to tree hazards; creek nearby
1,823.0 (alt.)	6,890	N42° 56' 01.3560" W122° 10' 49.7280"	2	Lightning Springs Camp	0.75 mile off alternate route; springs nearby
1,823.0 (alt.)	6,609	N42° 59' 27.5516" W122° 07' 48.2131"	2	Grouse Hill Camp	
1,828.6	5,494	N42° 56' 18.9018" W122° 13' 31.9803"	2	Bybee Creek Camp	Water nearby
1,835.3	6,259	N42° 59' 40.2811" W122° 11' 14.4626"	2	Red Cone Springs Camp	May be closed due to tree hazards; spring nearby
1,835.9 (alt.)	5,190	N43° 07' 58.1160" W122° 08' 49.9200"	118	Broken Arrow Campground	Flush toilets, potable water, showers, picnic table, fire grill
1,835.9 (alt.)	5,190	N43° 08' 12.5556" W122° 08' 30.6240"	5	Diamond Lake hiker/biker camp	Free; flush toilets, potable water, picnic table, fire grill

WEATHER TO GO

The lake's rim receives a yearly average of 48 feet of snowfall, and the resulting snowpack can make hiking difficult before mid-July.

SUPPLIES

There are no on-route supply points, but one alternate route we recommend takes you past the Crater Lake Post Office (97604), which is found in the same building as the park headquarters. This building is about 55.5 trail miles north of Fish Lake Resort, in northern Section B, and about 25 miles south of Diamond Lake Resort, in southern Section D. On your mailed parcels, mark your estimated time of arrival because the post office does not like to hold mail indefinitely. Below the post office is Mazama Village, which has an inn, campground, store, coin-operated laundry, and showers. Above the post office is the Rim Village, with meals and limited supplies.

PERMITS AND SPECIAL RESTRICTIONS

To camp in the Crater Lake National Park backcountry, you'll need a wilderness permit. It doesn't matter whether you are on foot, horseback, or skis, or whether you are entering on a popular summer weekend or in the dead of winter—they are still required. Free of charge, permits must be picked up in person at either Canfield Ranger Station or the Steel Visitor Center. Note that if you're trekking north or south through the park, you need only to sign the trail registers at the park boundaries.

There are specific camping restrictions at the park. No camping is allowed within 1 mile of any paved road, nature trail, or developed area, and none is allowed within 0.25 mile of Sphagnum Bog or Boundary Springs. As in any wilderness area, no camping is allowed in meadows or within 200 feet of any water source. The size of each backcountry party is limited to a maximum of 12 persons and 8 head of stock.

WATER

Crater Lake National Park lacks both ponds and flowing streams. However, snowpack near the lake's rim provides drinking water through early August. From midsummer onward, the stretch from Red Cone Springs to Section D's Thielsen Creek, a 20.6-mile stretch, may be dry.

SPECIAL CONCERNS

Sky Lakes Wilderness is an area of abundant precipitation and abundant lakelets. Both combine to ensure a tremendous mosquito population that will ruin your hike if you're caught without a tent. However, by mid-July the mosquito population begins to drop, and by early August a tent may not be necessary. Crater Lake National Park also has moist, mosquito-bearing ground through most of July.

OR 140 NEAR FISH LAKE TO OR 138 NEAR THE CASCADE CREST

>>>THE ROUTE

ALTERNATE ROUTE (continued from Section B) Some hikers may have taken Section B's alternate route/resupply access that guides them first to Lake of the Woods Resort for supplies and then north to OR 140. The following description takes them on an 11.2-mile route north back to the Red Lake Trail junction with the PCT. This stretch, 2.7 miles shorter than the comparable stretch of PCT, provides you with a lower, lake-dotted alternate route from OR 140.

To reach the trailhead, start from the north end of Lake of the Woods's east-shore Forest Service Road 3704, which ends at OR 140. Walk 0.2 mile west on the highway, and then branch north onto a pole-line road. (The power lines, on timber poles, are right next to the trees and so are hard to see from the highway. If you're eastbound on the highway, you'll find this road about 250 yards east of Billie Creek.) You go but 15 yards northwest on the road and then branch right, 60 yards directly north of the trailhead, located just before the pole line. Your mileage begins from here.

Rye Spur Trail 3771 starts west and in 0.4 mile quickly meets the Billie Creek Trail, which continues west for a loop around a part of Billie Creek. You continue on Rye Spur Trail, which switchbacks steeply north and then climbs 0.5 mile at an easier pace to FS 3633. Walk northwest up this low ridge to a short bridge across the Cascade Canal; in early summer the canal flows swiftly, but by August it can be bone dry.

VIEWS   The Rye Spur Trail continues climbing 1.2 miles north until it reaches the first of three clustered outcrops. Here you get some fine views of the scenery from Pelican Butte to the northeast, across to Mountain Lakes Wilderness to the southeast.

Beyond the outcrops, your views disappear, and you hike 3.3 miles at a leisurely pace to a recrossing of the Cascade Canal at 5,730 feet. This point is just 30 yards down the canal's road from a parking area by Fourmile Lake's dam. Had you hiked north along the canal road to this point, rather than taking the Rye Spur Trail, you would have saved yourself 0.2 mile distance and about 500 feet of climbing effort.

CAMPING   If evening is approaching and you're ready to set up camp, you can mosey west 0.5 mile to the lake's campground, then on the next day either continue on the alternate route or take Twin Ponds Trail a rolling 2.3 miles over to the PCT.

Keeping to the alternate route, you walk 30 yards east down the canal's road to the start of Badger Lake

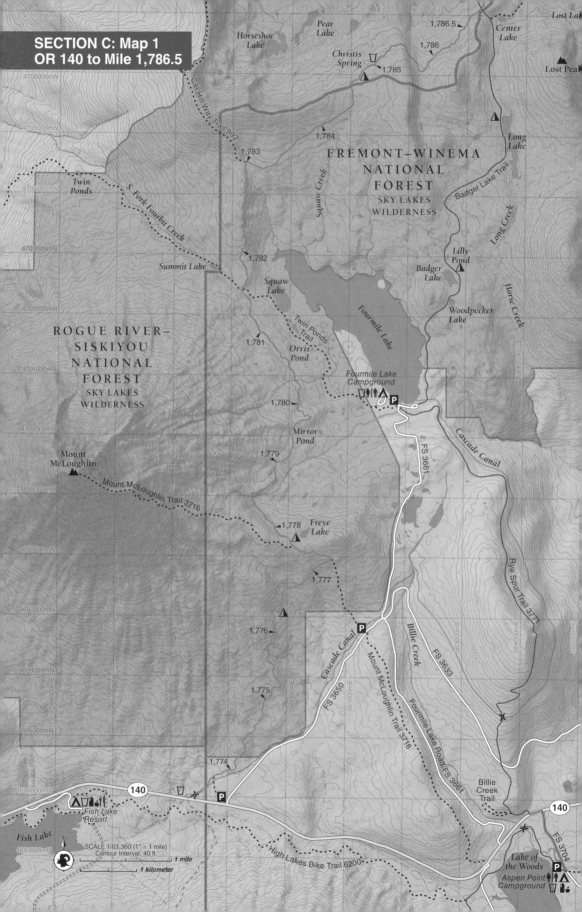

Horseshoe Lake

Pear Lake

Christis Spring

1,786.5

1,786

Center Lake

Lost La

Lost Pea

Long Lake

Cat Hill Way Trail 992

1,785

1,784

1,783

FREMONT–WINEMA NATIONAL FOREST

SKY LAKES WILDERNESS

Twin Ponds

S. Fork Fourbit Creek

Squaw Creek

Badger Lake Trail

Long Creek

Summit Lake

1,782

Squaw Lake

Fourmile Lake

Badger Lake

Lilly Pond

Horse Creek

ROGUE RIVER–SISKIYOU NATIONAL FOREST

SKY LAKES WILDERNESS

1,781

Twin Ponds Trail

Orris Pond

Woodpecker Lake

1,780

Fourmile Lake Campground

P

Mirror Pond

1,779

Mount McLoughlin

Mount McLoughlin Trail 3716

FS 3661

Cascade Canal

1,778

Freye Lake

1,777

Rye Spur Trail 3771

1,776

P

Cascade Canal

Billie Creek

FS 3633

1,775

FS 3650

Mount McLoughlin Trail 3716

Fourmile Lake Road/FS 3661

Billie Creek Trail

1,774

140

P

Fish Lake Resort

Fish Lake

140

FS 3704

High Lakes Bike Trail 6200

Lake of the Woods

P

Aspen Point Campground

SCALE 1:63,360 (1" = 1 mile)
Contour Interval: 40 ft.

1 mile

1 kilometer

Trail. This trail visits two of Fourmile Lake's bays, filled with lodgepole snags, and presents views of Mount McLoughlin and its avalanche-prone lower slopes. Now entering Sky Lakes Wilderness, you climb 0.5 mile to Woodpecker Lake, which is mostly less than chest deep.

CAMPING In 0.25 mile you reach more appealing Badger Lake, with better fishing and swimming than its neighbor; look for a fairly nice camp-site by the lake's northeast edge. Most hikers want a nice vista of the lake, and that usually doesn't include other hik-ers' tents. Set up your tent in an estab-lished site where possible and at least 200 feet from the water.

Next the trail passes knee-deep Lilly Pond and then passes a marshy meadow, both of interest to wildflower enthusiasts. Northward, there's sea-sonally boggy terrain to traverse, and then you climb 0.5 mile northeast to a junction with a trail that winds 0.3 mile east to a junction near the south shore of Long Lake.

CAMPING From it, another aban-doned trail departs south down Long Creek, while a spur trail shoots east to a good south-shore campsite. The lake is quite shallow, though deep enough to support trout and to offer some fair swimming.

Back on the alternate route, you begin a 0.5-mile easy descent north-east to the west shore of Long Lake and then continue north along it to a junction by the lake's north shore.

CAMPING Eastward, a spur trail goes over to a site spacious enough for group camping. Be aware that mosquitoes can plague the area as late as early August.

North of Long Lake, this fault-line trail crosses an unnoticeable gen-tle divide and then descends past a marshy meadow on its way down to a junction, 1 mile past Long Lake, with unmaintained Lost Creek Trail. This trail skirts the east side of Center Lake, which is knee-deep in its prime but only a grassy meadow in late summer.

Just after the Lost Creek Trail junc-tion, Badger Lake Trail 3759 ends and Red Lake Trail 987 begins. Climb over an adjacent ridge and in 0.2 mile, intersect the PCT (1,786.8–6,035').

On the official PCT, at the beginning of Sec-tion C, a large trailhead parking lot is provided for those hikers who plan to leave their vehicles along OR 140. A signed road to this lot begins 0.4 mile east of the PCT's highway crossing. From the sign, you go 15 yards north on FS 3650, turn left, and parallel the highway west to the nearby lot. From the lot's northwest corner a trail goes 0.2 mile north to the PCT. Don't park at the small space where the PCT crosses the highway.

This description begins where the PCT starts north from OR 140 (1,773.4–4,970'), just 0.2 mile west of the Jackson–Klamath County line and 40 yards east of the Cascade Canal.

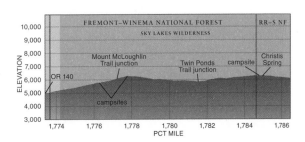

Just after you start up this trail, you bridge this seasonally flowing canal and then parallel it northeast to a junction (1,773.8–5,094') with the short trail back to the large trailhead parking lot. Just past this junction, the PCT almost touches the canal before it angles away and ascends open slopes that provide a view south toward Brown Mountain and its basalt flows. As the PCT climbs, it enters Sky Lakes Wilderness (1,774.2–5,221'), where it crosses lava flows, and then it enters a white-fir forest and continues up to a junction with Mount McLoughlin Trail 3716 (1,777.2–6,095') in a forest of red firs and mountain hemlocks.

SIDE TRIP Southeast, this heavily used trail descends 1 mile to a trailhead at FS 3650, which descends 3 additional miles to OR 140. Those hiking the last part of Section B along Lake of the Woods's west shore could take this trail to regain the PCT.

On the PCT, which briefly doubles as the Mount McLoughlin Trail, climb briefly west on an easier grade. Freye Lake, a shallow, semistagnant body of water, lies about 0.25 mile off the trail if you need water; your next available water source is Christis Spring, 7.5 miles away. Walk about 0.3 mile west on the PCT (1,777.7–6,251').

| VIEWS | **SIDE TRIP** Here, the Mount McLoughlin Trail takes its leave, climbing 3.5 miles west to the summit of this dormant stratovolcano. The views you get from it are among the best from any peak near the tristate PCT. If you have good weather, don't pass up the opportunity to climb it. Drop your heavy pack nearby, and take 2–3 hours to reach the often snowy summit. On your return, you can

sometimes use tempting snowfields to speed your descent, but be forewarned that these can lead you astray, as they diverge south-southeast from the east-heading trail.

Leaving Mount McLoughlin Trail, the PCT quickly tops a ridge, then winds slowly down through the forest, not once offering a view, and comes to a junction with the Twin Ponds Trail (1,781.5–5,840'). This junction lies between two shallow ponds that by late summer are no more than dry, grassy meadows.

| CAMPING | Summit Lake lies 0.4 mile northwest down the Twin Ponds Trail, but beyond the lake, the trail becomes very brushy. To the southeast the path winds 2.5 miles to a trailhead at the west end of Fourmile Lake Campground.

From the junction the PCT starts northeast, quickly veers north past a stagnant pond, climbs steadily up a ridge, and then descends slightly to a crest traverse, Cat Hill Way Trail 992 (1,783.0–6,079').

Your trail heads north to a ravine that is snowbound until late June and then veers east up to a gentle slope before curving northeast and climbing to a broad saddle. The route now contours across a slope forested with mountain hemlock, red fir, and western white pine.

WATER ACCESS

In 0.3 mile watch for an important spur trail leading north to Christis Spring (1,784.9–6,290').

You round a north ridge and descend southeast to another saddle. You bear northeast down toward a saddle to reach the PCT's southern junction with Red Lake Trail 987 (1,786.8–6,035'), where the alternate route from Section B rejoins the official PCT.

You're immediately confronted with a choice between following the official PCT and another alternate route, which the author recommends.

ALTERNATE ROUTE This rewarding and view-filled alternate has you continue along Red Lake Trail. You first make a moderate 0.2-mile descent to the east end of Blue Canyon Trail 982. CAMPING Westward, you can follow it 0.4 mile to a good spur trail that goes 130 yards north to Island Lake's most abundant campsites. Secluded ones lie above the lake's west shore. Good Leave No Trace practice encourages hikers to use well-established sites and eschews creating new sites.

Onward, Red Lake Trail heads 0.5 mile through huckleberry bogs to the northeast corner of Island Lake. From an adjacent campsite, a use trail goes 0.4 mile west to pleasing Dee Lake. Dee is an excellent lake for swimming—shallow enough to have warm water yet deep enough that it isn't an oversize swamp like the north half of Island Lake, which is mostly less than waist-deep.

CAMPING Beyond Island Lake your boggy, huckleberry-laden route north passes several ponds that are more suited to mosquitoes than to humans and then arrives at large but grassy and extremely shallow Red Lake, with possible camping and fishing. After another 0.5-mile walk north past this lake, you reach a junction. Ahead, the old Red Lake Trail is abandoned,

so climb another 0.5 mile east moderately up the new Red Lake Trail to rejoin the PCT (1,789.5–6,067′).

From its southern junction with the Red Lake Trail, the PCT makes a quite level, easy trek north, staying close to a fault-line crest, until it reaches its northern junction with the Red Lake Trail (1,789.5–6,067′).

With the official PCT and the alternate route rejoined at this junction, the PCT makes an easy, viewless, uneventful climb northeast to the start of another lake-studded route, the southwest end of Sky Lakes Trail 3762 (1,790.4–6,158′). At this junction, you have a choice of routes, the official PCT or several recommended alternate routes that begin on the Sky Lakes Trail, all described below.

ALTERNATE ROUTES Compared with the PCT, these optional routes add 2–3 miles to your hiking distance. CAMPING Start northeast on the Sky Lakes Trail. Soon you crest a broad divide and then make a moderate 0.25-mile diagonal trek down a fault escarpment before leveling off near mostly shallow Deer Lake. Some folks camp here, but far better camping, fishing, and swimming lie ahead.

Eastward 0.4 mile, you arc past a pond to a junction with Cold Springs Trail 3710. Next, your trail winds 0.3 mile northeast to a junction with Isherwood Trail 3729.

Diverting to Isherwood Trail: The 1.5-mile Isherwood Trail is 0.8 mile longer than its Sky Lakes Trail counterpart, but it passes five lakes and a greater number of campsites.

CAMPING Just a stone's throw over a low ridge, the Isherwood Trail comes to Lake Notasha. This lake, with a camp above its east shore, is the deepest of the five lakes and the only one stocked with both rainbow and brook trout. Resist the urge to create a new site where none existed. If the tent sites are filled, look for a site farther ahead.

Another low ridge separates Notasha from Elizabeth, which is shallow enough for warm swimming yet deep enough to sustain trout.

CAMPING Next you drop to the brink of a fault escarpment along the west shore of Isherwood Lake. From a horse camp midway along the escarpment, you can walk due west to adjacent, chest-deep Lake Liza, which has marginal appeal.

Beyond Isherwood, the trail winds north to a meadow and then veers east to the north tip of northern Heavenly Twin Lake. The Isherwood Trail ends at the Sky Lakes Trail just southwest of shallow Deep Lake.

Staying on Sky Lakes Trail: If you shun the Isherwood Trail, your Sky Lakes Trail soon passes between the Heavenly Twin Lakes, the smaller, deeper southern one being far less attractive than the northern one. By these two lakes, you reach a junction with South Rock Creek Trail 3709. Sky Lakes Trail turns north, skirts along the east shore of northern Heavenly Twin Lake, and in 0.4 mile meets the northeast end of Isherwood Trail.

Sky Lakes and Isherwood Trails rejoin: From this junction, you continue north past chest-deep Deep Lake and its seasonal satellites and reach Sky Lakes Cutoff Trail 3728. Shallow, uninviting Lake Land lies just below the trail's east end. The lake at best provides some warm swimming; however, you'd be better off visiting Wizzard Lake, a fairly deep lake just 200 yards northeast

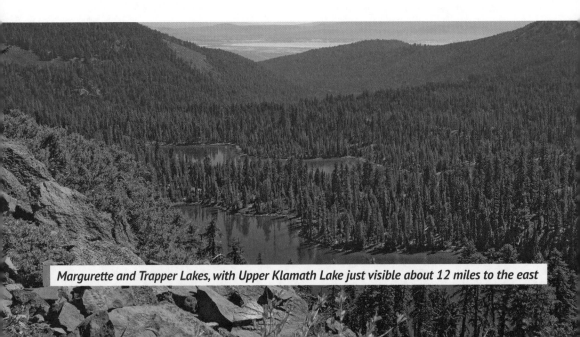

Margurette and Trapper Lakes, with Upper Klamath Lake just visible about 12 miles to the east

below Lake Land's outlet. You soon pass a knee-deep pond on the right and then, past a low ridge, two waist-deep lakelets.

CAMPING The south shore of Trapper Lake lies just ahead, and from the point where you see it, you could go 250 yards cross-country southeast to 38-foot-deep Lake Sonya, easily the basin's deepest lake. More likely, you'll want to camp at the east-shore sites of scenic Trapper Lake. Follow Leave No Trace principles and set up your tent no closer than 200 feet to the lake. This way your tent will not be centered in another hiker's pictures.

By this lake's outlet, you meet Cherry Creek Trail 3708, which descends 4.8 miles to a trailhead at FS 3550. This road in turn descends 1.9 miles to heavily traveled County Road 531, should you need to vacate the wilderness. From the upper end of the Cherry Creek Trail, you walk just a minute north along Trapper Lake to its northeast corner, where you meet Donna Lake Trail 3734.

Diverting to Donna Lake Trail: This 0.9-mile trail makes an initial ascent northeast before curving past Donna Lake and another Deep Lake and then climbing back to the Sky Lakes Trail.

CAMPING **Staying on Sky Lakes Trail:** The Sky Lakes Trail next climbs 0.2 mile west to a ridge junction with the Divide Trail 3717 at 6,010 feet, just above Margurette Lake. You'll find a couple of camps both north and south of this junction.

VIEWS **Diverting to the Divide Trail to Luther Mountain and the PCT:** Starting southwest, the well-graded, 2.6-mile Divide Trail 3717 is your first route back to the PCT. It ends at a junction with the PCT on a saddle immediately west of Luther Mountain (7,153'). That peak, which is the throat of an old volcano, is well worth climbing. Scramble east up to the summit to get a commanding view of the entire Sky Lakes Area plus a view down Cherry Creek canyon.

Staying on Sky Lakes Trail: Beyond the Divide Trail, the Sky Lakes Trail skirts past attractive Margurette Lake. With a prominent cliff for a tapestry and Luther Mountain for a crown, this deep lake reigns as queen of the Sky Lakes. You quickly pass two lakelets and then meet the northwest end of Donna Lake Trail 3734.

Sky Lakes and Donna Lake Trails rejoin: Ahead, you top out near chilly, unseen Tsuga Lake, just west of the trail, and then descend past a lower pair of Snow Lakes, which have a scenic but chilly backdrop. The descent ends at nearby, waist-deep Martin Lake, and then you go 0.4 mile to a junction with Nannie Creek Trail 3707, a 3.9-mile trail that is popular on summer weekends.

Back to the PCT on the Sky Lakes–Snow Lakes Trail: Northeastward, you're climbing on what is now called Snow Lakes Trail 3739, which makes an exhausting start that abates in 0.4 mile, where it turns southwest. Your

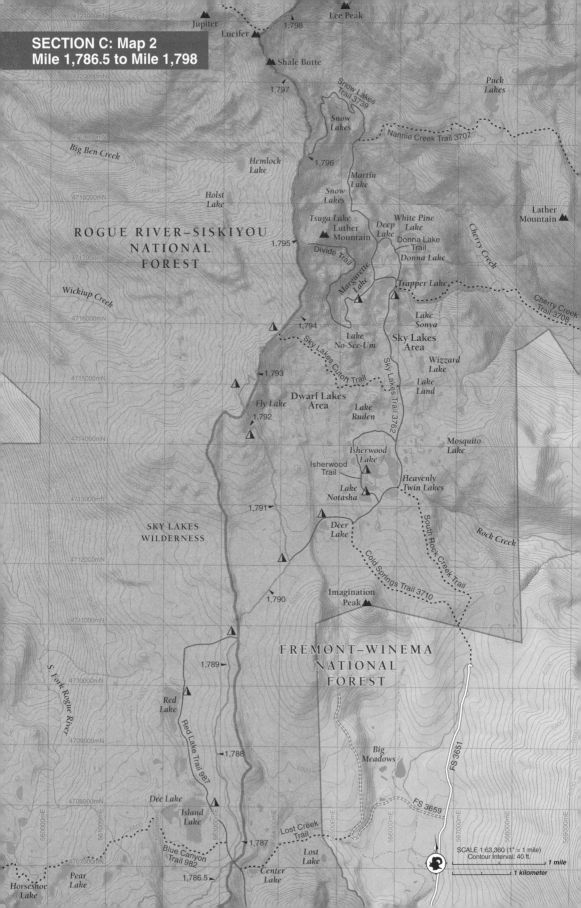

Jupiter

Lucifer

Lee Peak

1,798

Shale Butte

Puck Lakes

1,797

Snow Lakes Trail 3739

Snow Lakes

Nannie Creek Trail 3707

Big Ben Creek

Hemlock Lake

1,796

Martin Lake

Snow Lakes

Holst Lake

Lather Mountain

Tsuga Lake
Luther Mountain

Deep Lake

White Pine Lake

ROGUE RIVER–SISKIYOU NATIONAL FOREST

1,795

Donna Lake Trail

Donna Lake

Divide Trail

Cherry Creek

Wickiup Creek

Marguerite Lake

Trapper Lake

Cherry Creek Trail 3708

1,794

Lake No-See-Um

Lake Sonya

Sky Lakes Area

Sky Lakes Cutoff Trail

Wizzard Lake

Lake Land

1,793

Dwarf Lakes Area

Sky Lakes Trail 3762

Lake Ruden

Fly Lake

1,792

Mosquito Lake

Isherwood Lake

Isherwood Trail

Lake Notasha

Heavenly Twin Lakes

1,791

SKY LAKES WILDERNESS

Deer Lake

Rock Creek

South Rock Creek Trail

1,790

Cold Springs Trail 3710

Imagination Peak

FREMONT–WINEMA NATIONAL FOREST

1,789

Red Lake

S. Fork Rogue River

Red Lake Trail 987

1,788

Big Meadows

FS 3651

Dee Lake

Island Lake

FS 3659

Lost Creek Trail

1,787

Blue Canyon Trail 982

Lost Lake

Horseshoe Lake

Pear Lake

1,786.5

Center Lake

SCALE 1:63,360 (1" = 1 mile)
Contour Interval: 40 ft.

1 mile

1 kilometer

trail switchbacks up a ridge before switchbacking up to the top of a cliff. On it lie the upper Snow Lakes; just 0.2 mile past the southwest lake, your lake-blessed alternate route rejoins the PCT (1,796.0–6,693').

Where Sky Lakes Trail departs from the PCT toward the escarpment above Deer Lake, the PCT heads north-northwest in a forest of lodgepole pines and mountain hemlocks, ascends a gentle slope past several nearby ponds, and then reaches an open forest as it approaches a cliff above the Dwarf Lakes Area. Glaciated Pelican Butte (8,036') is the prominent summit in the southeast; the more subdued Cherry Peak (6,623') is directly east. You can't see the lakes below because the area is so forested. The trail switchbacks slightly up to avoid the cliff, switchbacks slightly down the west side, and soon encounters a 100-yard spur trail (1,792.9–6,619') to an overlook with a view that encompasses most of the rolling hills to the west. Now you switchback several times up to a small summit before descending the ridgeline to a saddle and an intersection with the Sky Lakes Cutoff Trail (1,793.7–6,580'), which heads east to meet the Sky Lakes Trail.

PLANTS The PCT now takes you northeast up to a ridge where the views east of the Sky Lakes Basin really begin to open up. Along the trail segment that crosses a barren slope of volcanic blocks, you are likely to find, sprouting in the thin volcanic soil, numerous creamy-white western pasqueflowers (also called anemones), which are readily identified by their finely dissected leaves, hairy stems, and dozens of stamens. By August, their flowers are transformed into balls of silky plumes.

The trail contours north-northeast to the west edge of a saddle and reaches Divide Trail 3717 (1,794.9–6,815'). If you have the time, climb nearby Luther Mountain for stupendous views of the Sky Lakes Area; see the end of "Diverting to the Divide Trail to Luther Mountain and the PCT" in the alternate routes, page 107. It passes virtually every body of water in the vicinity.

From the Divide Trail saddle, you descend moderately to a ridge and follow it north as it gradually levels off. After starting up the crest, you soon meet Snow Lakes Trail 3739 (1,796.0–6,693'). This junction is the end of the highly recommended alternate route; it also offers those who've stayed on the official PCT a 0.2-mile side trip to the first of a pair of Snow Lakes.

GEOLOGY With the official PCT and the alternate routes rejoined, you climb again, snaking up a ridge, and then obtain views of Mount McLoughlin to the south as you round the west slopes of Shale Butte. Not shale or even slate, Shale Butte is really a highly fractured andesite-lava flow.

Next the trail traverses the east slope of Lucifer (7,474') to a long saddle, on which you meet Devils Peak Trail 984 (1,797.7–7,232').

SIDE TRIP This heads 1.3 miles northwest to Seven Lakes Trail 981, on which you can go 2.5 miles east, first descending past South, Cliff, Middle, and Grass Lakes and then climbing briefly back to the PCT. On summer weekends, the Seven Lakes Basin receives heavy use, and it should be avoided then.

Just 100 yards after you leave the saddle's northeast end, you'll spot an abandoned segment of the Devils Peak Trail.

Elevation profile — horizontal axis PCT MILE from 1,788 to 1,798; vertical axis ELEVATION 3,000–10,000. Labels: ROGUE RIVER–SISKIYOU NATIONAL FOREST; FREMONT–WINEMA NATIONAL FOREST; RR–S NF; FREMONT–WINEMA NATIONAL FOREST. Red Lake Trail junctions; Sky Lakes Trail 3762 junction; campsites; Divide Trail junction; Snow Lakes Trail junction; Devils Peak Trail 984 junction.

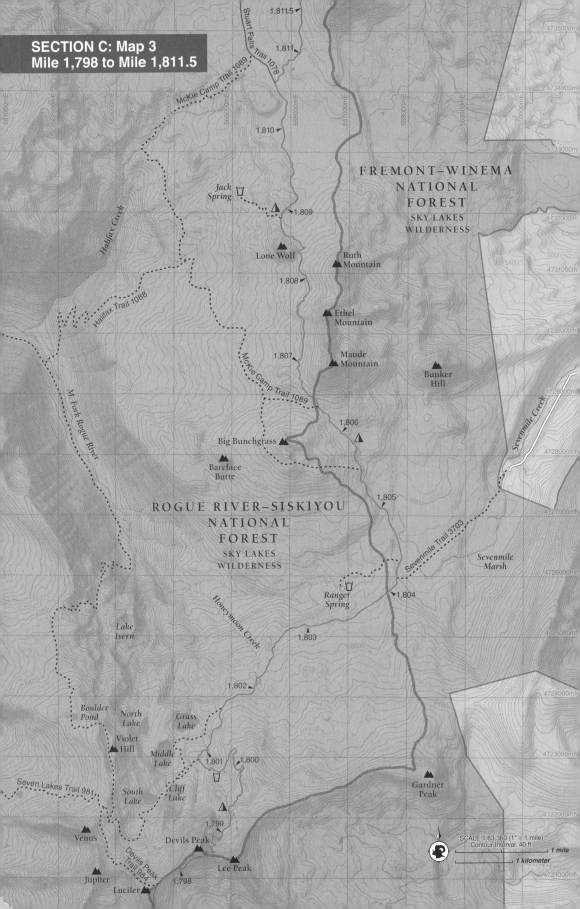

Stuart Falls Trail 1078

McKie Camp Trail 1089

1,811.5

1,811

1,810

FREMONT–WINEMA
NATIONAL
FOREST
SKY LAKES
WILDERNESS

Jack Spring

1,809

Halifax Creek

Lone Wolf

Ruth Mountain

1,808

Halifax Trail 1088

Ethel Mountain

McKie Camp Trail 1089

1,807

Maude Mountain

Bunker Hill

M. Fork Rogue River

1,806

Big Bunchgrass

Barcface Butte

Sevenmile Creek

1,805

ROGUE RIVER–SISKIYOU
NATIONAL
FOREST
SKY LAKES
WILDERNESS

Sevenmile Trail 3703

Sevenmile Marsh

Ranger Spring

1,804

Honeymoon Creek

1,803

Lake Ivern

1,802

Boulder Pond

North Lake

Grass Lake

Violet Hill

Middle Lake

1,801

1,800

Seven Lakes Trail 981

South Lake

Cliff Lake

Gardner Peak

1,799

Venus

Devils Peak

Devils Peak Trail 984

Jupiter

1,798

Lee Peak

Lucifer

SCALE 1:63,360 (1" = 1 mile)
Contour Interval: 40 ft.

1 mile

1 kilometer

GEOLOGY SIDE TRIP The abandoned trail segment makes a 0.5-mile, no-nonsense climb to the summit, from which you can make an even steeper 300-yard descent to the Devils Peak–Lee Peak saddle. Devils Peak is the remnant of an old volcano, and its summit vistas are well worth the effort. To the north, views include some of the Seven Lakes plus a good chunk of the Middle Fork canyon, including Boston Bluff. On the northern horizon is pointed Union Peak, the resistant plug of an eroded volcano. Immediately west of Union Peak, you see Mount Bailey (8,363'), which, like pointed Mount Thielsen (9,182'), is a hefty 36 miles away. Mount Scott (8,926') is the easternmost and highest of the Crater Lake environs peaks. On most days, you also see Mount Shasta (14,162'), 85 miles due south. Mount McLoughlin (9,495') is the dominating stratovolcano 15 miles south-southwest.

Those who don't visit the summit have a leisurely climb to the Devils Peak–Lee Peak saddle, where they meet hikers who climbed Devils Peak. The descent from the saddle is often a snowy one, and it can be impassable to pack and saddle stock even as late as August.

Early-summer backpackers generally slide or run down the snowpack until they locate the trail in the mountain-hemlock forest below. Those ascending this north slope on foot will find the climb strenuous but safe.

WATER ACCESS

The PCT switchbacks north down this slope; crosses a cascading, bubbling creek; and then in 0.25 mile passes a meadow. Cross its outlet creek, switchback downward, recross the outlet creek plus the earlier, cascading creek, and soon arrive at a junction (1,800.8–6,246').

SIDE TRIP Southwest, a trail goes 0.3 mile over to Seven Lakes Trail 981, along which you can walk 0.1 mile to Cliff Lake. Along the lake's east shore, by the edge of a large talus slope, you'll find a small, bedrock cliff that makes a perfect platform for jumping into the lake.

Beyond the Cliff Lake lateral, head northeast, cross a creek, and then make a steepening descent to another junction with the Seven Lakes Trail 981 (1,801.5–6,159'). Southwestward, this trail drops to overused Grass Lake.

Northeast, the PCT rambles down to usually flowing but often muddy Honeymoon Creek (1,802.1–5,992'). Past it, you undulate across generally viewless slopes and hear Ranger Spring, unseen below, as you approach a junction where you meet Sevenmile Trail 3703 (1,804.2–5,811').

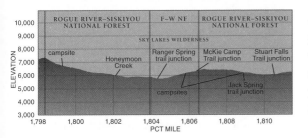

SECTION C

WATER ACCESS

The PCT descends quickly to a flat, broad saddle, where it meets Middle Fork Basin Trail (1,804.3–5,763'), which winds southwest 0.8 mile gradually down to the sonorous, tumultuous Ranger Spring. Northbound, water is scarce, so tank up at these pristine springs unless you plan to visit out-of-the-way Stuart Falls. If you don't visit remote and unreliable Jack Spring and don't take the alternate route to Stuart Falls, you then have about an 18-mile trek to Annie Spring (along the alternate Crater Lake route) or an 18.9-mile trek to Dutton Creek (along the PCT).

Now bound for Crater Lake, you first cross a dry flat and then reach McKie Camp Trail 1089 (1,806.4–6,327') as you approach a meadowy saddle.

CAMPING SIDE TRIP This trail goes 2.7 miles down to a junction with Halifax Trail 1088. Solace Cow Camp lies about 90 yards down that trail. Just north from the Halifax Trail junction is a usually flowing creek with an adjacent hikers' camp. Northbound on the McKie Camp Trail, you reach the McKie Camp environs in 1.5 miles, and it, too, has a usually flowing creek. You can then take the trail 1.7 miles northeast up to the Stuart Falls Trail, reaching it just under 0.5 mile northwest of the PCT. Hikers would take this described

route only if they really needed water, for it is quite a bit out of the way. However, the route may appeal to equestrians, as Solace and McKie Camps are popular horse camps.

From the saddle between Big Bunchgrass and Maude Mountain, the PCT climbs to the latter's west spur, from which it heads north along western slopes past Ethel and Ruth Mountains to a saddle just east of Lone Wolf. CAMPING Now the trail starts east but quickly switchbacks northwest and descends 0.5 mile through a snow-harboring fir-and-hemlock forest before curving north to a flat. Here, where others have camped, you spy the Jack Spring spur trail (1,808.9–6,205').

WATER ACCESS

This trail heads west to a low saddle from which it drops steeply 0.5 mile northwest to Jack Spring. Due to the steepness of this descent, plus the difficulty some folks have finding bucket-size Jack Spring, you should take this trail only if you really need water.

GEOLOGY Your route now winds gently down to the Oregon Desert, which holds a reservoir of water, all of it underground. The landscape has been buried in pumice and ash deposited from the final eruptions of Mount Mazama circa 5700 BC, eruptions that led to the stratovolcano's collapse and the subsequent formation of Crater Lake in the resulting depression. Most of the area's streams were buried under ash and pumice, and the trekker faces water-shortage problems all the way to Thielsen Creek in Section D, some 47 trail miles away.

SECTION C

You traverse the west edge of the "desert," which in reality is an open lodgepole-forest flat. Leaving the "desert" behind, you top a low, adjacent saddle and then meet the south end of Stuart Falls Trail 1078 (1,810.5–6,061'). Once the snow melts, you won't find any water on or near the PCT all the way north to OR 62, some 10.4 miles away. And from there you'll have to walk about 0.5 mile east to Annie Spring or 0.5 mile farther to Mazama Campground. Unless you have enough water to make this stretch, you will have to take the Stuart Falls Trail, given as an alternate route below.

ALTERNATE ROUTE In just under 0.5 mile, Stuart Falls Trail meets the north end of McKie Camp Trail 1089, which was briefly described earlier. Walk an easy 1.25 miles north, and then descend moderately northwest to a junction with the Lucky Camp Trail 1083.

The Stuart Falls Trail passes three creeks of variable staying power before it crosses always-reliable Red Blanket Creek to reach the upper end of the Red Blanket Falls Trail.

CAMPING Now you stroll up along Red Blanket Creek to a spur trail that takes you less than 0.5 mile to Stuart Falls Camp. This large, flat area near the base of Stuart Falls is for humans only. If you have stock animals, you must picket them immediately north of the Stuart Falls Trail, not down at the camp.

The next day, tank up on water and start up the Stuart Falls Trail. In about 0.3 mile, you enter Crater Lake National Park near a ravine with a seasonal creek. From it, your route is an old, abandoned road that faithfully guides you northeast back to the PCT (1,816.0–6,311').

Meanwhile, from the south end of the Stuart Falls Trail, PCT devotees start northeast from the fork. The PCT heads toward the crest, once again thwarting your hopes for water. It climbs north across the lower slopes of Goose Egg, reaches the crest just beyond that peak, and then stays very close to the crest as it descends to a crossing of an old, closed road only a few

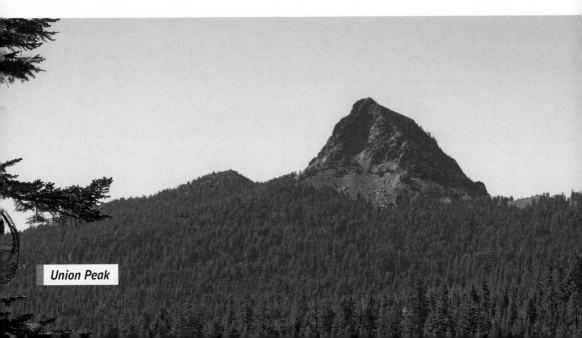

Union Peak

SECTION C

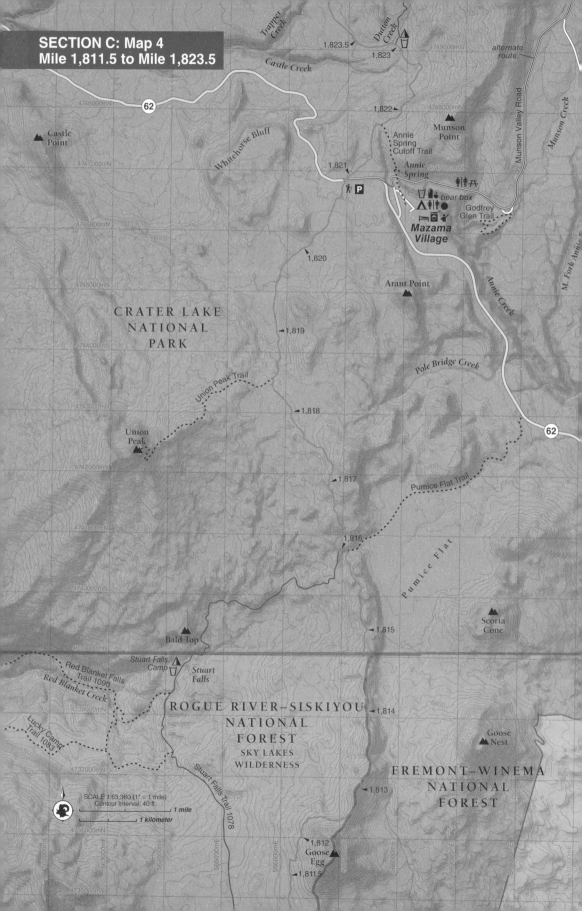

Trapper Creek

Dutton Creek

1,823.5

1,823

alternate route

Castle Creek

62

1,822

Munson Valley Road

Munson Creek

Annie Spring Cutoff Trail

Munson Point

Castle Point

Whitehorse Bluff

Annie Spring

bear box

1,821

P

Mazama Village

Godfrey Glen Trail

1,820

Arant Point

Annie Creek

M. Fork Annie C.

CRATER LAKE NATIONAL PARK

1,819

Pole Bridge Creek

Union Peak Trail

1,818

62

Union Peak

Pumice Flat Trail

1,817

1,816

Pumice Flat

Scoria Cone

1,815

Bald Top

Stuart Falls Camp

Stuart Falls

1,814

Goose Nest

Red Blanket Falls Trail 1090

Red Blanket Creek

ROGUE RIVER–SISKIYOU NATIONAL FOREST

FREMONT–WINEMA NATIONAL FOREST

Lucky Camp Trail 1083

SKY LAKES WILDERNESS

Stuart Falls Trail 1078

1,813

SCALE 1:63,360 (1" = 1 mile)
Contour Interval: 40 ft.

1 mile

1 kilometer

1,812

Goose Egg

1,811.5

yards before the trail tread ends at a second old, closed road (1,816.0–6,311') where the alternate route rejoins it.

SIDE TRIP Northeast, the first closed road, as the Pumice Flat Trail, goes 2.8 monotonous miles to OR 62. Southwest, the second route descends 2.5 miles to Stuart Falls Camp, reversing the last leg of the aforementioned alternate route.

With the official PCT and alternate routes rejoined, you head deeper inland, already a solid mile within Crater Lake National Park, progressing along the second old, closed road. Ramble onward, gaining slightly in elevation; enter an oval, open flat; and then top out at the south end of a long but narrow, open flat (1,818.4–6,503').

SIDE TRIP From this end another closed road—the Union Peak Trail—meanders 2.6 miles west to the steep summit. Weather permitting, you should not pass up the opportunity to scale this prominent landmark. Drop your heavy pack at the end of the old road and scramble, sometimes using your hands, up to Union Peak's tiny summit.

The PCT traverses the narrow, open flat and then takes you down through a dense, viewless forest that contains some of the finest specimens of mountain hemlocks you'll find anywhere. Before mid-July, this shady stretch can be quite snowbound. Finally you come to a small trailhead parking area along the south side of OR 62 (1,820.9–6,177').

Three options await you across OR 62: The first is the official PCT, which begins as a trail on the other side of the highway and makes a long arc around Crater Lake's west rim, generally staying 2–3 miles away from the lake and 1,000–2,500 feet below it. Equestrians must take the official PCT. You have no resupply options on the official PCT because it bypasses the park's post office. The second option starts on the official PCT but branches off in 2.1 miles. In the 1990s, the National Park Service constructed a hiker-only PCT rim route that branches off at the Dutton Creek Trail. This "hikers' PCT" also bypasses the park's post office, but it does go through Rim Village, which has lodging, a cafeteria, and a gift store but no grocery store. We describe this alternate hikers' PCT beginning on page 121. The third option, for long-distance hikers who need to resupply, is the "Alternate Route and Resupply Access from OR 62" described on page 116. This route passes near Mazama Village, which has a hike-in campground and a store, among other amenities. The route also visits park headquarters, where you'll find the post office, and it goes through the facilities at Rim Village before linking up with the hikers' PCT.

TRAIL INFO The official PCT avoids the lake's rim because one of the criteria for the PCT is that it bypass heavily traveled routes—and the Rim Drive surely is one of them. However, another good reason to route the trail low is that the rim accumulates a lot of snow, which can last well into July and sometimes into August, and equestrians wouldn't be able to use it until then.

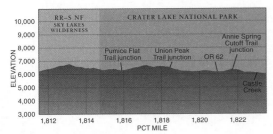

ALTERNATE ROUTE AND RESUPPLY ACCESS FROM OR 62

From where the PCT crosses OR 62 at a level stretch 0.8 mile west of the highway's junction with the park's south-rim access road, you start east along the highway. In 0.3 mile, the highway bends southeast, and you leave it, descending 0.25 mile east on the old highway's abandoned roadbed. This ends at the base of a ravine, up which the Annie Spring Cutoff Trail climbs 0.5 mile north back to the PCT. Your route heads south-southeast about 300 yards over to the Crater Lake south-rim access road. This is about midway between Annie Spring and the entrance to Mazama Campground.

CAMPING Because you won't have a legal camping opportunity anywhere along the park's roads, you might as well head 250 yards south to the campground's entrance road and then 0.4 mile to the campground proper. If you've started your day's hike from Stuart Falls by 7 a.m., you'll reach the campground by 3 p.m., even if you've taken the side trip to Union Peak. The campground is often full by 5 p.m., though on weekends it can fill much earlier. It is in Mazama Village, which also includes a store, an inn, a gas station, and coin-operated showers and laundry. A hiker/biker walk-in area is also available, and most PCT hikers take advantage of its casual layout. The visible burn damage is the result of 2017's

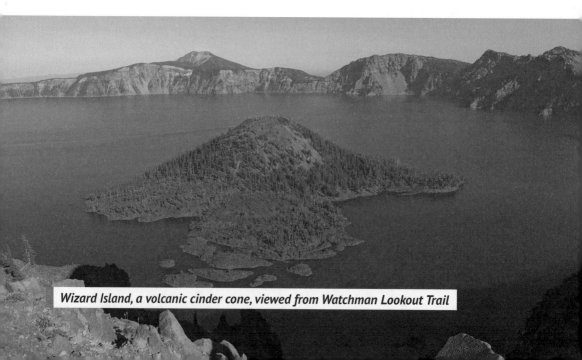

Wizard Island, a volcanic cinder cone, viewed from Watchman Lookout Trail

catastrophic High Cascades Complex fires.

The next morning, retrace your steps to where you first met the south-rim access road, and curve 0.1 mile along the road and over to a bridge that spans Annie Creek. You'll see copious Annie Spring—the source of the creek—just upstream from the bridge. Eastbound, you pass Goodbye Creek Picnic Area (with water) in 0.8 mile and reach a curve north in 0.4 mile. From the curve, the Godfrey Glen Trail makes a 1-mile loop out to vertical-walled Annie Creek canyon and back. You have almost an hour's trek north up Munson Valley along the viewless access road, and you pass ranger residences before reaching Crater Lake's West Rim Drive in 2.2 miles. Still well below the rim, you start north, only to meet park headquarters and its post office in another 600 feet. Pick up whatever packages you've mailed to yourself. You can also get information on weather, wildflower conditions, and the like; get a wilderness permit to camp in the park's backcountry (such as at Lightning Springs or Red Cone Springs); and buy books and pamphlets about the park and the Cascade Range.

From the park headquarters, head north up West Rim Drive, which in 0.7 mile bends south.

You wind in and out of a couple of gullies and, upon reaching the westernmost one, have the option of hiking 0.3 mile due north up it to Crater Lake Lodge. Otherwise, head southwest 0.6 mile on West Rim Drive up to Munson Ridge and then north 1 mile to the Rim Village junction. Just 60 yards before this junction, you'll see the top end of the Dutton Creek Trail. This alternate route's distance to here, including a 1-mile detour to Mazama Village, is 7.6 miles. Those taking the alternate hikers' PCT (page 121) will meet you here. GEOLOGY Your reaction to your first view of this 1,932-foot-deep lake may be disbelief, as your memory tries to recollect a similar feature. As the deepest lake in the United States and the seventh-deepest in the world, Crater Lake is a pristine ultramarine blue on a sunny day, and the 900-foot height of this Rim Village vantage point deepens the color.

From the Rim Village junction, you can walk east through the "village," which has a complex with a gift shop, a cafeteria, and a restaurant. Behind this complex are rustic cabins for rent, usually on a daily basis. Just past the complex is a small visitor center, from which stairs drop to the Sinnott Memorial, which provides one of the best views of the lake. Crater Lake

SECTION C

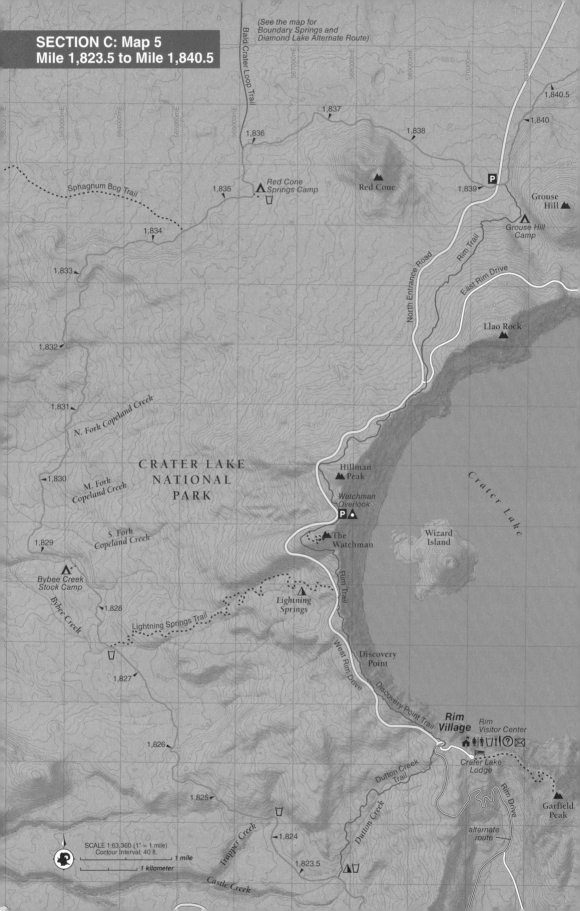

(See the map for
Boundary Springs and
Diamond Lake Alternate Route)

Bald Crater Loop Trail

1,837

1,838

1,840.5

1,836

1,840

Red Cone

Grouse
Hill

Sphagnum Bog Trail

1,835

Red Cone
Springs Camp

P

1,839

Grouse Hill
Camp

1,834

Rim Trail

1,833

North Entrance Road

East Rim Drive

Llao Rock

1,832

CRATER LAKE
NATIONAL
PARK

N. Fork Copeland Creek

1,831

1,830

M. Fork
Copeland Creek

Hillman
Peak

Crater Lake

Watchman
Overlook

1,829

S. Fork
Copeland Creek

P

The Watchman

Wizard
Island

Bybee Creek
Stock Camp

Lightning
Springs

Rim Trail

Bybee Creek

1,828

Lightning Springs Trail

1,827

West Rim Drive

Discovery
Point

1,826

Discovery Point Trail

Rim
Village

Rim
Visitor Center

Crater Lake
Lodge

1,825

Dutton Creek
Trail

Garfield
Peak

Trapper Creek

1,824

Dutton Creek

Rim Drive

alternate
route

SCALE 1:63,360 (1" = 1 mile)
Contour Interval: 40 ft.

1,823.5

1 mile

1 kilometer

Castle Creek

Lodge, open only during summer, looms above the end of the Rim Village road, and from it the Garfield Peak Trail climbs 1.8 miles to a scenic view of Crater Lake.

To resume your journey, start just above the top end of the Dutton Creek Trail, at the Rim Village junction. If snow abounds, you'll have to take the paved West Rim Drive 5.8 miles to North Entrance Road and then 2.6 miles down it to the signed PCT's small trailhead parking area. The hikers' PCT is slightly longer.

From the Rim Village junction (alternate-route mile 7.6) to Discovery Point, no camping is allowed. Take the rim-hugging, often snow-patched Discovery Point Trail northwest, reaching signed Discovery Point at the second saddle. You then climb up and down 1.4 miles to the third saddle, at the top end of the Lightning Spring Trail. At each of the scenic saddles, there's parking for tourists taking West Rim Drive, as is true with saddles ahead.

CAMPING About 0.75 mile down the 4.2-mile Lightning Spring Trail is a short spur trail heading south to campsites among the two Lightning Springs.

The hikers' PCT leaves Discovery Point, climbing north toward The Watchman, a lava flow that formed on Mount Mazama's flank about 50,000 years ago. When slopes get too steep, your trail veers west, crosses The Watchman's west ridge, and then descends 1.4 miles northeast to a prominent saddle with ample parking, the Watchman Overlook. This descent is across often snowy slopes, which can bury the route. About 0.5 mile before the overlook, the Watchman Lookout Trail starts a 0.5-mile climb to the summit. If you have the time and energy, don't pass up the opportunity to take in the commanding views.

Beyond the Watchman Overlook, the hikers' PCT starts north toward Hillman Peak, and then, as before, the trail rounds the peak's west slopes and descends northeast to the Crater Lake rim. For about a mile, you have a true crest experience as you descend to the West Rim Drive's junction with

SECTION C

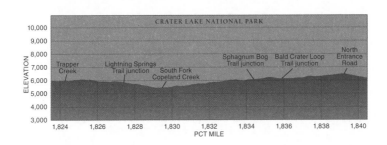

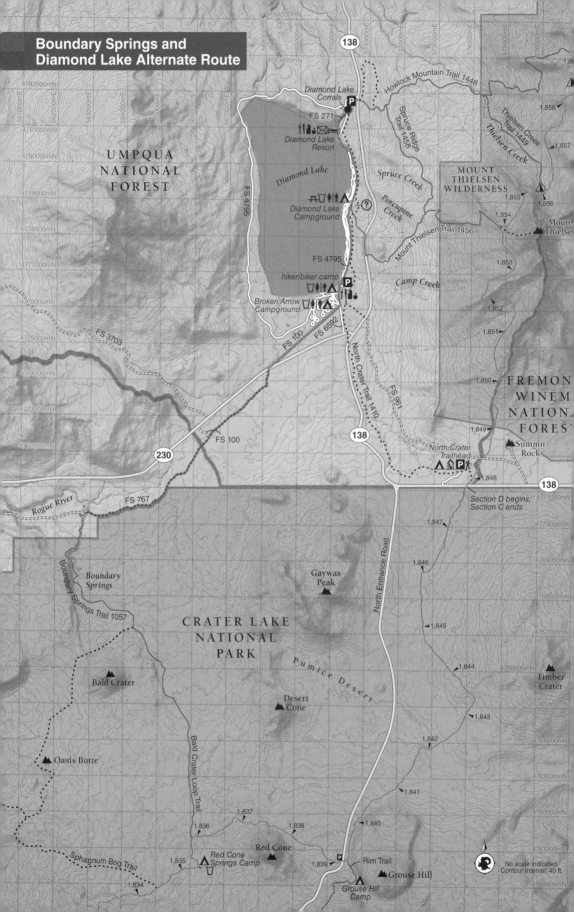

Boundary Springs and Diamond Lake Alternate Route

138

UMPQUA NATIONAL FOREST

Diamond Lake Corrals

FS 271

Diamond Lake Resort

Diamond Lake

Spruce Ridge Trail 1458

Spruce Creek Trail 1458

Howlock Mountain Trail 1448

Thielsen Creek Trail 1449

Thielsen Creek

1,858

1,857

MOUNT THIELSEN WILDERNESS

1,855

1,856

Moun Thielse

1,854

Diamond Lake Campground

FS 4795

Spruce Creek

Porcupine Creek

Mount Thielsen Trail 1456

1,853

FS 4795

hiker/biker camp

P

Camp Creek

1,852

1,851

Broken Arrow Campground

FS 100

FS 6592

North Crater Trail 1410

FS 961

1,850

FREMON WINEM NATION FORES

138

1,849

Summit Rock

230

FS 100

North Crater Trailhead

P

1,848

138

Rogue River

FS 767

Section D begins; Section C ends

1,847

Boundary Springs Trail 1057

Boundary Springs

Gaywas Peak

1,846

1,845

CRATER LAKE NATIONAL PARK

Pumice Desert

1,844

Bald Crater

Desert Cone

1,843

Timber Crater

Bald Crater Loop Trail

North Entrance Road

1,842

Oasis Butte

1,841

1,837

Red Cone

1,840

Sphagnum Bog Trail

1,836

1,838

Red Cone Springs Camp

P

1,839

Rim Trail

Grouse Hill

1,835

Grouse Hill Camp

1,834

No scale indicated. Contour Interval: 40 ft.

North Entrance Road. Follow the eastern border of the parking lot, and cross East Rim Drive at the north end of its parking lot. Angle northwest past this junction, and head north, splitting the distance between East Rim Drive and North Entrance Road. Now you make an increasingly forested descent in and out of minor ravines down to the official (equestrians') PCT, just east of North Entrance Road (1,839.2–6,491'). The total mileage of your alternate route, starting from OR 62, is 15.6 miles. If you joined the alternate route via the Dutton Creek Trail, then it is 11.4 miles.

The PCT route, for both hikers and equestrians, from OR 62 over to North Entrance Road is about 2.7 miles longer than the alternate route via Mazama Village and Rim Village. However, it involves a lot less climbing and therefore less effort. From OR 62, this entirely viewless section begins by climbing, part of it up a fault-line ravine. Then it descends momentarily east to the head of a second fault-line ravine (1,821.7–6,336'). Southward, the Annie Spring Cutoff Trail heads down it, ending in a flat just west of Annie Spring.

WATER ACCESS

On the PCT, start northeast and soon pass three seasonal tributaries of Castle Creek before turning west and passing a fourth (1,822.7–6,134)', which is year-round in some years.

About 2 minutes past it, you'll find the Dutton Creek Trail (1,823.0–6,093'), on which you can connect with the alternate route called the hikers' PCT. It's described below; no stock animals are allowed on the hikers' PCT route.

ALTERNATE ROUTE ("HIKERS' PCT") This route climbs 2.4 fairly hard miles on the Dutton Creek Trail to the vicinity of Crater Lake's Rim Village junction. If you take this route or the "Alternate Route and Resupply Access from OR 62," you'll reach about 7,700 feet elevation as you round The Watchman, and this locale then will be your highest PCT elevation in Oregon and Washington. For those on the official PCT, the highest PCT elevation will be near Tipsoo Peak, north of pointed Mount Thielsen, in the southern part of Section D. Pick up the rest of the hikers' PCT route at "To resume your journey" in "Alternate Route and Resupply Access from OR 62," page 116.

CAMPING From the Dutton Creek Trail junction, the official PCT, which equestrians must take, soon reaches very reliable Dutton Creek (1,823.1–6,075'), with a spur trail southwest down to some close-by campsites. These comprise the first of three official camping areas along the park's PCT. The two others are at Bybee Creek and Red Cone Springs, the latter being your last source of water until well into Section D.

WATER ACCESS

Your trail descends 1.25 miles to two-forked Trapper Creek, passing two seasonal creeks on the way.

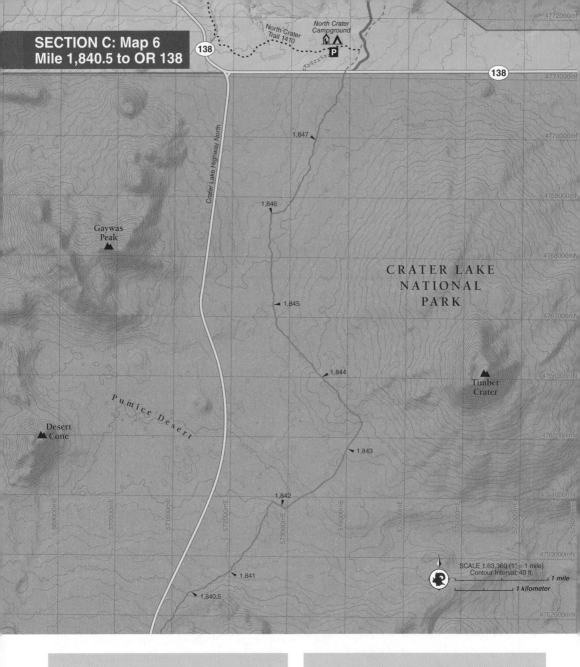

138

North Crater
Trail 1410

North Crater
Campground

P

138

1,847

1,846

Gaywas
Peak

CRATER LAKE
NATIONAL
PARK

1,845

1,844

Timber
Crater

Pumice Desert

Desert
Cone

1,843

1,842

1,841

1,840.5

SCALE 1:63,360 (1" = 1 mile)
Contour Interval: 40 ft.

1 mile

1 kilometer

Trapper Creek flows most of the summer, but later on you'll have to go downstream to find it flowing.

Ahead, you ramble about 1.25 miles over to a divide and then make a noticeable descent north to four forks of South Fork Bybee Creek. The first three flow most of the summer, but the fourth is vernal. Past the fourth, the road briefly rises and then descends 0.5 mile to lasting Bybee Creek.

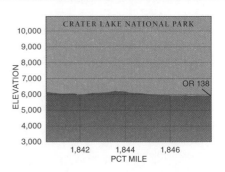

CRATER LAKE NATIONAL PARK

OR 138

ELEVATION

10,000
9,000
8,000
7,000
6,000
5,000
4,000
3,000

1,842   1,844   1,846
PCT MILE

CAMPING Immediately beyond it, an old road, the Lightning Spring Trail (1,827.4–5,869'), begins a 4.2-mile climb to Rim Drive. You can wind on down to another junction (1,828.6–5,608') from which an old, closed spur road descends 0.2 mile west to stock camps along a tributary of Bybee Creek. If the tributary is dry, look for water just downstream.

Beyond the spur road, the PCT soon turns west and then descends. Your route turns north and soon crosses the fairly reliable South (1,829.5–5,458') and Middle (1,829.7–5,485') Forks of Copeland Creek.

Open, lodgepole-punctuated meadows stretch 0.25 mile beyond the Middle Fork, and these, like the meadows north of them, are favorite browsing spots for elk. From the second set of meadows, you climb 2.6 miles to a ridge, follow it briefly east, and then continue 1 mile east up gentle slopes to a junction with Sphagnum Bog Trail (1,834.4–6,088').

WATER ACCESS

CAMPING Next you climb to a very important junction (1,835.3–6,240'), where a spur trail heads 150 yards east-southeast to Red Cone Springs and several adjacent camps. If you plan to avoid any side trips to the Diamond Lake Recreation Area, your next on-trail water will be at Thielsen Creek, about 20 miles away. And if you plan to visit the recreation area, you will have similar water problems. Obviously, you don't drop to Diamond Lake to get water, since you could reach Thielsen Creek just as fast; rather, you visit it to resupply or enjoy its amenities. Prepare yourself for a long, dry day, unless you are

hiking before mid-July, in which case you're likely to encounter trailside snow patches.

If you find the thought of a long, waterless stretch too distressing, you do have a water-blessed option. And you have to hike a total of only about 12 miles to reach Broken Arrow Campground, above the south shore of Diamond Lake. To take this route, first continue north on the PCT down to a junction with the Bald Crater Loop Trail (1,835.9–6,129'), where you can continue on the official PCT or take an alternate route to Boundary Springs and Diamond Lake.

ALTERNATE ROUTE On this route you leave the eastbound PCT adherents as you descend dry, viewless, monotonous Bald Crater Loop Trail 4 miles north to a junction with the westbound portion of the loop to Oasis Butte. You continue north on Boundary Springs Trail 1057, then northwest, 1.7 miles down to voluminous Boundary Springs. No camping is allowed within 0.25 mile of the springs, so continue north down the Rogue River canyon, leaving Crater Lake National Park in about 1 mile, bridging the Rogue River, and then reaching FS 767 in another 0.7 mile.

On FS 767, head 2.8 miles east-northeast to a junction from which a short road (FS 100) winds 0.3 mile northwest to busy OR 230. Just before you reach the highway, you continue 2.3 miles northeast on an abandoned road whose end is blocked off by a newer section of OR 230. Cross the highway, relocate the abandoned road, and follow it 0.25 mile north to FS 100. Southbound hikers, note that this road begins about 100 yards east of Horse Lake; if you reach that lake, you've walked a bit too far.

CAMPING On FS 100 head northeast 0.8 mile to its end at FS 6592. Anywhere along this stretch, you can head north over to the adjacent, giant Broken Arrow Campground. On FS 6592, you head 0.25 mile north to a junction with FS 4795, which circles Diamond Lake. Starting on a northbound segment of FS 4795, you walk briefly over to a day-use parking area to the west and the old Mount Thielsen Trail to the east. From the parking area, you can take a path briefly southwest over to a hiker/biker camp with five sites, tap water, and flush toilets. Just above the southeast corner of Diamond Lake, this is the ideal place to spend the night.

Continue north on FS 4795. For further directions, see Section D's first alternate route, on page 134, which continues north from here.

PCT adherents ignore the Boundary Springs alternate route and make a generally uphill, usually easy traverse. Most of it is through an open lodgepole-pine forest, and you'll round avalanche-prone Red Cone about 1.5 miles before you reach a small trailhead parking area alongside North Entrance Road (1,839.2–6,496').

Just a few yards ahead, near where the PCT turns north, the hikers' PCT—the author's recommended route described in "Alternate Route and Resupply Access from OR 62," descending north from the Crater Lake rim—meets the official route.

GEOLOGY You begin your viewless, waterless trek by walking east over to the nearby base of Grouse Hill. This huge mass of rhyodacite lava congealed just before Mount Mazama erupted and collapsed to create the Crater Lake caldera. The eruptions, occurring about 7,700 years ago, "sandblasted" the top of Grouse Hill.

With the official PCT and the alternate route/resupply access rejoined, hikers and equestrians tread northeast between road and flow, which gradually diverge before you reach a short stretch of former road at the northeast corner of the shining pumice desert. On it, you walk 260 yards east to a turn northeast (1,842.0–5,996'). On a former road, you climb gently toward Timber Crater and, where the road becomes steeper, angle northwest (1,843.3–6,146'). You climb just 0.25 mile before continuing northwest on a long, viewless, snaking descent.

Heading toward OR 138, the PCT first strikes east and then traverses north-northeast to reach the Crater Lake National Park boundary immediately before OR 138 (1,847.8–5,923'). The PCT crosses the highway just 70 yards west of a broad, low crest pass of the Cascade Range. You won't find any parking here, so continue 230 yards from the highway to a junction, from which North Crater Trail 1410 descends 0.25 mile west to a well-developed trailhead parking area.

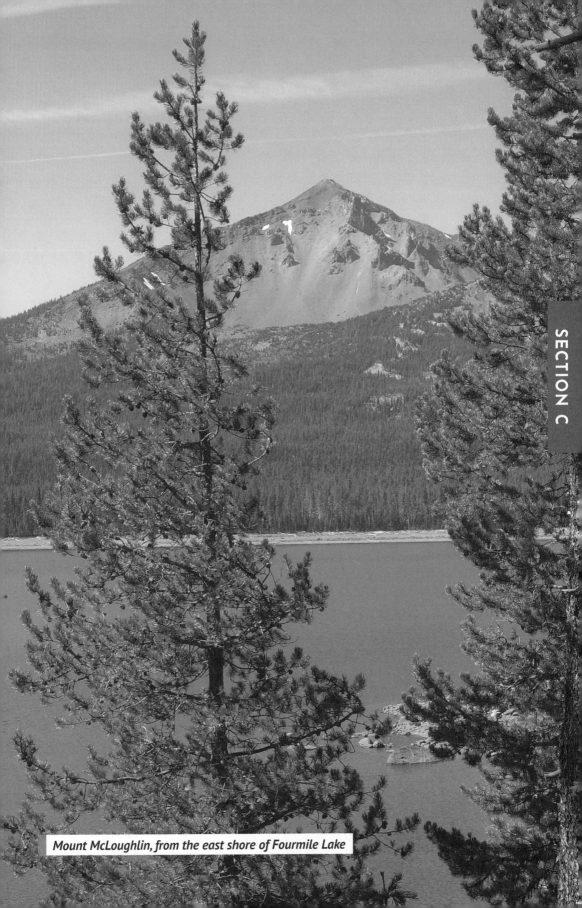

Mount McLoughlin, from the east shore of Fourmile Lake

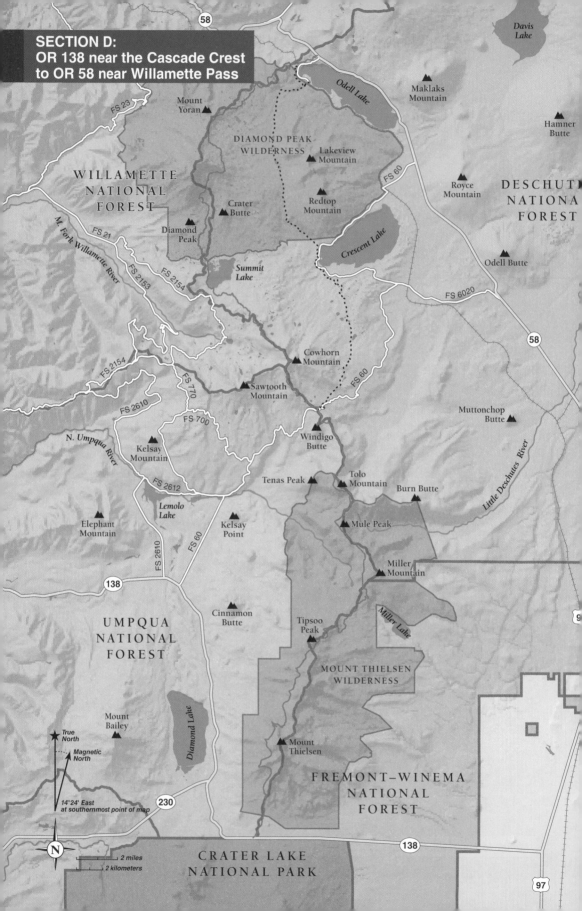

SECTION D:
OR 138 near the Cascade Crest
to OR 58 near Willamette Pass

58

Davis Lake

FS 23

Mount Yoran ▲

Odell Lake

Maklaks Mountain ▲

Hamner Butte ▲

DIAMOND PEAK WILDERNESS

Lakeview Mountain ▲

FS 60

Royce Mountain ▲

DESCHUTE NATIONA FOREST

WILLAMETTE NATIONAL FOREST

Crater Butte ▲

Redtop Mountain ▲

FS 21

Diamond Peak ▲

Crescent Lake

Odell Butte ▲

FS 2153

FS 2154

M. Fork Willamette River

Summit Lake

FS 6020

58

FS 2154

Cowhorn Mountain ▲

FS 60

Muttonchop Butte ▲

FS 770

Sawtooth Mountain ▲

FS 2610

FS 700

N. Umpqua River

Windigo Butte ▲

Little Deschutes River

Kelsay Mountain ▲

FS 2612

Tenas Peak ▲

Tolo Mountain ▲

Burn Butte ▲

Lemolo Lake

Mule Peak ▲

Elephant Mountain ▲

FS 60

Kelsay Point ▲

FS 2610

Miller Mountain ▲

9

138

Cinnamon Butte ▲

Tipsoo Peak ▲

Miller Lake

UMPQUA NATIONAL FOREST

MOUNT THIELSEN WILDERNESS

★ *True North*

Magnetic North

Mount Bailey ▲

Diamond Lake

Mount Thielsen ▲

14° 24' East
at southernmost point of map

230

FREMONT–WINEMA NATIONAL FOREST

N

2 miles

2 kilometers

CRATER LAKE NATIONAL PARK

138

97

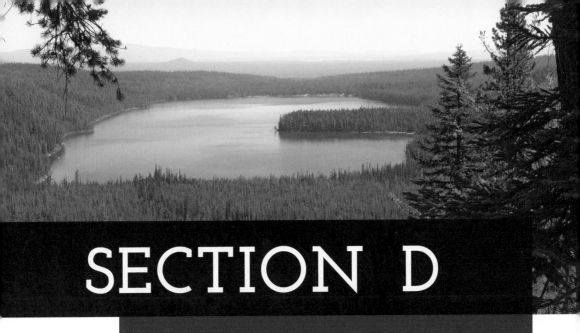

SECTION D

OR 138 near the Cascade Crest to OR 58 near Willamette Pass

NEEDLE-POINTED MOUNT THIELSEN, approached early on this hike, is this section's star attraction; its terrain is even more spectacular than that seen along the Pacific Crest Trail (PCT) through this section's Diamond Peak Wilderness. When the PCT was finally completed through this section around 1977, its route, now more faithful to the crest, replaced its predecessor, the Oregon Skyline Trail (OST). The OST touched on enjoyable Diamond Lake, which most long-distance PCT hikers still visit by taking the North Crater Trail, and passed Maidu Lake, both good camping areas when mosquitoes aren't biting. Maidu Lake is an important water source, and it is just a mile off the PCT. Some hikers may be interested in the old OST route through this section, especially if they're seeking more lakes or less snowpack, so the original route is described here as well as the new one.

This section of the PCT is well graded and has interesting, if not dramatic, views of Mount Thielsen, Sawtooth Ridge, Cowhorn Mountain,

Above: Miller Lake is inviting, but it's an hour away from the PCT.

Diamond Peak, and Mount Yoran. All are easily accessible to peak baggers, but Mount Yoran should be left for experienced mountaineers. The only significant lake along the official PCT route is Summit Lake. Like Diamond Lake, it is a worthy place to spend a layover day.

DECLINATION 14°24'E

USGS MAPS

Pumice Desert East, OR	Emigrant Butte, OR
Tolo Mountain, OR	Miller Lake, OR
Mount Thielsen, OR	Diamond Peak, OR
Cowhorn Mountain, OR	Burn Butte, OR
Diamond Lake, OR (alternate route)	Willamette Pass, OR

POINTS ON THE TRAIL, SOUTH TO NORTH

	Mile	Elevation in feet	Latitude/Longitude
OR 138 near the Cascade crest	1,847.8	5,923	N43° 05' 20.0308" W122° 05' 30.5370"
North Crater Trail junction	1,848.0	5,898	N43° 05' 26.9100" W 122° 05' 22.7800"
Mount Thielsen Trail junction	1,853.9	7,334	N43° 09' 12.6969" W122° 04' 50.7862"
Thielsen Creek Trail junction	1,856.2	6,950	N43° 09' 44.5279" W122° 03' 50.4817"
Howlock Mountain Trail junction	1,859.1	7,291	N43° 11' 46.2873" W122° 02' 55.5844"
Oregon/Washington high point	1,860.8	7,572	N43° 12' 42.7205" W122° 02' 16.2825"
Maidu Lake Trail junction	1,865.9	6,203	N43° 14' 32.1337" W121° 59' 38.7896"
Windigo Pass	1,878.3	5,821	N43° 22' 03.0256" W122° 01' 59.4407"
FS 380 near Summit Lake Campground	1,890.7	5,604	N43° 27' 48.7527" W122° 08' 05.3126"
Lils Lake	1,901.8	6,020	N43° 33' 45.5816" W122° 06' 28.6070"
Midnight Lake	1,904.8	5,386	N43° 35' 02.3012" W122° 04' 29.5296"
Pengra Pass	1,906.2	5,021	N43° 35' 28.9617" W122° 03' 27.9341"
OR 58 near Willamette Pass	1,907.9	5,088	N43° 35' 49.7619" W122° 02' 01.3060"

CAMPSITES AND BIVY SITES

Mile	Elevation in feet	Latitude/ Longitude	Number of tents	Feature	Notes
1,848.0 (alt.)	5,930	N43° 05' 19.8024" W122° 07' 00.4548"	2	North Crater Campground	Vault toilet, picnic table, fire ring, hitching posts
1,848.0 (alt.)	5,190	N43° 07' 58.1160" W122° 08' 49.9200"	118	Broken Arrow Campground	Flush toilets, potable water, showers, picnic table, fireplace
1,848.0 (alt.)	5,190	N43° 08' 12.5556" W122° 08' 30.6240"	5	hiker/biker camp	Free; flush toilets, potable water, picnic table, fireplace
1,848.0 (alt.)	5,190	N43° 09' 33.4800" W122° 07' 59.1240"	238	Diamond Lake Campground	Flush toilets, potable water, showers, picnic table, fireplace
1,853.9 (alt)	6,877	N43° 09' 52.5800" W122° 03' 59.3100"	4	Thielsen Creek Camp	0.2 mile off PCT near mile marker 1,856.2; water

SECTION D

CAMPSITES AND BIVY SITES *(continued)*

Mile	Elevation in feet	Latitude/ Longitude	Number of tents	Feature	Notes
1,858.4	7,133	N43° 11' 18.7526" W122° 03' 13.6002"	2		On left; fire ring
1,865.9	6,002	N43° 15' 10.6000" W121° 59' 59.9100"	4	Maidu Lake	0.9 mile off PCT, water
1,872.1	6,218	N43° 18' 17.5023" W122° 00' 09.4753"	>4	Tolo Camp	Six Horse Spring nearby
1,878.3 (alt)	5,726	N43° 23' 13.9624" W122° 00' 37.3309"	2	Nip and Tuck Lakes	Flat spot near trail on left
1,878.3 (alt)	4,850	N43° 28' 22.8360" W122° 01' 58.2960"	73	Spring Campground	0.6 mile off alternate trail; vault toilet, drinking water
1,878.3 (alt)	5,764	N43° 31' 42.1075" W122° 04' 13.6571"	>4	Diamond View Lake	
1,878.3 (alt)	4,800	N43° 34' 57.4680" W122° 02' 41.1720"	32	Trapper Creek Campground	Vault toilet; drinking water sometimes available
1,878.3 (alt)	4,819	N43° 34' 57.3096" W122° 02' 32.3628"	5	Shelter Cove Resort PCT camp	Toilets, water, showers, laundry
1,889.3	5,574	N43° 26' 47.7875" W122° 07' 57.8620"	>4	Summit Lake	Flat spot near trail in trees, water
1,890.6	5,564	N43° 27' 45.1027" W122° 07' 59.7126"	3	Summit Lake Campground	Vault toilet, picnic table, fire ring
1,892.5	5,888	N43° 28' 51.1207" W122° 08' 31.2211"	2	Pond	Flat spot near trail in trees, water
1,897.8	6,932	N43° 31' 39.9492" W122° 07' 11.4899"	2		Flat spot near trail in trees

SUPPLIES

Because there are no on-route supply points, most long-distance PCT hikers take one of the alternate routes north to Diamond Lake. The store at Diamond Lake Lodge is one of the best anywhere near the PCT. This resort also has a post office (97731) and serves good meals at reasonable prices.

Near Section D's north end, you can leave the PCT at Pengra Pass and descend 1.5 miles to Shelter Cove Resort. The resort accepts mailed packages but can only hold them about two weeks. Send them by UPS only to Shelter Cove Resort, West Odell Lake Road, OR 58, Crescent Lake, OR 97425.

SECTION D

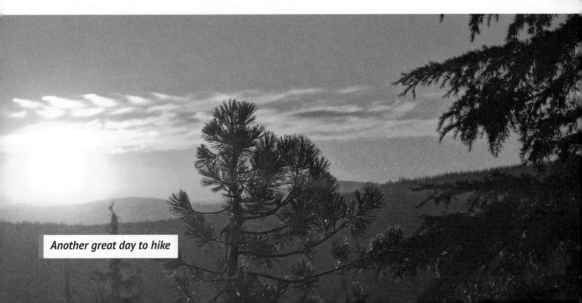

Another great day to hike

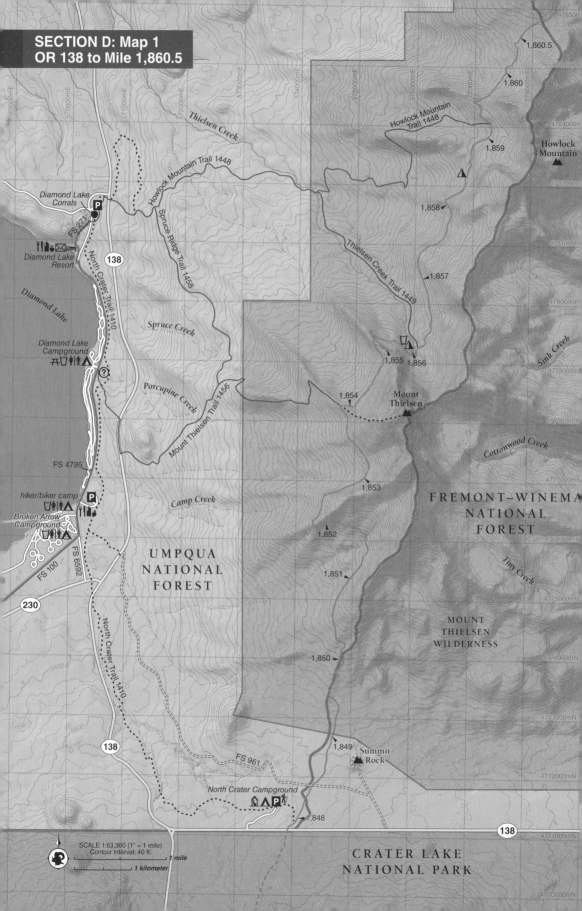

Thielsen Creek

Howlock Mountain Trail 1448

1,860.5

1,860

1,859

Howlock Mountain

1,858

Diamond Lake Corrals

Howlock Mountain Trail 1448

Spruce Ridge Trail 1458

FS 2715

North Crater Trail 1410

Thielsen Creek Trail 1449

Diamond Lake Resort

138

Sink Creek

1,857

Spruce Creek

1,855 1,856

Diamond Lake

Diamond Lake Campground

Porcupine Creek

1,854

Mount Thielsen

Mount Thielsen Trail 1456

Cottonwood Creek

FS 4795

1,853

FREMONT–WINEMA
NATIONAL
FOREST

Camp Creek

hiker/biker camp

1,852

Broken Arrow Campground

FS 6592

1,851

Tiny Creek

FS 100

UMPQUA
NATIONAL
FOREST

MOUNT
THIELSEN
WILDERNESS

230

1,850

North Crater Trail 1410

138

1,849

Summit Rock

FS 961

North Crater Campground

138

1,848

SCALE 1:63,360 (1" = 1 mile)
Contour Interval: 40 ft.

1 mile

1 kilometer

CRATER LAKE
NATIONAL PARK

OR 138 NEAR THE CASCADE CREST TO
OR 58 NEAR WILLAMETTE PASS
>>>THE ROUTE

This section's hike begins at OR 138 (1,847.8–5,923') just 70 yards west of the almost flat watershed divide in this locale of the Cascade Range. Trailhead parking is available just north of OR 138 and west of the PCT. The short road that goes northeast to the trailhead starts from OR 138 just 0.5 mile west of the Cascade divide and 0.8 mile east of Crater Lake's north-rim access road.

From OR 138, the PCT heads northeast 230 yards to a junction with the south end of North Crater Trail 1410 (1,848.0–5,898'). Just 3 minutes into the hike, you're faced with a decision—the first of several routes leaving the PCT for the Diamond Lake environs. The North Crater Trail doesn't go to any crater; rather, it descends toward Diamond Lake, runs north above its east shore, and then in 9.3 miles ends at the Diamond Lake Corrals, which are situated about 0.5 mile northeast of Diamond Lake Resort. If you want the quickest, easiest route to Diamond Lake, start along this trail.

RESUPPLY ACCESS

North Crater Trail 1410 reaches the trailhead parking area in 0.25 mile and then continues. In 60 yards, it reaches an old southwest-descending road that dies out in both directions. Go just 200 yards down this road and then fork right

(northwest) onto a broad path that descends to a ravine. From here a snowmobile route climbs northeast, leading eastbound hikers astray. Westward you cross, in 0.5 mile, an old road, which was referred to at the end of Section C. Just 0.6 mile later, the trail tread joins that road again, where it loops into a ravine. Follow the road 0.75 mile down to where it curves west and flattens out. Leave the road and take a trail that starts north along a crest between two gullies.

Your route ahead should now be obvious, and you parallel OR 138 for 2.5 miles until it diagonals across your path. Dash across the busy highway and follow a short trail segment 0.2 mile over to OR 230. You could continue north along the North Crater Trail, but because that route is largely viewless, you might miss a number of lakeside attractions. Therefore, walk 100 yards west on

SECTION D

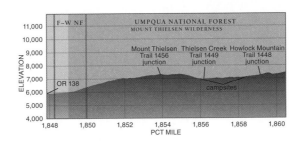

OR 230 to a junction with east-shore Forest Service Road 6592. Just under 0.5 mile north on it, you meet a straight, southwest-heading road—the old OR 230, today's FS 100—along which Section C's Boundary Springs Trail alternate route joins your route. As in that route, you head 0.25 mile north to a junction with Diamond Lake's loop road, FS 4795.

CAMPING Anywhere along this last stretch, you could have walked west to the east side of nearby Broken Arrow Campground. Also, a momentary walk west on the road takes you to a path that goes 100 yards north to a hiker/biker camp, with five sites, tap water, and flush toilets—an ideal place to spend the night. From it a path goes north momentarily to another path on which you can walk about a minute northeast over to FS 4795.

If you didn't head over to the camp, then at the junction of FS 4795 and FS 6592, start north on FS 4795 and momentarily pass the trail over to the camp, starting southwest. Opposite it is a short trail east back to Trail 1410, which you recently left. Immediately ahead, you reach a private campground on your right and soon arrive at South Shore. If you've been living for days out of your pack, you'll certainly welcome this store and its café.

CAMPING Just north of the store is the south end of 2-mile-long Diamond Lake Campground, which is sandwiched between the lake and FS 4795. You can drop to it anytime you desire.

Midway along the lake's east side, you reach an intersection with the campground's entrance to the left (west) and the Diamond Lake Information Center to the right (east). From that center, a spur trail goes to the North Crater Trail. Onward, you pass more of the campground; then, from its north end, you can hop onto a trail that parallels your road and the lakeshore for over a mile to Diamond Lake Resort's entrance road.

Head 0.3 mile over to the complex, resupply at its well-stocked general store, pick up your mailed parcels at the post office, and/or enjoy a hearty meal at the restaurant. If you're well funded, rent a fishing boat and catch a couple of rainbow trout, which grow considerably larger here than in the lakes of Sky Lakes Wilderness. Some long-distance hikers may even be desperate enough for civilization's amenities to stay at the resort's lodge.

After your stay, however brief or long, start north up the road immediately west of the gas station. This road climbs back to FS 4795, reaching it in only a minute's walk. To the east of this junction is the entrance road to Diamond Lake Corrals. Walk east to the road's far end, and beside it you'll find a tread. Northward, Howlock Mountain Trail 1448 swings east, spinning off Spruce Ridge Trail 1458 (which goes over to Mount Thielsen Trail 1456) and Thielsen Creek Trail 1449. All take you back to the PCT and will be described in the pages to come. Southward, North Crater Trail snakes 9.3 miles to the PCT, ending just north of Section D's start, OR 138.

From the North Crater Trail 1410 junction, those taking the PCT route have an easy climb to the old, abandoned Summit Rock Road/ Forest Service Road 961 (1,848.4–5,946').

SIDE TRIP This road, which is a ski route in winter, also provides a route—albeit inferior—to Diamond Lake. The road curves 4.2 miles over to the new OR 138, along whose shoulder you walk 0.4 mile and then follow the defunct Mount Thielsen Trail 0.5 mile west over to FS 4795, at the lake's southeast corner.

Onward, the PCT climbs gently north for 0.6 mile and enters the Mount Thielsen Wilderness (1,849.0–6,004'); soon the gradient steepens, and the trail makes a few open switchbacks up a ridge before it curves northwest around the ridge. Now you make a long but comfortable ascent, rounding Mount Thielsen's southwest ridge before traversing across a

glaciated bowl to a trail junction on the peak's west ridge. Here you meet Mount Thielsen Trail 1456 (1,853.9–7,334'). To the east, this trail leads to the summit of Mount Thielsen (9,182').

SIDE TRIP Sometimes called the lightning rod of the Cascades, Mount Thielsen is easily accessible and should not be bypassed. When you ascend it, however, leave your pack behind; it has what may be one of the steepest trails in existence—more of a climb than a hike. The trail quickly exits above treeline and then climbs increasingly loose pumice slopes. The last 200 feet are especially difficult, so use extreme caution.

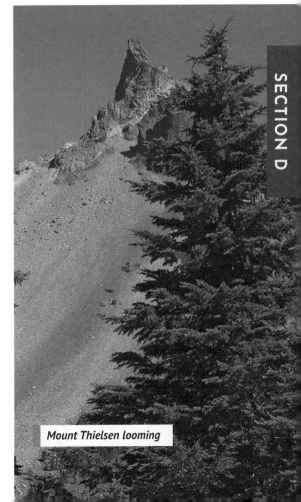

Mount Thielsen looming

SECTION D

VIEWS   The view from the summit area is spectacular and worth the effort. You can see north 107 miles to Mount Jefferson (10,462') and south 120 miles to Mount Shasta (14,117').

Back at the junction with the PCT, you can also take the Mount Thielsen Trail 1456 west to Diamond Lake.

ALTERNATE ROUTE If you want to drop to Diamond Lake for recreation or supplies, start west down Mount Thielsen Trail 1456, and in just 2.5 miles you arrive at a junction with Spruce Ridge Trail 1458. You can take either route to Diamond Lake, but to maximize scenery, make a loop.

On the waterless Mount Thielsen Trail, descend 1.7 miles to a trailhead on OR 138. Unfortunately, the trail doesn't continue west to the lakeshore road, so hike 0.5 mile north on OR 138 to where it begins to curve northeast. Drop west about 200 yards cross-country to North Crater Trail 1410. Walk 0.25 mile north on it to where a trail heads west over to a U.S. Forest Service information center.

CAMPING   Continue west to quickly reach east-shore FS 4795, which is opposite the entrance to Diamond Lake Campground.

Now follow the resupply access route on page 131 for 1.2 miles north to Diamond Lake Resort's entrance road, 0.3 mile over to the resort, 0.5 mile up a minor road back to FS 4795, and then 0.1 mile east through Diamond Lake Corrals to the Howlock Mountain Trailhead.

Howlock Mountain Trail 1448 heads northeast, joining another trail from the corrals immediately before passing through a horse tunnel under OR 138. From the far side of the tunnel, a trail heads north, but you climb southeast up the slopes of a lateral moraine.

GEOLOGY   The glacier that carried this morainal debris originated on the north slopes of Mount Mazama, a towering volcano that collapsed about 7,700 years ago at the site now occupied by Crater Lake.

Immediately beyond the crest of the moraine, you meet a second minor trail, which heads north down a ravine. You then switchback to the crest of a higher moraine and on it meet Spruce Ridge Trail 1458, which is the first of three options back to the PCT:

1. Spruce Ridge Trail: If you went to Diamond Lake as a side trip, take this return option if you don't want to miss a foot of the PCT. The waterless Spruce Ridge Trail starts southeast along a minor ridge and makes an easy, spruce-free, generally viewless ascent 2.6 miles south to the Mount Thielsen Trail. Up it, turn left (east) and retrace your steps to where you left the PCT, on the west ridge of Mount Thielsen.

2. Thielsen Creek Trail: Continue 1.9 miles east on the Howlock Mountain Trail, passing in 0.3 mile the seasonal west fork of Thielsen Creek, later skirting Timothy Meadows, and then reaching Thielsen Creek and adjacent Thielsen Creek Trail 1449. Take this moderately climbing trail, which parallels its namesake, southwest back up to the PCT.

CAMPING You'll pass a short spur trail over to Thielsen Creek Camp about 100 yards before reaching the junction with the PCT.

3. Howlock Mountain Trail: From the lower end of the Thielsen Creek Trail, continue straight (east) 3.2 miles up Howlock Mountain Trail, which can have snow patches in mid-July but can be waterless by early August. You'll see Howlock Mountain, rising 1,000 feet above you, just before you reach the PCT.

You will likely see many day hikers and climbers here as they ready themselves to embark along the west ridge toward the rocky summit. Initially, hikers head along the forested border southeast up to about 8,000 feet, overlooking the steepening scree field to the north and slipping off to the south side of the ridge as the trail takes a northeastern route before turning north about 125 feet below the peak.

If you stayed on the PCT instead of visiting Diamond Lake, from the Mount Thielsen Trail 1456 junction, the PCT crosses the open, view-packed northwest slopes of Mount Thielsen to the peak's northwest ridge (1,854.9–7,370'). From here you can see your next major peak—bulky, snowy Diamond Peak—to the north.

WATER ACCESS

The trail now makes long switchbacks down from the ridge, then descends southeast to Thielsen Creek (1,856.1–6,925'). Over this last mile of trail, snow sometimes lingers through late July. Thielsen Creek is your first source of permanent water since Red Cone Spring, 20.8 miles back, or Crater Lake Rim Village, 26.2 miles south. Your next on-route, permanent source of water is at Summit Lake, a whopping 34 miles ahead, so many hikers stop at out-of-the-way Maidu Lake, a good camping area only 9.8 miles ahead. Six Horse Spring, in 16 miles, may also have water.

Just past the Thielsen Creek crossing, you reach Thielsen Creek Trail 1449 (1,856.2–6,950'), where you meet the Thielsen Creek Trail return option from Diamond Lake.

CAMPING You can descend about 100 yards on Thielsen Creek Trail to a spur trail that leads 100 yards west down to Thielsen Creek Camp. Because this is the first PCT campsite with water since Red Cone Springs, it can be overcrowded. When space is limited, it's important to practice Leave No Trace etiquette and set your tent 200 feet away from the trail and out of sight of other tents. Expanded campsites degrade very quickly.

CAMPING Leaving the Thielsen Creek area, the PCT makes a winding contour north to an open bowl, Pumice Flat (1,858.4–7,133'). The PCT heads east just above it into a stand of mountain hemlocks. If you are hiking through this area in early season, you might want to camp under a cluster of hemlocks and lodgepoles near the low summit 0.25 mile west of you. You can obtain early-season water from the seasonal creek just north of it or from nearby snow patches.

After the PCT heads east into the hemlocks, it quickly starts an ascending, counterclockwise traverse around the bowl. Just past a meadow where the trail turns from north to northwest, you'll reach a junction (1,859.1–7,291') with well-used Howlock Mountain Trail 1448. The last Diamond Lake alternate route, described earlier, ends here.

The PCT now makes an obvious climb to a crest saddle (1,859.5–7,415') that lies on a western spur of the ragged, severely glaciated Sawtooth Ridge. Leaving the crest saddle, you may encounter lingering snowbanks before you reach your first meadow. The meadows usually have posts through them to help PCT hikers stay on track. On this stretch, on the southeast flank below Tipsoo Peak, you reach the high point—in elevation—of the Oregon/Washington PCT (1,860.8–7,572').

SIDE TRIP Tipsoo Peak, due north, is an easy 20-minute climb for peak baggers, and its summit views are second only to Thielsen's for providing an overview of this region.

On the lower south slopes of Tipsoo Peak, just north of a broad saddle, the PCT starts a descent northeast. About halfway to a saddle, the trail bends north across an open ravine and then hugs the forested lower slopes of Tipsoo Peak as it continues northeast to that saddle

(1,861.6–7,300'). Here you can inspect the severely glaciated north face of red-black Tipsoo Peak.

From this saddle, hikers used to zip northeast straight down to Maidu Lake, but the route has been changed so that you now make a long, counterclockwise traverse around a flat, volcanic summit. This route provides three scenic viewpoints that reveal Red Cone and Miller Lake; then the trail veers northeast across the county-line crest to a switchback and makes a long, winding, viewless descent to the west end of a broad saddle on which you cross Maidu Lake Trail 1446 (1,865.9–6,203').

WATER ACCESS

CAMPING Here the Maidu Lake Trail starts north, proceeds to cross the county-line saddle, and then descends a gully to the south shore of shallow, semiclear Maidu Lake. Most hikers will want to make the 0.9-mile trek down to this lake's relatively warm waters, for the next PCT campsite with near-water access is the sometimes overcrowded Tolo Camp, 6.2 miles farther. The lakeshore has abundant space for camping, though until early August a tent is necessary to provide refuge from the myriad mosquitoes. An easy way to stay clear of mosquitoes is

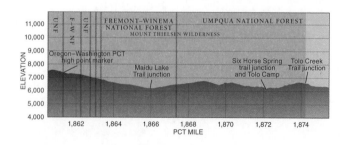

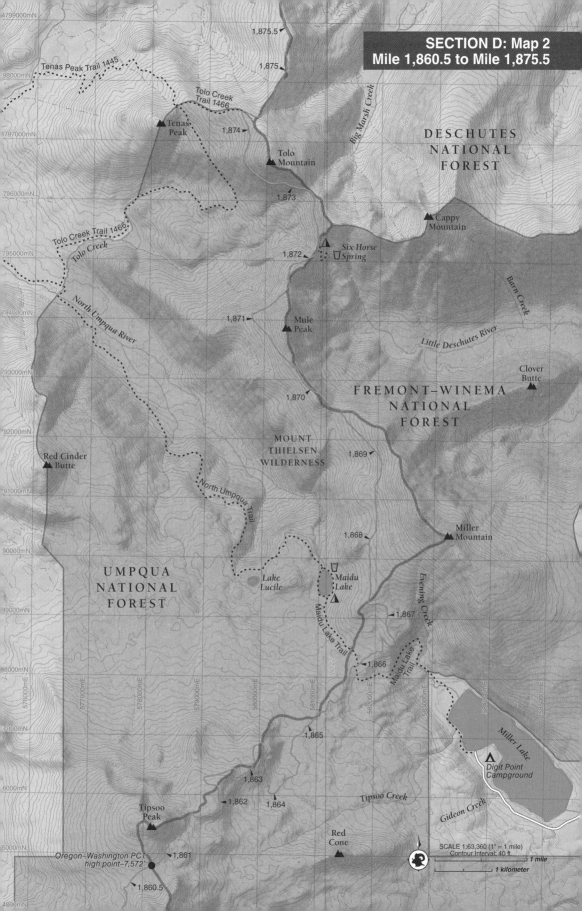

Tenas Peak Trail 1445

Tolo Creek
Trail 1466

1,875.5

1,875

1,874 ►

Big Marsh Creek

**DESCHUTES
NATIONAL
FOREST**

▲ Tenas
Peak

Tolo
Mountain

1,873 ►

▲ Cappy
Mountain

Tolo Creek Trail 1466

Tolo Creek

Six Horse
Spring

1,872 ►

Barn Creek

North Umpqua River

Mule
▲ Peak

1,871 ►

Little Deschutes River

1,870 ►

**FREMONT–WINEMA
NATIONAL
FOREST**

Clover
Butte ▲

Red Cinder
▲ Butte

**MOUNT
THIELSEN
WILDERNESS**

1,869 ►

North Umpqua Trail

1,868 ►

Miller
▲ Mountain

**UMPQUA
NATIONAL
FOREST**

Lake
Lucile

Maidu
Lake

Evening Creek

1,867 ►

Maidu Lake Trail

1,866 ►

Maidu Lake Trail

W1422

Miller Lake

1,865 ►

Digit Point
Campground

1,863 ►

1,862 ►   1,864

Tipsoo Creek

Tipsoo
▲ Peak

Red
Cone ▲

Gideon Creek

SCALE 1:63,360 (1" = 1 mile)
Contour Interval: 40 ft.

◄ 1,861

Oregon–Washington PCT
high point–7,572'

1 mile

1 kilometer

► 1,860.5

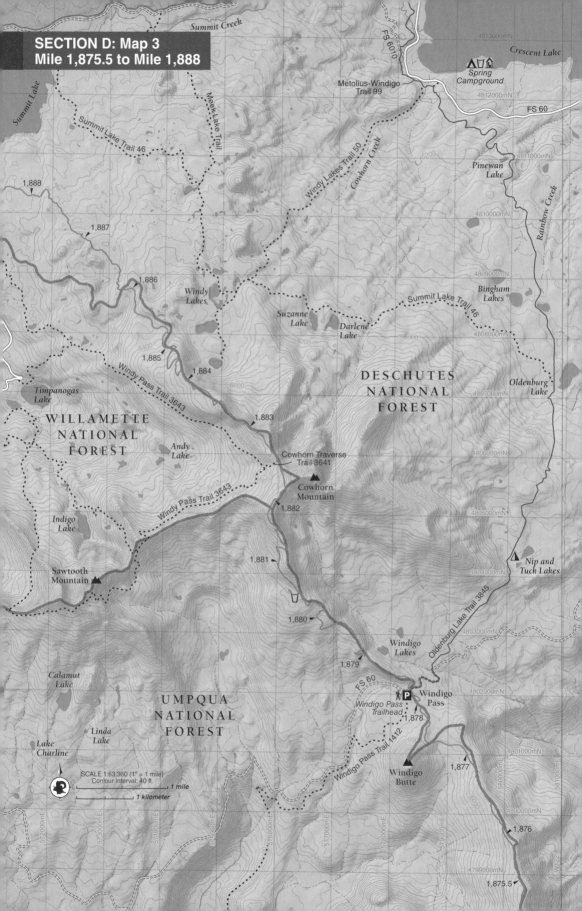

Summit Creek

FS 6010

Crescent Lake

Spring Campground

Metolius-Windigo Trail 99

FS 60

4813000mN

4812000mN

Summit Lake

Meek Lake Trail

Summit Lake Trail 46

Windy Lakes Trail 50

Cowhorn Creek

Pinewan Lake

4811000mN

Rainbow Creek

1,888

1,887

1,886

Windy Lakes

Suzanne Lake

Darlene Lake

Summit Lake Trail 46

4810000mN

Bingham Lakes

4809000mN

4808000mN

1,885

1,884

DESCHUTES NATIONAL FOREST

Oldenburg Lake

4807000mN

Timpanogas Lake

Windy Pass Trail 3643

1,883

WILLAMETTE NATIONAL FOREST

Andy Lake

Cowhorn Traverse Trail 3641

Cowhorn Mountain

1,882

4806000mN

4805000mN

Indigo Lake

Windy Pass Trail 3643

1,881

Oldenburg Lake Trail 3845

Nip and Tuck Lakes

4804000mN

Sawtooth Mountain

1,880

Windigo Lakes

4803000mN

Calamut Lake

UMPQUA NATIONAL FOREST

1,879

FS 60

P

Windigo Pass Trailhead

Windigo Pass

4802000mN

1,878

Linda Lake

Windigo Pass Trail 1412

1,877

4801000mN

Lake Charline

Windigo Butte

4800000mN

SCALE 1:63,360 (1" = 1 mile)
Contour Interval: 40 ft.

1 mile

1 kilometer

1,876

1,875.5

4799000mN

572000mE

573000mE

574000mE

575000mE

576000mE

577000mE

578000mE

579000mE

580000mE

581000mE

to set up your tent no closer to the shore than 200 feet (apparently mosquitoes can't breathe past this point so you'll be safe, some say).

The PCT leaves the Maidu Lake Trail, quickly crosses that trail's former tread, and then climbs to a spur-ridge view of Miller Lake. After enjoying several views of the lake, you cross the spur ridge and follow it north to a crossing of the main, county-line ridge (1,867.3–6,515'). Beyond it you climb gently to an auxiliary saddle; then, with an equal climb, you top out at a junction from which the abandoned OST once descended southwest to Maidu Lake. The PCT now contours 0.25 mile and then begins a gradually steepening descent to a crest saddle (1,869.6–6,525'). The trail now climbs to the long Mule Peak crest, crosses it, diagonals northwest down the peak's west slopes, and then diagonals northeast to a saddle.

WATER ACCESS

CAMPING Continuing this crest route, you descend to a second saddle, where lies Tolo Camp (1,872.1–6,218'), with camping space for about four hikers. From the camp, Trail 1411 switchbacks east 0.3 mile down to Six Horse Spring, which has no available camping space. From Tolo Camp, there will

be no reliable water until Summit Lake, 17 miles farther. However, you'll find near-trail water at several places north of Windigo Pass.

From the Tolo Camp saddle, travel over to another saddle, and then cross the south and west slopes of Tolo Mountain to the Mount Thielsen Wilderness boundary and Tolo Creek Trail 1466 (1,874.2–6,605'), which starts west down a ridge to connect with the Tenas Peak Trail 1445. Now outside Mount Thielsen Wilderness, the PCT turns east, descends to the ridgecrest, and then follows it more than 2.5 miles before swinging west across a broad, low saddle to the lower north slopes of a pyroclastic cone called Windigo Butte (6,420'). Now descend less than 0.25 mile along the butte's north spur, and then curve northwest over to a junction with a spur trail (1,877.9–5,845') that goes 300 yards west to the Windigo Pass Trailhead parking area.

North from the junction, the PCT quickly drops into a ravine, climbs over a low ridge, and reaches Forest Service Road 60 only 140 yards east of Windigo Pass (1,878.3–5,821'). The old road, which starts by the trail's west side, takes you 0.25 mile southwest to the Windigo Pass Trailhead parking area, used by north- and southbound hikers alike. From this junction with FS 60, you have the choice of staying on the PCT or taking an alternate route, which used to be the OST. The author recommends the alternate route with the caution that this trail is not officially maintained to be a PCT alternate route.

SECTION D

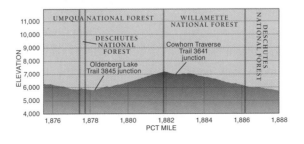

ALTERNATE ROUTE Some hikers still prefer to take the old OST route, which closely approaches Odell Lake and which has more lakes where you can camp. These lakes, of course, have mosquito issues, at least before August, so before then you can choose between mosquitoes on the alternate route and snow patches on the PCT.

If you decide to hike the alternate route, turn right and hike 0.7 mile northeast down FS 60 to a trailhead, just 15 yards past a seasonal but obvious creek. The trail's name has been changed to Oldenburg Lake Trail, which is part of Metolius-Windigo Trail 99, and on it you start northeast, contour 1.7 miles across gentle slopes of manzanita and sparse forest cover, and then descend slightly to the Nip and Tuck Lakes spur trail.

CAMPING This trail heads east-southeast for a level 200 yards to the two lakes, which are only one lake in early summer. The peninsula that juts between the two lobes makes an excellent campsite, and the warm, shallow lake water is very inviting.

The Oldenburg Lake Trail heads north-northeast and climbs gently at first but then makes a somewhat sunny, moderate-to-steep 1-mile climb to a ridge, providing you with only one reward—a view south of Mount Thielsen. The path ahead is now downhill almost all the way to Crescent Lake.

Now you start moderately down and head 1.3 miles north to the west shore of Oldenburg Lake and then north 1.1 miles past two of the Bingham Lakes to a junction with a west-northwest trail to the third. This third Bingham Lake, at the end of the 100-yard spur trail, is the largest and perhaps the clearest of all the shallow lakes between Maidu Lake and Crescent Lake. Continuing 2 miles north along the route, you pass through an area of sparse lodgepoles, and then descend gradually and cross a seasonal creek whose luxuriant green vegetation contrasts vividly with the surrounding sparsely needled lodgepoles. The trail rounds a low ridge and then reaches the northeast end of murky, man-made Pinewan Lake, which is often dry in late summer. Here and for a short distance west, the trail follows the Emigrant Road built and used by the Elliot Wagon Train in October 1853.

Go about 100 yards before the trail forks right (northwest) from the road and winds 0.25 mile down to a ravine. Ahead it wraps around a minor ridge and then descends 0.25 mile to a junction with an abandoned trail. The route then goes just 80 yards northwest to a ravine and turns northeast, dying out before reaching nearby FS 60.

CAMPING If you were to walk 0.25 mile west on that road, you'd reach FS 260, which descends 0.5 mile to Crescent Lake's Spring Campground.

From the junction, you head west on the Metolius-Windigo Trail 99. It rapidly reaches a ravine, curves around a minor ridge, and then weaves northwest down to a junction after 0.9 mile.

CAMPING Northeastward, a spur trail heads 150 yards over to FS 60 and then continues just beyond it to a trailhead parking area for the Oldenburg Lake and Windy Lakes Trails. Just 0.25 mile southeast up FS 60, you'd find Spring Campground's road, FS 260.

Westward, go about 220 yards before meeting southwest-climbing Windy Lakes Trail 50. Onward, the Metolius-Windigo Trail almost touches FS 60 as it travels from northwest to north over to Summit Lake Road 6010. Cross it, parallel it 100 yards north, walk 100 feet up the road, and find the trail starting from the road's east side. In 0.5 mile you wind down to the boggy environs of Whitefish Creek and then, 200 yards past it, reach FS 220 only 60 yards west of its junction with FS 60. Follow this road north through Whitefish Horse Camp, and in 0.3 mile reach a campground loop that has a vault toilet and piped water, which for late-season trekkers could be the last reliable water until Diamond View Lake, 5.5 miles away.

Branch left and locate the Whitefish Creek Trail 3842 trailhead along the northwest part of the loop. From the loop's north part, the Metolius-Windigo Trail heads northeast.

You head northwest on Whitefish Creek Trail 3842, enter Diamond Peak Wilderness in about 0.5 mile, and then climb rather gently 1.6 miles to a fairly reliable tributary of Whitefish Creek. The trail remains within earshot of Whitefish Creek—when it's running—as you climb 3.1 miles northwest and then north up to a flat and a linear pond at an intersection with Crater Butte Trail 3844, 4 miles due east of Diamond Peak (8,744').

CAMPING From the junction, your trail heads 0.7 mile north past several shallow, somewhat stagnant ponds before arriving at large but shallow Diamond View Lake. Photographs are best here when the peak is snow-clad, which, unfortunately, is when the lake is mosquito-clad. You pass campsites and then leave the lake behind as you make tracks north through swampy lodgepole flatlands to the headwaters of Trapper Creek.

This creek remains unseen and unheard for 2 miles until the trail reaches slopes above the creek, where the latter cascades north down toward a marsh. In the third mile, the trail reaches the creek, more or less follows it to the marsh, and then goes east through a shady mountain-hemlock forest. To avoid the creekside's wet ground, the trail generally stays on the lower slopes just south of the creek. Follow the creek as it meanders east and then cascades northeast down past a small, breached dam. Almost immediately after this concrete structure, you reach a trail junction where an access trail continues northeast but your trail turns north.

The access trail leads to Trapper Creek Campground and Shelter Cove Resort. It descends 240 yards past the Diamond Peak Wilderness boundary and railroad tracks and crosses the tracks 20 yards west-northwest of a huge, steel overhead signal. Head east across the railroad tracks and under the overhead signal to a dirt road that descends 150 yards to FS 5810 along the west shore of Odell Lake (4,788').

HISTORY This lake was named for William Holden Odell, who, with B. J. Pengra, surveyed the military wagon road up the Middle Fork of the Willamette in 1865. On July 26, Odell climbed a butte and set eyes on this lake; both butte and lake now bear his name.

CAMPING If you walk 0.25 mile northwest on FS 5810, you'll reach the entrance to Trapper Creek Campground. If you walk 250 yards southeast on FS 5810, you'll reach Shelter Cove Resort, which has a small store, coin-operated showers, and a relatively inexpensive campsite fee for PCT hikers. As was mentioned at the beginning of this chapter, the resort holds parcels mailed via UPS.

After backtracking to the Trail 42 junction (by the breached dam), you curve west 150 yards down to a bridge that crosses Trapper Creek only 35 yards below the dam. Leaving this creek behind, contour the slopes 0.5 mile and reach an intersection with Yoran Lake Trail 3849. This trail

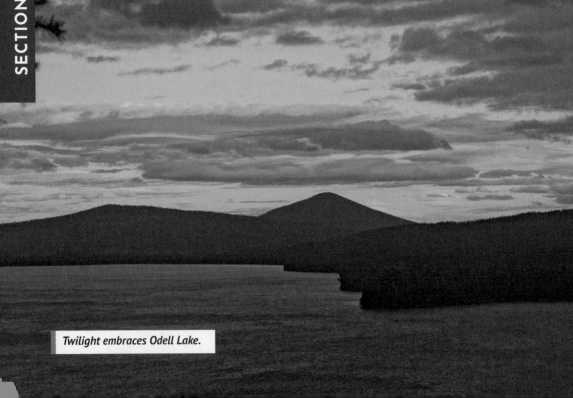

Twilight embraces Odell Lake.

goes northeast moderately to steeply 250 yards down to the railroad tracks, from which you follow a dirt road 70 yards to FS 5810. You can follow FS 5810 east to the campground and a bit farther east to the resort.

North of the intersection, Yoran Lake Trail parallels the railroad tracks below and passes seasonal creeklets before reaching, after 0.7 mile, a spur road that climbs northwest 0.4 mile to Pengra Pass. Start along this road from a point 70 yards west of the tracks, and follow it up 80 yards around a bend to a resumption of the trail, which branches right and ascends 130 yards northwest to a small creek under the shade of a Douglas-fir forest.

PLANTS Here you find shooting stars, bluebells, bunchberries, and Oregon grapes, which are typically associated with this type of forest.

The trail now climbs gently 0.5 mile northeast and reaches a junction with the PCT. Midway up this short ascent, you meet the upper end of a shorter, steeper trail (an alternate route) that starts where the railroad tracks enter a tunnel.

From Windigo Pass on FS 60, the PCT begins a northwesterly route to Willamette Pass that is 7.8 miles longer than the alternate route. It climbs 0.5 mile to a crest crossing from which, for reliable water, you could head due north 0.25 mile, staying east of the crest as you descend to the southwestern Windigo Lake, about 130 feet below you. Avoiding water, the PCT closely follows the crest about 1 mile and then climbs 400 vertical feet on a winding course to a minor crest saddle (1,880.5–6,588').

WATER ACCESS

From here you can traverse 200 yards northwest across relatively flat terrain to an unseen lakelet with acceptable water.

Beyond the unseen lakelet, the PCT climbs the crest over to a saddle (1,882.2–7,100') by the southwest ridge of pointed Cowhorn Mountain.

SIDE TRIP The short, rewarding climb to the top of this miniature Mount Thielsen is an obvious though steep one.

The trail now descends northwest along the crest, eventually switchbacking down to the edge of a forested bowl. About 0.5 mile beyond the forested bowl, you start a diagonal descent across a considerable escarpment and soon reach amorphous terrain on which you cross an imperceptible crest.

WATER ACCESS

A little over 3 miles of meandering brings you close to Summit Lake's south shore (1,889.2–5,577'), and a short traverse west brings you to FS 6010 (1,889.4–5,570'), at the lake's southwest corner.

Cross this road three times as you follow the PCT north along it to a crossing of Emigrant Pass Road/FS 380 and entry to the Diamond Peak Wilderness (1,890.7–5,604').

CAMPING From here you can head 200 yards over to Summit Lake Campground, above the lake's northwest corner. This lake is a good one for a layover day

SECTION D

because, like large Cascade Range lakes, it has clear water and relatively few mosquitoes.

WATER ACCESS

CAMPING From the intersection of FS 380 and FS 6010, the trail starts northeast, and you enter Diamond Peak Wilderness as the route winds northwest past a series of seven ponds and lakelets shown on the map and even more smaller, unmapped ones. After leaving the west shore of the last mapped one (1,891.8–5,670'), the trail winds north up a relatively dry stretch to a slope above the south shore of one of the few accessible lakes (1,892.5–5,888'), near which adequate camps can be found. The trail curves down to the lake's east shore and then, in 0.3 mile, crosses a spring from an unseen pond only 30 yards from the trail.

Continuing north, you wind up to a junction with the Crater Butte and Rockpile Trails (1,893.7–6,184'). Beyond it, you climb north and then northwest easily up to a switchback (1,895.0–6,600'), from which you get one of several forthcoming views of stunning, steep-sided Mount Thielsen. The trail

northeast climbs gently to moderately across the imperceptible Lane–Klamath County line and levels off in a glaciated bowl just east of Diamond Peak.

SIDE TRIP Hikers wishing to climb this peak can scramble west from here up Class 2 rubble slopes.

Leaving the bowl, you traverse east and catch a view in the south of Crater Lake's rim framed between Mount Thielsen (9,182') on the left and Mount Bailey (8,363') on the right. Closer, in the southeast, is large Crescent Lake. You round the curving, northeast ridge of Diamond Peak and soon exchange southern views for northern ones.

VIEWS In open areas in the mountain-hemlock forest, you may see— if weather permits—South Sister (10,358'), Middle Sister (10,047'), Mount Washington (7,794'), and very distant Mount Jefferson (10,497'). Closer by stand two imposing monoliths, Mount Yoran (7,100') and Peak 7,138; you'll traverse below the latter.

Before that northeast traverse, however, the winding course makes a broad arc to the north, passing some reliable creeklets and then tiny tarns before commencing a steady descent past Peak 7,138.

Leaving the ridge slopes behind, you descend to lake-and-pond-dotted slopes and arrive above the north shore of Lils Lake (1,901.8–6,020'), one of the most attractive lakes until the Rosary Lakes, north of OR 58.

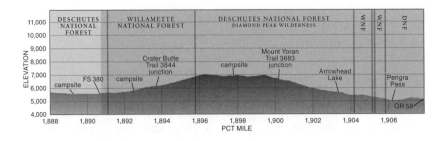

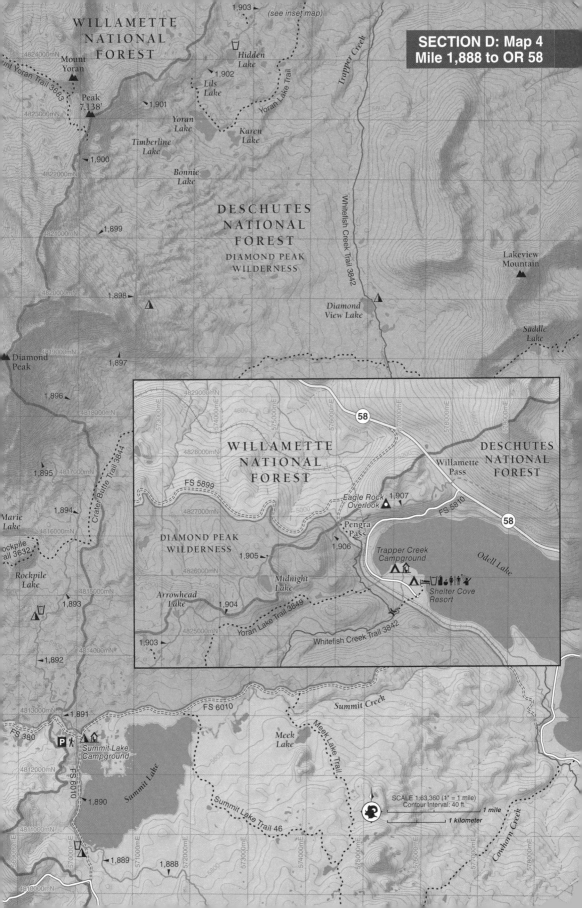

WILLAMETTE
NATIONAL
FOREST

Mount Yoran

Peak 7,138'

Mount Yoran Trail 3683

Yoran Lake

Timberline Lake

Bonnie Lake

1,903

(see inset map)

Hidden Lake

Lils Lake

Karen Lake

Yoran Lake Trail

Trapper Creek

DESCHUTES
NATIONAL
FOREST
DIAMOND PEAK
WILDERNESS

Whitefish Creek Trail 3842

Diamond View Lake

Lakeview Mountain

Saddle Lake

Diamond Peak

Crater Butte Trail 3844

Marie Lake

Rockpile Trail 3632

Rockpile Lake

Inset Map (Section D: Map 4)

WILLAMETTE
NATIONAL
FOREST

DIAMOND PEAK
WILDERNESS

FS 5899

Eagle Rock Overlook 1,907

Pengra Pass

1,906

1,905

Midnight Lake

Arrowhead Lake

1,904

Yoran Lake Trail 3849

Whitefish Creek Trail 3842

1,903

58

Willamette Pass

DESCHUTES
NATIONAL
FOREST

FS 5810

58

Odell Lake

Trapper Creek Campground

Shelter Cove Resort

FS 6010

Summit Creek

Meek Lake

Meek Lake Trail

1,891

FS 380

P

Summit Lake Campground

FS 6010

Summit Lake

Summit Lake Trail 46

1,890

1,889

1,888

SCALE 1:63,360 (1" = 1 mile)
Contour Interval: 40 ft.

1 mile

1 kilometer

Cowhorn Creek

WATER ACCESS

Not too far beyond Lils Lake, you see even larger Hidden Lake to the east through the trees, and the trail descends to within about 100 feet of its northwest corner (1,902.4–5,854').

Beyond this lake, you descend 1.25 miles past shallow, mosquito-infested ponds before angling southeast and descending to a broad flat of silver fir, mountain hemlock, and western white pine. A bend northward takes you up to a low saddle, from which you descend to within 70 yards of fairly well-hidden Midnight Lake (1,904.8–5,386'). You may wish to stop for water here or at a nearby pond 0.25 mile farther along the route. Beyond both bodies of water, you cross a saddle and then descend steadily to a closed road at Pengra Pass (1,906.2–5,021'), just 80 yards southeast of its junction with FS 5899.

RESUPPLY ACCESS

To get food or mailed packages at Shelter Cove Resort (mentioned in the alternate route on page 140), follow this road 0.5 mile southeast down to FS 5810, and then follow that road southeast 1 mile over to the resort. To return to the PCT, either backtrack or follow the last part of the alternate route, a maintained section of the defunct OST.

At Pengra Pass, you leave the wilderness and contour right (east) to the junction (1,906.6–5,066') at which the alternate route ends. Here you'll also find an old trail that descends steeply south 0.25 mile to FS 5810.

The PCT now climbs to a small bluff, where the Eagle Rock Overlook provides the only good view of Odell Lake along the route. The trail climbs a few yards beyond the viewpoint, contours over to a pond on the right, and then makes a short, switchbacking descent to OR 58 (1,907.9–5,088'), which you reach 0.25 mile southeast of Willamette Pass.

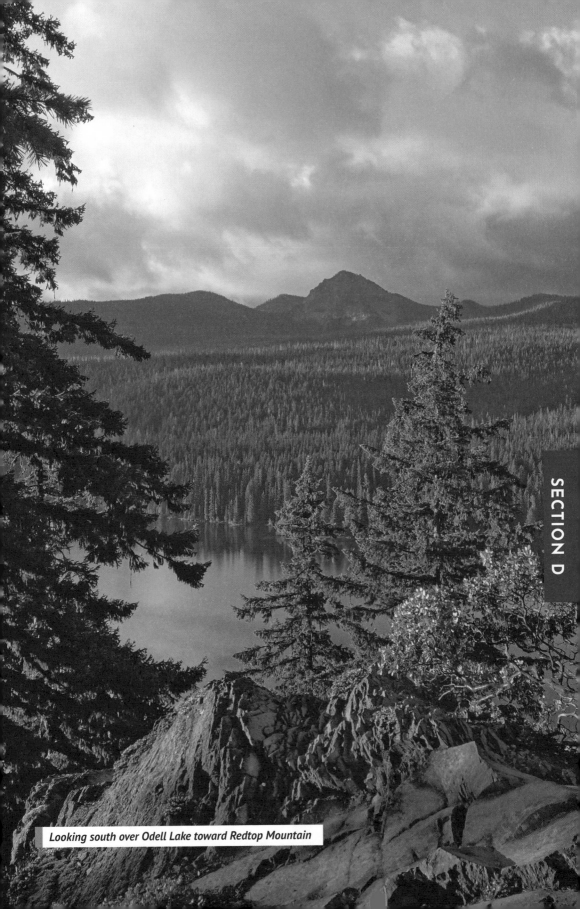

Looking south over Odell Lake toward Redtop Mountain

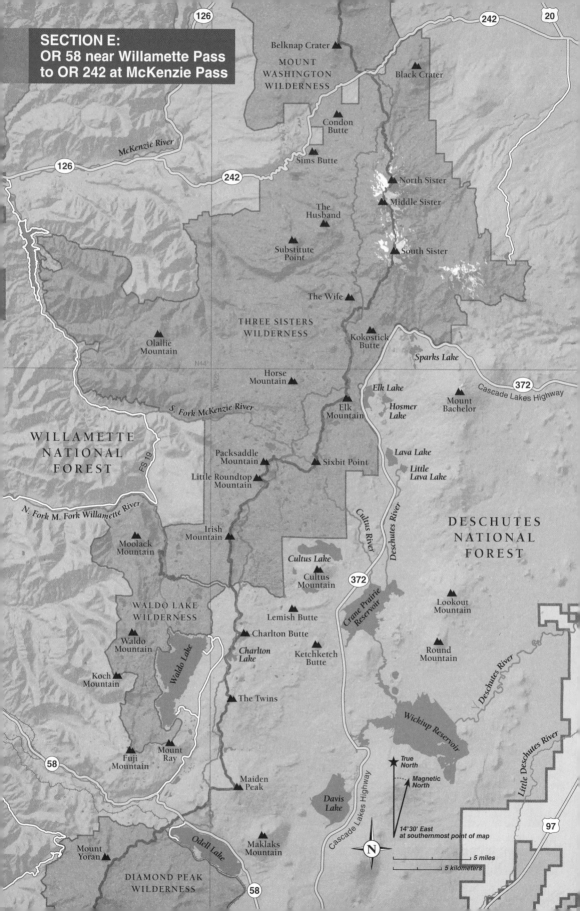

126

242

20

Belknap Crater

MOUNT
WASHINGTON
WILDERNESS

Black Crater

McKenzie River

126

242

Condon
Butte

Sims Butte

North Sister

Middle Sister

The
Husband

Substitute
Point

South Sister

The Wife

THREE SISTERS
WILDERNESS

Kokostick
Butte

Sparks Lake

Olallie
Mountain

N44

Horse
Mountain

Elk Lake

Hosmer
Lake

Mount
Bachelor

Cascade Lakes Highway

372

S. Fork McKenzie River

Elk
Mountain

Lava Lake

WILLAMETTE
NATIONAL
FOREST

Packsaddle
Mountain

Sixbit Point

Little
Lava Lake

Little Roundtop
Mountain

FS 19

N. Fork M. Fork Willamette River

Irish
Mountain

DESCHUTES
NATIONAL
FOREST

Moolack
Mountain

Cultus Lake

Cultus River

Deschutes River

Cultus
Mountain

372

WALDO LAKE
WILDERNESS

Lemish Butte

Crane Prairie Reservoir

Lookout
Mountain

Waldo
Mountain

Waldo Lake

Charlton Butte

Charlton
Lake

Ketchketch
Butte

Round
Mountain

Koch
Mountain

Deschutes River

The Twins

Little Deschutes River

Fuji
Mountain

Mount
Ray

Wickiup Reservoir

58

Maiden
Peak

True
North

Magnetic
North

Davis
Lake

Maklaks
Mountain

Cascade Lakes Highway

14°30' East
at southernmost point of map

97

Mount
Yoran

N

5 miles

DIAMOND PEAK
WILDERNESS

5 kilometers

58

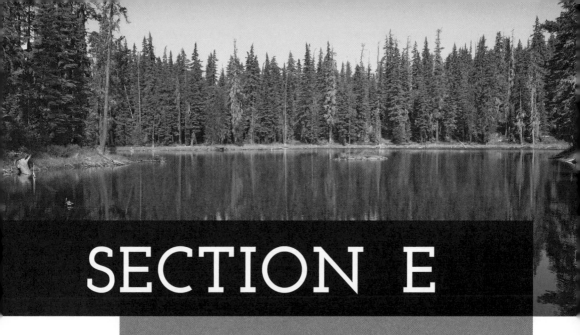

SECTION E

OR 58 near Willamette Pass to OR 242 at McKenzie Pass

IN SECTION E, the Pacific Crest Trail (PCT) traverses three types of terrain. The first third of this section's PCT traverses slopes mostly under canopy, with an old burn area providing some views. On the middle third, which starts at Irish Lake, the trail crosses flatter land that is peppered with enjoyable lakes (once the mosquito population dwindles). On the northern third, the trail skirts the Three Sisters, and views abound of glacier-draped peaks and spreading, sinister lava flows. Like Section C's Sky Lakes Wilderness, Three Sisters Wilderness, which dominates most of this section, is flooded with weekend hikers. And for good reason—it is very scenic and readily accessible.

DECLINATION 14°30'E

Above: Island Lake offers a cool respite at midday.

USGS MAPS

Elk Lake, OR	South Sister, OR
Irish Mountain, OR	The Twins, OR
Mount Washington, OR	Waldo Lake, OR
North Sister, OR	Willamette Pass, OR
Packsaddle Mountain, OR	

POINTS ON THE TRAIL, SOUTH TO NORTH

	Mile	Elevation in feet	Latitude/Longitude
OR 58 near Willamette Pass	1,907.9	5,088	N43° 35' 49.7619" W122° 02' 01.3060"
Lower Rosary Lake	1,910.7	5,720	N43° 35' 56.7876" W121° 59' 56.0383"
Moore Creek Trail junction to Bobby Lake	1,917.6	5,469	N43° 39' 45.1215" W121° 59' 16.2584"
Charlton Lake Trail junction	1,925.1	5,737	N43° 44' 39.3897" W121° 58' 44.9246"
FS 600 at Irish Lake	1,930.6	5,563	N43° 48' 29.8009" W121° 57' 48.9486"
Junction with Cliff Lake and Porky Lake Trails	1,944.2	5,152	N43° 56' 02.4921" W121° 53' 44.2747"
Island Meadow Trail junction to Elk Lake	1,952.6	5,250	N43° 58' 55.1544" W121° 49' 30.8224"
Red Hill Trail junction	1,958.6	6,002	N44° 02' 17.0822" W121° 49' 46.5139"
North Fork of Mesa Creek	1,962.9	5,700	N44° 04' 46.2346" W121° 49' 04.8171"
Glacier Way Trail junction	1,973.0	6,399	N44° 10' 44.4532" W121° 49' 05.2776"
Minnie Scott Spring	1,976.2	6,681	N44° 11' 46.0806" W121° 47' 33.5841"
South Matthieu Lake	1,979.7	6,023	N44° 13' 53.8113" W121° 46' 23.4469"
Junction with trail to Lava Camp Lake	1,982.6	5,287	N44° 15' 27.1200" W121° 47' 23.9670"
OR 242 at McKenzie Pass	1,983.8	5,309	N44° 15' 35.4103" W121° 48' 18.7279"

CAMPSITES AND BIVY SITES

Mile	Elevation in feet	Latitude/ Longitude	Number of tents	Feature	Notes
1,911.5	5,848	N43° 36' 29.5736" W122° 00' 01.4276"	>4	Middle Rosary Lake	
1,914.4	6,039	N43° 37' 55.3536" W122° 00' 12.6426"	15	Maiden Peak Shelter	100 yards northeast of PCT
1,920.8	6,402	N43° 42' 00.8954" W121° 59' 40.9156"	3	The Twins	
1,925.3	5,723	N43° 44' 38.3400" W121° 58' 40.6800"	>2	Charlton Lake	
1,930.6	5,560	N43° 48' 33.5664" W121° 57' 33.9840"	6	Irish Lake Campground	0.25 east of PCT; vault toilet, picnic table, fire pit
1,933.3	5,672	N43° 50' 17.1150" W121° 56' 51.4742"	>4	Brahma Lake	
1,934.3	5,857	N43° 50' 43.1981" W121° 57' 22.2314"	2	Jezebel Lake	
1,935.3	6,057	N43° 51' 15.3761" W121° 57' 53.3832"	2	Stormy Lake	Flat spot near trail on left; vista
1,942.3	5,115	N43° 55' 13.5792" W121° 54' 38.0934"	>4	Mac Lake	

CAMPSITES AND BIVY SITES *(continued)*

Mile	Elevation in feet	Latitude/ Longitude	Number of tents	Feature	Notes
1,943.4	5,048	N43° 55' 23.1275" W121° 53' 43.5257"	>4	Horseshoe Lake	
1,944.2	5,161	N43° 56' 00.9600" W121° 53' 38.7600"	>4	Cliff Lake	Shelter and sites above cliff on northwest shore of lake
1,947.2	5,527	N43° 57' 26.0821" W121° 52' 54.0430"	>4	Dumbbell Lake	
1,952.6 (alt.)	4,900	N43° 58' 47.0316" W121° 48' 34.1964"	19	Elk Lake Campground	Vault toilets, drinking water, picnic table, fire ring
1,958.8	6,003	N44° 02' 26.0142" W121° 49' 35.6891"	>4	Sisters Mirror Lake	
1,962.8	5,719	N44° 04' 40.8561" W121° 49' 01.8669"	4	Creek nearby	
1,974.9	6,512	N44° 11' 21.9823" W121° 48' 08.9414"	2	White Branch	Shaded bivy
1,979.3	6,063	N44° 13' 32.2496" W121° 46' 31.7375"	4		Flat spot near edge of Yapoah lava flow
1,982.6	5,282	N44° 15' 39.6360" W121° 47' 12.2640"	12	Lava Camp Lake Campground	0.6 mile off-trail; vault toilet, picnic table, fire pit, water

SUPPLIES

No on-route supplies are available, but at mile 1,952.6 you can make a 1.25-mile detour to Elk Lake Resort, which has a café and a small store that caters to anglers. The resort also holds PCT packages (Elk Lake Resort, 60000 Century Dr., Bend, OR 97701). Before mailing packages, contact the resort (541-489-7378) to verify that it still offers this free service.

While off your beaten path, the towns of Sisters and Bend are within easy reach at the end of this section, especially considering the friendly demeanor of Oregonians toward hikers. Both towns offer full services; however, if you need a nationally known outdoor recreation equipment dealer, Bend has one you'll recognize.

PERMITS

If you're section hiking, you will need to obtain a Central Cascades Wilderness Permit to enter the Three Sisters and Mount Washington Wilderness areas from the Friday before Memorial Day through the last Friday in September. For more information, visit fs.usda.gov/detail/willamette /passes-permits/recreation/?cid=fseprd688355.

SPECIAL CONCERNS

Long-distance PCT hikers seem to agree that the trail's worst concentrations of mosquitoes are found either in Sky Lakes Wilderness in Section C or in the lake-and-pond-dotted south half of Three Sisters Wilderness. Therefore, bring a tent and plenty of mosquito repellent if you are hiking through this section before August.

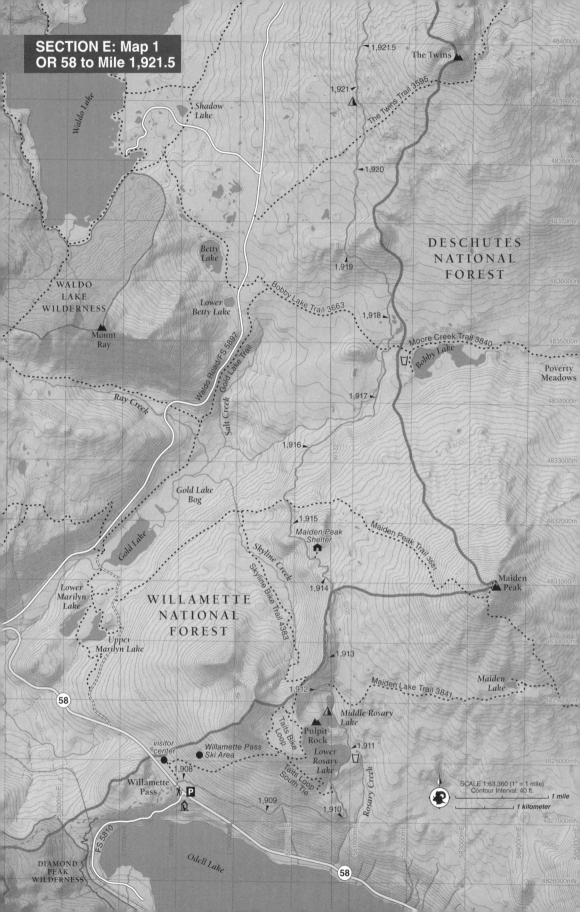

Waldo Lake

Shadow Lake

← 1,921.5

The Twins ▲

▲ 1,921

The Twins Trail 3595

← 1,920

Betty Lake

DESCHUTES NATIONAL FOREST

1,919 ▼

WALDO LAKE WILDERNESS

Lower Betty Lake

Bobby Lake Trail 3663

1,918 ◄

Moore Creek Trail 3840

▲ Mount Ray

Waldo Road FS 5897

Gold Lake Trail

Bobby Lake

Poverty Meadows

Ray Creek

Salt Creek

1,917 ◄

1,916 ◄

Gold Lake Bog

1,915 ◄

Maiden Peak Trail 3681

Gold Lake

Skyline Creek

Maiden Peak Shelter

Skyline Bike Trail 4383

1,914 ◄

▲ Maiden Peak

Lower Marilyn Lake

WILLAMETTE NATIONAL FOREST

1,913 ◄

Maiden Lake Trail 3841

Maiden Lake

Upper Marilyn Lake

1,912 ◄

Tails Bike Loop

Middle Rosary Lake

58

Pulpit Rock

1,911 ◄

visitor center

Willamette Pass Ski Area

Lower Rosary Lake

Tails Loop South Tie

Rosary Creek

1,908

Willamette Pass

P

1,909 ▼

1,910 ▼

SCALE 1:63,360 (1" = 1 mile)
Contour Interval: 40 ft.

——— 1 mile

——— 1 kilometer

FS 5810

58

DIAMOND PEAK WILDERNESS

Odell Lake

OR 58 NEAR WILLAMETTE PASS TO OR 242 AT MCKENZIE PASS

>>>THE ROUTE

Where southeast–northwest OR 58 reaches broad Willamette Pass, you'll find a visitor information center and ski area immediately north of it. About 0.4 mile southeast on OR 58, you'll reach Forest Service Road 5810, branching southwest, and just 100 yards before it is a short spur road branching northeast and then turning east, becoming a dirt road. At its end is trailhead parking, and from there an 80-yard spur trail goes north to the PCT, which crosses OR 58 about 0.1 mile northwest of the trailhead's road.

Starting from OR 58 (1,907.9–5,088'), follow the PCT past a northwest-heading trail leading to the ski area and continuing as it curves east behind the Highway Commission's long cinder-storage building. Then meet the trailhead-parking spur trail (1,908.1–5,132') immediately past it.

The PCT now climbs steadily east through a forest of Douglas-fir, western white pine, and mountain hemlock to a saddle and then curves north to pass a junction with the Taits Loop (1,910.5–5,669') and then a 100-foot-high rock jumble before reaching the ridge above Lower Rosary Lake (1,910.7–5,720').

WATER ACCESS

This clear lake is deep in early summer, and in this it contrasts strongly with the other lakes its size that you've seen so far along the entire route. By late summer, however, the lake level can fall more than 20 feet due to seepage through the porous volcanic rocks, leaving its eastward drainage channel high and dry.

CAMPING Now climb northwest to the southeast corner of deep, blue-green Middle Rosary Lake (1,911.4–5,830'), which is even more impressive than the south lake because it lies at the base of 400-foot-high Pulpit Rock. On a weekend, you're likely to see climbers scaling this rock. Walk alongside the lake, and then pass the low dividing ridge between the middle and north lakes, where you'll find excellent camping (1,911.5–5,848'). Try to choose a site that's neither too close to the trail nor the water, without expanding into new areas. Wherever you choose to set up camp, do it on a durable surface such as dirt.

You reach shallower North Rosary Lake, and then follow the trail as it climbs west above the lake's north shore before switchbacking east-northeast up to a junction with Maiden Lake Trail 3841 (1,912.1–5,994'), which descends east-southeast and then contours east toward that lake.

Continue east 130 yards and then switchback west up to a saddle at the Willamette National Forest boundary (1,912.6–6,173'), but not before getting one last glance back at Pulpit

SECTION E

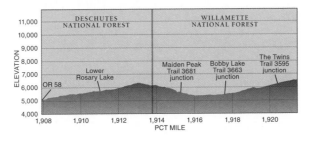

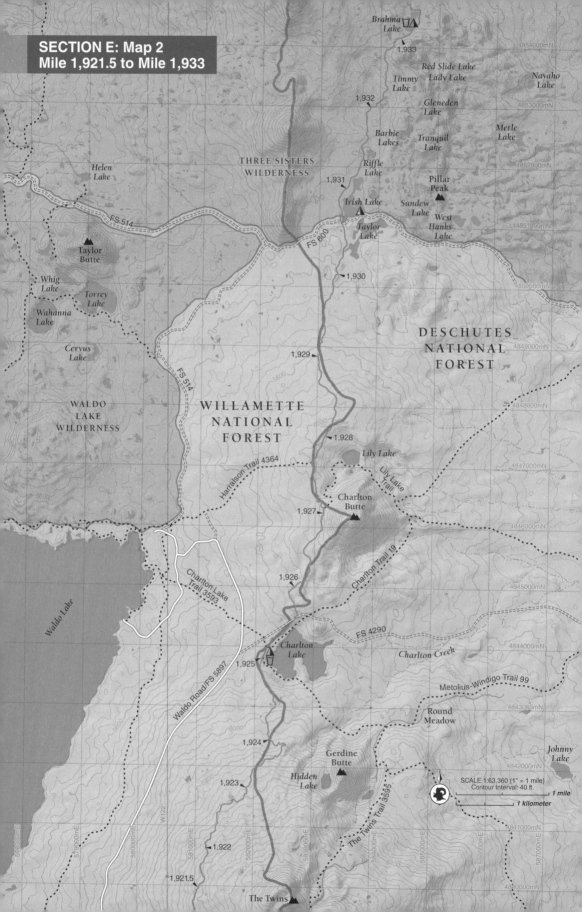

Brahma
Lake
1,933

Red Slide Lake
Timmy   Lady Lake   Navaho
Lake   Lake
1,932
Gleneden
Lake
Barbie   Tranquil   Merle
Lakes   Lake   Lake

Riffle
Helen   Lake   Pillar
Lake   Peak

THREE SISTERS
WILDERNESS   1,931
Irish Lake   Sundew
FS 514   Lake   West
Taylor   Hanks
FS 800   Lake   Lake

1,930

Taylor
Butte

Whig
Lake   DESCHUTES
Torrey   NATIONAL
Lake   1,929   FOREST
Wahanna
Lake

Cervus
Lake   FS 514
1,928

WALDO   Lily Lake
LAKE   WILLAMETTE
WILDERNESS   NATIONAL   Lily Lake
FOREST   Trail

1,927   Charlton
Butte

Harralson Trail 4364

Charlton Trail 19
1,926

Charlton Lake
Trail 3593   FS 4290

Charlton Creek
Waldo Lake   Charlton
1,925   Lake

Metolius-Windigo Trail 99
Waldo Road/FS 5897

Round
Meadow

1,924
Gerdine   Johnny
Butte   Lake
1,923
Hidden
Lake

SCALE 1:63,360 (1" = 1 mile)
Contour Interval: 40 ft.
1 mile
The Twins Trail 3595
1 kilometer
1,922

1,921.5

The Twins

Rock; Rosary Lakes; and, in the distance, Odell Lake, Odell Butte, and Crescent Lake.

After heading north along the east-facing slopes of a linear ridge, a stretch that offers Maiden Peak views, the newer stretch crosses the ridge at a minor saddle and then soon descends moderately to an intersection of Maiden Peak Loop Snow Trail (1,914.4–6,039').

CAMPING Northeast, this trail leads 100 yards to the Maiden Peak Shelter. There's no water here, but it sleeps 15 people and is a great spot to seek refuge from a storm.

The PCT continues northwest, first dropping moderately 0.75 mile, passing a junction with Maiden Peak Trail 3681 (1,915.3–5,634'), and then traversing northeast about a mile before curving north across wet meadows up to a junction with Bobby Lake Trail 3663 and Moore Creek Trail 3840 (1,917.6–5,469'). To the west, the Bobby Lake Trail travels about 2 miles to paved Waldo Road/FS 5897.

WATER ACCESS

It's best now to head east 0.25 mile on Moore Creek Trail to the west end of large, clear Bobby Lake (5,408'), for the next reliable source of water is Charlton Lake, about 7.5 miles farther.

On the PCT, head north past two large ponds, climb northwest to a saddle, curve northeast down from it, and then climb to an intersection with The Twins Trail 3595 (1,920.4–6,264').

About a mile north from this junction, you can walk 70 yards west across rock slabs for an unobstructed view west, from Diamond Peak north to Waldo Lake. With nearly 10 square miles of water surface and a depth of 420 feet (second deepest in Oregon to Crater Lake), Waldo Lake is the eighth-largest natural lake in Oregon and one of the purest lakes in the world. The absence of a permanent inlet to bring nutrients into the lake accounts for its lack of plant life, which contributes to its purity. You can see to depths of 120 feet on a calm day.

The PCT shortly begins a gentle descent, crossing one ravine after another. You pass above one small pond and soon reach a cluster of three ponds grouped around a small knob. The route descends northeast, reaches the watershed divide by a small pond, and then descends west a short distance before curving north toward gentler slopes above Charlton Lake (5,692').

WATER ACCESS

Head north through a forested flat area, reach the slopes above the lake, and descend to an intersection with Charlton Lake Trail 3593 (1,925.1–5,737'), about 100 yards north of a small pond. The lakeshore is 100 yards southeast; FS 5897 is 150 yards northwest, just beyond the pond. By heading northeast 0.1 mile, you reach a closed spur road heading southeast to the lake from FS 5897.

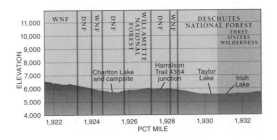

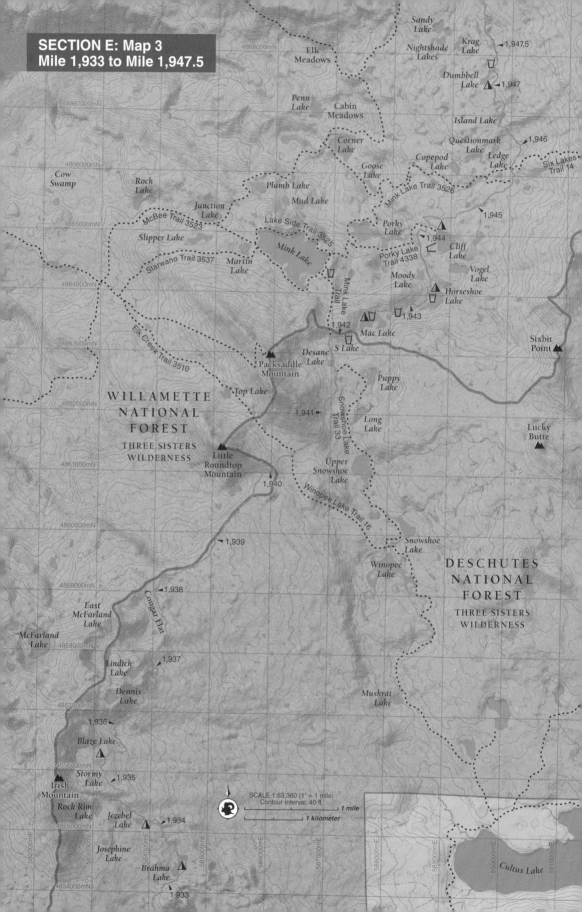

Sandy Lake

Nightshade Lakes

Krag Lake ← 1,947.5

Elk Meadows

Dumbbell Lake ◭ ← 1,947

Penn Lake

Cabin Meadows

Island Lake

Corner Lake

Questionmark Lake ← 1,946

Copepod Lake

Ledge Lake

Cow Swamp

Rock Lake

Goose Lake

Six Lakes Trail 14

Junction Lake

Plumb Lake

Mud Lake

Mink Lake Trail 3526

Porky Lake

McBee Trail 3523

Lake Side Trail 3525

← 1,945

Slipper Lake

◭ ← 1,944

Cliff Lake

Starwano Trail 3537

Martin Lake

Mink Lake

Porky Lake Trail 4338

Vogel Lake

Moody Lake

Horseshoe Lake

Elk Creek Trail 3510

Mink Lake Trail

Desane Lake

1,942

Mac Lake

1,943

S Lake

Sixbit Point ▲

Packsaddle Mountain

Puppy Lake

Top Lake

Snowshoe Lake Trail 33

WILLAMETTE
NATIONAL
FOREST

1,941

Long Lake

Lucky Butte ▲

THREE SISTERS
WILDERNESS

Little Roundtop Mountain

Upper Snowshoe Lake

1,940

Winopee Lake Trail 16

← 1,939

Snowshoe Lake

DESCHUTES
NATIONAL
FOREST

← 1,938

Winopee Lake

THREE SISTERS
WILDERNESS

East McFarland Lake

Cougar Flat

McFarland Lake

Lindick Lake 1,937

Dennis Lake

Muskrat Lake

1,936 ←

Blaze Lake ◭

Stormy Lake ← 1,935

Irish Mountain ▲

Rock Rim Lake

Jezebel Lake ◭ ← 1,934

SCALE 1:63,360 (1" = 1 mile)
Contour Interval: 40 ft.

1 mile

1 kilometer

Josephine Lake

Brahma Lake ◭

1,933

Cultus Lake

Then you diagonal north across the road to a broad trail that you follow north about 45 yards to where it bends northwest 40 yards to a roadside parking area. From this bend, the PCT heads east–northeast and climbs gently up the divide to a diagonal crossing of FS 5897 (1,925.6–5,799') at a 20° bearing.

After crossing FS 5897, the trail starts north into an area regenerating from a 1996 burn, climbs northwest to the low watershed divide, and then contours north past small ponds and Charlton Butte to a junction on the right (east) with Lily Lake Trail (1,927.0–6,006'), which descends about 0.75 mile to that isolated lake. Continuing north, you keep following the divide down a north slope to a small flat and then climb over two low mounds before reaching the southwest arm of shallow Taylor Lake (1,930.3–5,550').

CAMPING The trail immediately angles away from the lake, heads north past a pond on the left (west), and then reaches FS 600 at Irish Lake (1,930.6–5,563'). Popular Irish Lake Campground is 0.25 mile east on the road.

To pick up the trail again, go west 25 yards on the road and then north 50 yards along a spur road to the trailhead. You enter Three Sisters Wilderness (1,930.7–5,578') as the route heads north above the west shore of Irish Lake and then passes west of shallow but clear Riffle Lake (1,931.5–5,581'). *Note:* If you are section hiking, you must obtain a Central Cascades Wilderness Permit to enter the Three Sisters Wilderness (see page 151).

Now you climb a low ridge and descend slightly to a flat with two large lily-pad ponds before climbing to a higher ridge. The lakes and

ponds of this area are shallow and, like those in the Sky Lakes region, support an abundant mosquito population from late spring through mid-July.

WATER ACCESS

CAMPING Passing a number of stagnant ponds and small lakes in rapid succession, you descend to a nice campsite on the east shore of Brahma Lake (1,933.3–5,672'), which is distinguished by a forested island. Resist any temptation to increase the size of campsites. Once begun, this can become a site-destroying trend.

CAMPING The route continues north along the lakeshore, contours west, and then climbs moderately up slopes and through a miniature gorge before reaching the northeast corner of clear Jezebel Lake (1,934.3–5,857'). A campsite is perched on the low ridge south of this corner.

CAMPING Climbing northwest above the lake, you reach a shady glen from which a trail once climbed 0.3 mile west–southwest to Rock Rim Lake. Your trail rounds a linear ridge descending east, climbs west along its north slope, and then angles north past the outlet of Stormy Lake (1,935.3–6,057'). Sturdy causeways will keep your feet dry while traversing the boggy areas over this mile. The sight of the towering cliffs of Irish Mountain over this lake will leave you with a

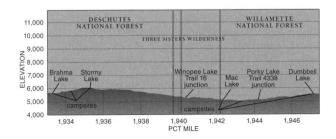

vivid memory of this choice spot. As always, Leave No Trace ethics advise setting up camp at least 200 feet from the shore. This helps preserve the lake's beauty as well as leaves a clear vista for other hikers.

Leaving this lake behind, you descend to smaller, slightly cloudy Blaze Lake (1,935.7–5,950') and then contour north past an abundance of ponds before the trail descends a ridge to a low divide just east of open Cougar Flat (1,937.8–5,750'). Your route winds down to Lake 5678 and then passes smaller water bodies as it follows the ridge northeast down to Tadpole Lake (1,939.9–5,340'), perched on a forested saddle. Traverse the lake's grassy north shore, and then descend north to a grassy pond and a junction with Elk Creek Trail 3510 and Winopee Lake Trail 16 (1,940.3–5,263').

SIDE TRIP Elk Creek Trail climbs left (northwest) over a low saddle and descends into the Elk Creek drainage; the Winopee Lake Trail curves right (southeast) around a knoll before descending to Winopee Lake.

Continue northeast across the lower slopes of Packsaddle Mountain (6,144'), walk north past an undesirable-looking lake to the east, and arrive at a junction with Snowshoe Lake Trail 33 (1,941.5–5,254'), which descends east.

WATER ACCESS

Now you hike north past Desane Lake and again enter Willamette National Forest as you cross a flat divide and descend into the Mink Lake Basin, where you meet a junction with Mink Lake Trail 3526 (1,941.9–5,160').

SIDE TRIP This 2.7-mile loop climbs northwest up a low, broad ridge before descending north to Mink Lake, stocked with eastern brook and rainbow trout. From there, the loop winds east, dropping to Porky Lake, with more eastern brook trout. You can then follow Porky Lake Trail 4338 east back to the PCT at the Cliff Lake outlet creek.

WATER ACCESS

The PCT follows a string of sparkling lakes that make an appropriate necklace for South Sister. In rapid succession you encounter S Lake (5,150'); Mac Lake (5,100'), with rainbow trout; Merrill Lake (5,080'); and Horseshoe Lake (5,039'), a shallow lake with both rainbow and eastern brook trout.

The trail curves around to the north shore of Horseshoe Lake and then reaches a spur trail (1,943.4–5,040') that bears 0.2 mile north to Moody Lake (5,020'). You cross the usually dry outlet of Horseshoe Lake and then continue north gently up and around a band of cliffs to a reunion with Porky Lake Trail 4338 (1,944.2–5,152') beside the Cliff Lake outlet creek.

CAMPING Just 130 yards southeast up a spur trail beside this creek is deep, green, rock-and-alder-lined Cliff Lake (5,161'). There are campsites atop the cliff along this popular lake's northwest shore, and should you be caught in foul weather, you can camp in comfort in the Cliff Lake shelter. Good eastern-brook-trout fishing, along with the opportunity for a lazy swim, justifies a stop at this lake.

PLANTS Backtracking from here, you pass bear grass blooming between boulders and, near the shelter, avoid stepping on delicate bunchberries and shooting stars that grow on the moist, shady forest floor.

Back at the loop-trail junction, you cross Cliff Lake's outlet creek, walk northwest, and then round a pile of large boulders and easily climb to a seasonal creek. Cross it, hike up a switchback, and then work up northeast to a junction with the other end of Mink Lake Trail 3526 and Six Lakes Trail 14 (1,945.7–5,354').

SIDE TRIP Mink Lake Trail heads west down toward a meadow and to Goose Lake, then turns south to reach Porky and Mink Lakes. Six Lakes Trail starts southeast to an unnamed lake, heads east to the divide, and then continues as Trail 14 east down to Cascade Lakes Highway.

On the PCT, head north, quickly descend to Reserve Meadow, and travel northeast along its edge before curving northwest away from its east end. You then climb to relatively deep Island Lake (1,946.5–5,443'), which has a patch of grass in its center.

WATER ACCESS

From this lake, you climb the trail to a rock pile, contour west past two stagnant ponds, and then hike north until you are just above a 50-yard-long peninsula that juts southwest into Dumbbell Lake (1,947.2–5,527'). From this rocky spur, you can fish or swim in the lake's warm, clear waters.

The trail now gradually climbs north past many ponds to a low divide and then descends to a junction (1,949.3–5,496') with the Red Hill Trail 3515, which heads 6.3 miles to Camelot Lake via popular Horse Lake.

From this junction 1.5 miles south of Horse Lake, the PCT branches right (east) and descends toward Island Meadow but stays within the forest's edge as you hike southeast along its southern border. You soon reach a bridge across a small creek. The trail strikes southeast again but shortly turns and follows a wandering route northeast before descending north to a mile-high meadow across which you traverse north-northeast to a junction with Sunset Lake Trail 3515.1 (1,951.3–5,284'), which passes that lake midway in its descent to the Red Hill Trail. Now go east-southeast on the PCT, enter forest, pass a large seasonal pond 50 yards south, and then snake east over an undetected drainage divide before descending to a junction with Island Meadow Trail 3 (1,952.6–5,250').

RESUPPLY ACCESS

The Island Meadow Trail makes a southeast descent 0.9 mile to a trailhead parking area, from which a road descends 270 yards to Cascade Lakes Highway. On this you can head south 70 yards to the Elk Lake Resort entrance. Down at the lakeside resort, you can obtain meals and limited supplies.

WILDLIFE If you visit the resort by early July, you'll likely see barn swallows nesting in the rafters above its entrance.

Rather than backtrack up the Island Meadows Trail, you can head north on the road 0.2 mile past its trailhead and start up Horse Lake

SECTION E

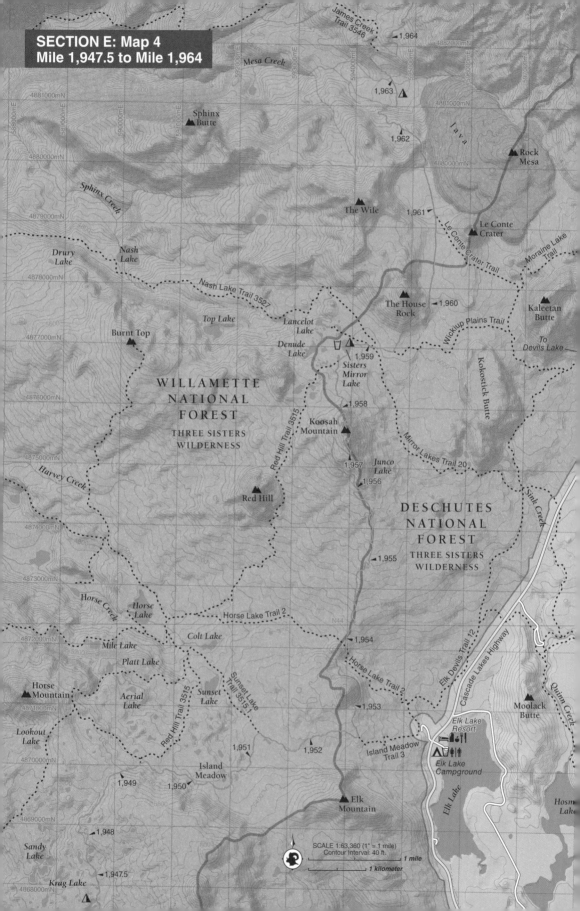

SECTION E: Map 4
Mile 1,947.5 to Mile 1,964

James Creek Trail 3546

1,964

Mesa Creek

1,963

1,962

Lava

Sphinx Butte

Rock Mesa

Sphinx Creek

The Wife

1,961

Le Conte Crater

Le Conte Crater Trail

Moraine Lake Trail

Drury Lake

Nash Lake

Nash Lake Trail 3527

The House Rock

1,960

Wickiup Plains Trail

Kaleetan Butte

Top Lake

Lancelot Lake

To Devils Lake

Burnt Top

Denude Lake

1,959

Sisters Mirror Lake

Kokostick Butte

WILLAMETTE NATIONAL FOREST

1,958

THREE SISTERS WILDERNESS

Red Hill Trail 3515

Koosah Mountain

Mirror Lakes Trail 20

Harvey Creek

1,957

Junco Lake

1,956

Red Hill

DESCHUTES NATIONAL FOREST

Sink Creek

THREE SISTERS WILDERNESS

1,955

Horse Creek

Horse Lake

Horse Lake Trail 2

1,954

Elk Devils Trail 12

Cascade Lakes Highway

Mile Lake

Colt Lake

Quinn Creek

Platt Lake

Horse Lake Trail 2

1,953

Moolack Butte

Horse Mountain

Aerial Lake

Sunset Lake

Red Hill Trail 3515

Sunset Lake Trail 3515.1

Elk Lake Resort

Lookout Lake

1,951

1,952

Island Meadow Trail 3

Elk Lake Campground

Island Meadow

Elk Lake

1,949

1,950

Hosm Lake

1,948

Elk Mountain

Sandy Lake

SCALE 1:63,360 (1" = 1 mile)
Contour Interval: 40 ft.

1 mile

1,947.5

1 kilometer

Krag Lake

Trail 2, which takes you 1.5 miles northwest up to the PCT.

CAMPING Large, 57-foot-deep Elk Lake (4,884') offers great trout fishing and is a nice place for a layover day at Elk Lake Campground, just south of the resort. Although the lake has no outlet and no permanent inlets, its water stays quite clear because fresh groundwater continues to seep into the lake at about the same rate that groundwater leaves it.

From the junction with the Island Meadow Trail, the PCT climbs north toward a cinder cone (5,676'), rounds its eastern half, and then heads north to a lesser summit before reaching an intersection on a saddle with Horse Lake Trail (1,953.9–5,300'). This trail descends southeast to the same trailhead parking area but takes 1.5 miles to reach it.

Following the divide, the PCT climbs gently north at first but steepens as it curves over to the western slope of Koosah Mountain (6,520'). Here the PCT makes a long switchback up to the ridge and then contours to its east slope, where, by stepping a few yards east, you can absorb an eastern panorama from Elk and Hosmer Lakes north past conical Bachelor Butte (9,065') and Broken Top (9,175') to South Sister (10,358'). Although you can't see Cascade Lakes Highway below, you can hear the rumble of logging trucks on it.

Hiking northwest, you encounter switchbacks down the north slope and then reach a flat and continue north to a junction at the south shore of placid, shallow Camelot Lake. Here, the Red Hill Trail heads southwest (1,958.6–6,002').

WATER ACCESS

After a brief hike northeast on the PCT, you reach the south edge of Sisters Mirror Lake (1,958.8–6,003'), from which you'll see South Sister mirrored in the lake when the water is calm.

CAMPING From here you can head along the west shore to some good camps on a rocky bluff along the lake's northwest shore. Some camps in this general vicinity may be closed, due to previous camper impact, and the U.S. Forest Service urges visitors to camp at lakes west of Camelot and Sisters Mirror Lakes. Fires are strictly prohibited here.

The PCT heads north along Sisters Mirror Lake's east shore, and along this short stretch you can climb to a low bench that offers small campsites. Next the trail turns east from the lake, and in about 300 yards it reaches a junction with the use trail heading west across a meadow toward the lake's rocky bluff. Near the east end of the meadow, about 130 yards past the junction, you'll come to a junction

SECTION E

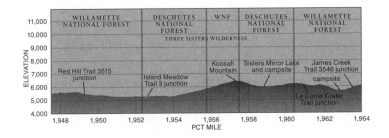

(1,959.0–5,989') with two official trails, Nash Lake Trail 3527 and Mirror Lakes Trail 20.

SIDE TRIP Nash Lake Trail 3527 starts north before turning northwest, while Mirror Lakes Trail 20 makes a long, mostly gentle descent south-southeast, reaching Cascade Lakes Highway in about 3.5 miles.

Now the route climbs slightly as it traverses east to an important junction with Wickiup Plains Trail (1,959.3–6,017').

SIDE TRIP From here, the well-graded Wickiup Plains Trail first rambles about 1.25 miles east across a fairly youthful lava flow to a junction with the southwest end of the Moraine Lake Trail. Then the Wickiup Plains Trail heads 0.5 mile east along the south edge of the Wickiup Plain to another junction. From it, a narrow trail goes 0.5 mile north to an intersection of the Moraine Lake Trail and then continues 1.3 miles northwest over to the PCT. The Wickiup Plains Trail leaves its namesake for a well-graded 2.2-mile descent to the Devils Lake area, with camping, picnicking, and fishing (this spring-fed lake is too cold for comfortable swimming). A large trailhead parking area lies just south of Tyee Creek, between the highway and the lake, and is quite heavily used by Bend's residents and visitors. Bend, the largest Oregon city east of the Cascades, lies about a half-hour's drive away.

From the west end of the Wickiup Plains Trail, the PCT heads north along a minor ridge to the south base of The House Rock and then traverses its wooded lower slopes up to an arm of the Wickiup Plain. The trail climbs north gently up this partly forested plain and after

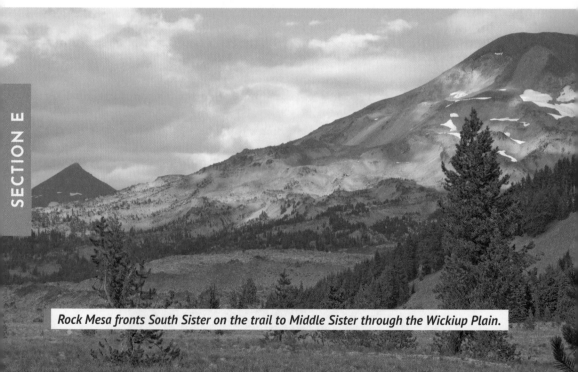

Rock Mesa fronts South Sister on the trail to Middle Sister through the Wickiup Plain.

SECTION E

0.5 mile crosses the broad county-line divide (1,960.5–6,218').

Now you begin to approach Le Conte Crater, a low cinder cone to the northeast. Due west from the crater's north base, you meet the Le Conte Crater Trail (1,960.9–6,160'), which goes 1.8 miles southeast to the Wickiup Plains Trail; starting near Devils Lake, that trail provides the fastest way in to the South Sister vicinity. Just north of Le Conte Crater, you see a vast, desolate, steep-sided jumble appropriately called Rock Mesa.

By now you've probably noticed The Wife (7,054'), a conspicuous summit off to the west, and you've probably observed that South Sister (10,358') is a redhead.

SIDE TRIP Should you wish to climb to the summit of South Sister, strike east from a point just south of Le Conte Crater, and then head northeast along the east margin of Rock Mesa. When you reach the peak's lower slope, climb north directly up it, and pass between Clark and Lewis Glaciers as you near the summit cone. When you top its rim, you'll find it crowned with a snow-clad lake (10,200'), which occupies a crater that may have been active in the last few thousand years.

WILDLIFE Back on the PCT, continue to the north end of Wickiup Plain. Newberry knotweed and scattered grass attest to the dryness of the pumice soil, but plentiful gopher mounds indicate that at least one mammal thrives here. At the north edge of the plain, the trail curves northwest over a low saddle and then descends to a creek that passes through a large meadow.

PLANTS In early July this meadow is a continuous field of yellow cinquefoil that contrasts sharply with the wintry chill of deep snow patches on the surrounding forested slopes.

You leave this island of sunshine behind and press onward northwest into the forest and down alongside a small ravine. The trail makes a switchback east and leads down to the south fork of Mesa Creek.

CAMPING Step across it, hike north into a large, grassy meadow, and then reach the north fork of Mesa Creek (1,962.9–5,700'). You'll find campsites both east and west of the meadow. Do not place your tent or bivy within 200 feet of the creek or in any meadow. It will destroy the vegetation in as few as three visits.

Past the north fork, you reach a tributary in 100 yards—a scenic lunch spot. Leaving the meadow and its sparkling creeks behind, you climb northwest to a junction with James Creek Trail 3546 (1,963.5–5,922'), which makes a gentle ascent west before curving north along the old Oregon Skyline Trail (OST) route.

On the PCT, you ascend east, curve north, and then round a murky lakelet just to the east. Continuing to climb north, the route tends to follow the break in the slope between the foot of South Sister to the east and the Separation Creek headwaters to the west. Along the course, you pass through numerous small meadows and beside a fine, 6-foot-diameter mountain hemlock before you descend slightly to cross Hinton Creek (1,965.7–6,282'). After hiking to the other side of the low divide, you descend past a cliff of a high-density, parallel-fractured, shalelike flow. Here you cross Separation Creek (1,966.2–6,400'), whose flow, like that of Hinton Creek, has usually sunk beneath the pumice by mid-August.

Now you come face-to-face with Middle Sister (10,047'), which you can easily climb its south or west slope. Continuing north, you follow posts and rock piles across a pumice flat and reach shallow, clear Reese Lake (1,966.5–6,460') where water can be gathered. The fragile timberline ecosystem here is very sensitive

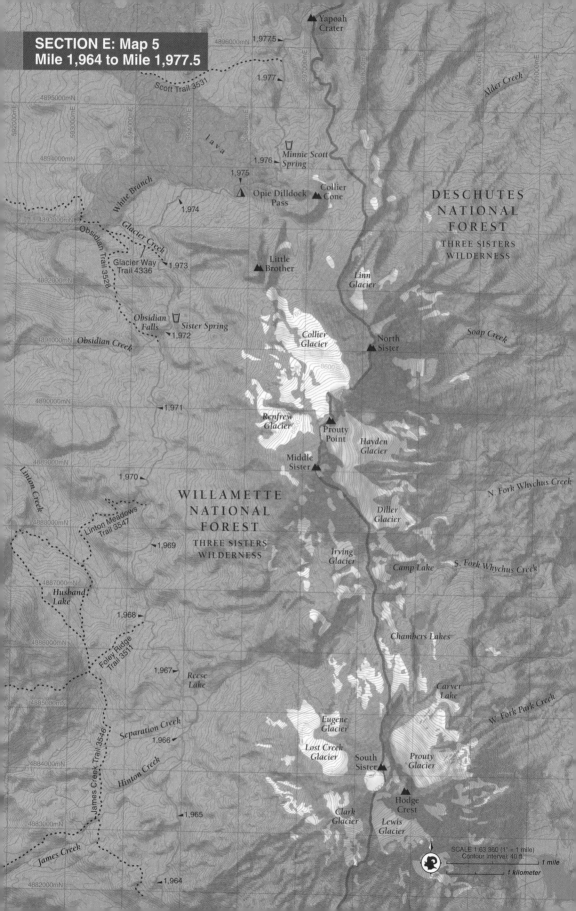

▲ Yapoah
Crater

4896000mN

1,977.5

Scott Trail 3531

1,977

Alder Creek

Iava

Minnie Scott
Spring

1,976

1,975

Opie Dilldock
Pass

△

▲ Collier
Cone

DESCHUTES
NATIONAL
FOREST

THREE SISTERS
WILDERNESS

White Branch

1,974

Glacier Creek

Obsidian Trail 3528

Glacier Way
Trail 4336

1,973

Little
Brother

▲

Linn
Glacier

Obsidian
Falls

Sister Spring

1,972

Collier
Glacier

North
Sister ▲

Soap Creek

Obsidian Creek

8600

Renfrew
Glacier

1,971

Prouty
Point ▲

Hayden
Glacier

Middle
Sister ▲▲

Diller
Glacier

N. Fork Whychus Creek

Linton Creek

1,970

WILLAMETTE
NATIONAL
FOREST

THREE SISTERS
WILDERNESS

Irving
Glacier

Camp Lake

S. Fork Whychus Creek

Linton Meadows
Trail 3547

1,969

Husband
Lake

4887000mN

Chambers Lakes

1,968

Foley Ridge
Trail 3511

Carver
Lake

1,967

Reese
Lake

W. Fork Park Creek

James Creek Trail 3546

Separation Creek

1,966

Eugene
Glacier

Lost Creek
Glacier

South
Sister ▲

Prouty
Glacier

Hinton Creek

Clark
Glacier

Hodge
Crest

1,965

Lewis
Glacier

James Creek

1,964

SCALE 1:63,360 (1" = 1 mile)
Contour Interval: 40 ft.

1 mile

1 kilometer

to human impact, so treat it gently. Consider gathering water, but camp elsewhere.

The route north now crosses half a dozen seasonal, step-across creeks as it descends toward Linton Creek and finally bends west down to a meadow; at its north end you meet Foley Ridge Trail 3511 (1,967.9–6,294'), which leads south-southwest down a slope.

GEOLOGY The Husband (7,524'), off to the west, is the resistant plug of an ancient volcano that once reigned over this area before the Three Sisters matured.

Just after you start north again, you reach a tributary of Linton Creek and then 70 yards farther reach a second tributary. From these seasonal creeks, the trail climbs gradually north through a hemlock forest to where it meets the Linton Meadows Trail 3547 (1,969.5–6,461') descending steeply southwest. The PCT ascends moderately northeast and then angles north to a gentle slope from which you can look south and identify, from east to west, the Mount Thielsen pinnacle (9,182'), the Mount McLoughlin pyramid (9,495'), and the Diamond Peak massif (8,744').

PLANTS Now follow an open, undulating pathway 2 miles north over loose slopes with trailside rose paintbrushes, yellow cinquefoils, pink heathers, and white pasqueflowers.

Just before traversing Middle Sister's forested west flanks, you will enter the Obsidian Area (1,971.5–6,536'). Note that this is a no-camping zone for thru-hikers. Cross a rocky meadow and descend to a junction with Obsidian Trail 3528 (1,971.8–6,469') just above Obsidian Creek.

SIDE TRIP Obsidian Trail 3528 takes you 5.2 miles down to OR 242.

Start hiking east moderately up to a slope, and then go northeast up to trickling, 50-foot-high Obsidian Falls, from which you top a small shelf and cross spring-fed Obsidian Creek.

WATER ACCESS

Next you'll reach Sister Spring (1,972.1–6,634'), which is usually flowing.

Now tread north on a trail that sounds and feels like glass. It is. The black obsidian is nature's own glass. This area has great cultural significance to American Indians, who traveled here from all over the Pacific Northwest to harvest obsidian for arrows and tools. Please don't take any souvenirs from this archaeologically sensitive area. The trail soon leaves the shelf, descends a ridge, and then turns east and intersects Glacier Way Trail 4336 (1,973.0–6,399').

GEOLOGY **SIDE TRIP** This path descends moderately 0.7 mile to the Obsidian Trail, which can be followed 3.4 miles to McKenzie Highway. An efficient mountaineering party can follow this route up from the highway, climb Middle and North Sisters via the Collier Glacier col, and return to

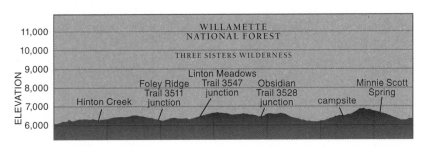

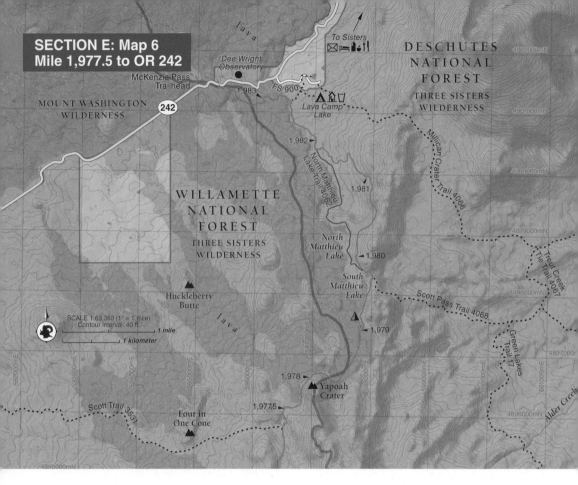

the trailhead late the same day. From the col, Middle Sister (10,047') can be climbed via its north ridge without any special equipment. Likewise, North Sister (10,085') can be climbed via its southwest ridge to the south arête, but the climb north along this sharp crest requires a safety rope. The view from Middle Sister is particularly instructional, for from it you can compare the degree of glaciation on all Three Sisters. North Sister, the oldest of the three, has suffered repeated periods of glaciation. South Sister (10,358'), the youngest, retains its symmetry, for it hasn't existed long enough to be eroded and reshaped as the other peaks have.

One hundred yards east of the Glacier Way intersection, you bridge Glacier Creek and then reach a pleasant, hemlock-shaded site where the Sunshine Shelter once stood. Climb briefly north over the western spur of Little Brother (7,810'), exiting the Obsidian Area here, and then descend slightly to the steep south slope above White Branch (1,974.9–6,512').

CAMPING After climbing along this creek, which can go dry in August, you eventually cross it; here, you can camp above its north bank on a flat called

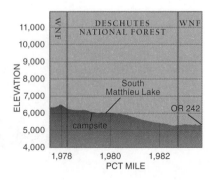

Sawyer Bar. Remember to set up your bivy site at least 200 feet away from the creek.

The trail bears north 200 yards partway across a basalt flow and then angles east up a ridge of solidified lava to the breached Collier Cone—the obvious source of this flow. Here, at Opie Dilldock Pass (1,975.5–6,900'), mountaineers' paths take off south up to Collier Glacier.

WATER ACCESS

You turn north and travel across several lava ridges before descending north to Minnie Scott Spring (1,976.2–6,681'), which is likely to be snowbound through mid-July.

The trail now makes a curving, counterclockwise descent almost to Minnie Scott Spring's creek, crosses a ridge, descends north to a large, grassy meadow, and shortly meets Scott Trail 3531 (1,977.2–6,277').

GEOLOGY SIDE TRIP Descending west to OR 242 in about 5 miles, the Scott Trail follows the narrow strip of land between the Four in One Cone (6,258') basalt flow on its north side and the Collier Cone (7,534') basalt flow on its south side. The age of these flows and of the Yapoah Crater (6,737') basalt flow immediately north of you is about 2,600 years.

The PCT now follows the Scott Trail north as it curves northeast and switchbacks up a northwest spur of the Ahalapam Cinder Field. The trail then curves around the slopes of Yapoah Crater and enters Deschutes National Forest. Yapoah Crater's lava flow—at least 400 years old—extends north to OR 242 and beyond. Looking north, you can see a row of

peaks: Mount Washington (7,794'), Three Fingered Jack (7,841'), and the snowy Mounts Jefferson (10,497') and Hood (11,235').

Now the PCT winds along and around ridges of the Yapoah lava flow, and you're thankful that the rocky trail exists, even when it is covered with snow patches. A cross-country hike across this material would be very exhausting! Reaching the edge of the flow, you parallel it north on a blocky cinder trail to a junction from which Scott Pass Trail 4068 descends east-southeast toward Trout Creek. Just 70 yards north down from this junction is Scott Pass and adjacent, diminutive South Matthieu Lake (1,979.7–6,023'). The area around South and North Matthieu Lakes is a no-camping zone for thru-hikers.

VIEWS   At this pass you get one of your best views east of central Oregon, which is drier than the west countryside because of the rainshadow cast by the Cascade Range.

Just above South Matthieu Lake's northwest corner, you come to a junction with the old OST route leading to North Matthieu Lake (1,979.8–6,050'); you can stay on the official PCT or take an alternate route with water on the former OST.

ALTERNATE ROUTE The old OST, now called North Matthieu Lake Trail 4062, descends to North Matthieu Lake. This alternate segment first winds 0.3 mile down to the southeast corner of appealing North Matthieu Lake, then in 0.25 mile leaves it at its northwest corner. From the lake, switchbacks guide you down steep slopes, and then you parallel the east edge of Yapoah Crater lava flow, passing a small pond on the east and then one on the west before rejoining the PCT.

From the junction near South Matthieu Lake, the PCT first crosses slopes of a fairly young cinder cone, which on a clear day offers you a far-ranging view of northern Oregon's higher Cascade Peaks: Mount Washington, Three Fingered Jack, Mount Jefferson, and Mount Hood. Then comes a fairly long, viewless, though mostly well-graded descent to another junction with North Matthieu Lake Trail 4062 (1,981.9–5,455'), where the alternate route rejoins the PCT.

Now, you have a gentle descent northwest along the east edge of the Yapoah Crater lava flow and soon come to a junction (1,982.6–5,287') with an important lateral trail.

WATER ACCESS

CAMPING This trail snakes 0.25 mile northeast to a large trailhead parking area that lies along the south side of FS 900, an OR 242 spur road that goes over to Lava Camp Lake. Because your next potential source of water is 12.5 miles away at Big Lake, you should consider camping at the lake's campground. You'll find the lake just northeast of the parking area, the two separated by a minor ridge. If the weather looks bad, look for a shelter above the southeast corner of the lake. The shallow lake's water is not pristine, so if you'd rather not treat it, you might get safe water from car campers.

From the lateral-trail junction, the PCT makes a zigzag course west over the blocky lava field and leaves Three Sisters Wilderness as you cross narrow OR 242 (1,983.8–5,309') 500 yards west of the Dee Wright Observatory, a lookout tower well worth visiting for its views. Just 0.2 mile west down this highway is a parking area with a trailhead for those starting their hike north from McKenzie Pass.

HISTORY This pass was named for the river that was explored in 1811 by Donald McKenzie, a member of John Jacob Astor's Pacific Fur Company. It was opened to travel in 1862 when Felix Scott and his party of 250 men chopped their way through the forest, building the road for their 106 ox-hauled wagons as they traveled. They crossed the divide via what is known as the Old Scott Trail, 2 or 3 miles south of the present road.

Having crossed the highway, you enter Mount Washington Wilderness, for which you need a Central Cascades Wilderness Permit to enter if you're section hiking. Due to the jumbled nature of the lava flow, the trail must take a twisted route over to the small trailhead parking area (1,984.1–5,210').

RESUPPLY ACCESS

Sisters, an upscale tourist town with restaurants, lodging, a small grocery store, and a post office, is 15 miles east on OR 242.

Just 23 miles southeast from Sisters on US 20 is the larger town of Bend, which offers lodging, restaurants, entertainment, hiking outfitters, grocery stores, and herbal-supply specialists.

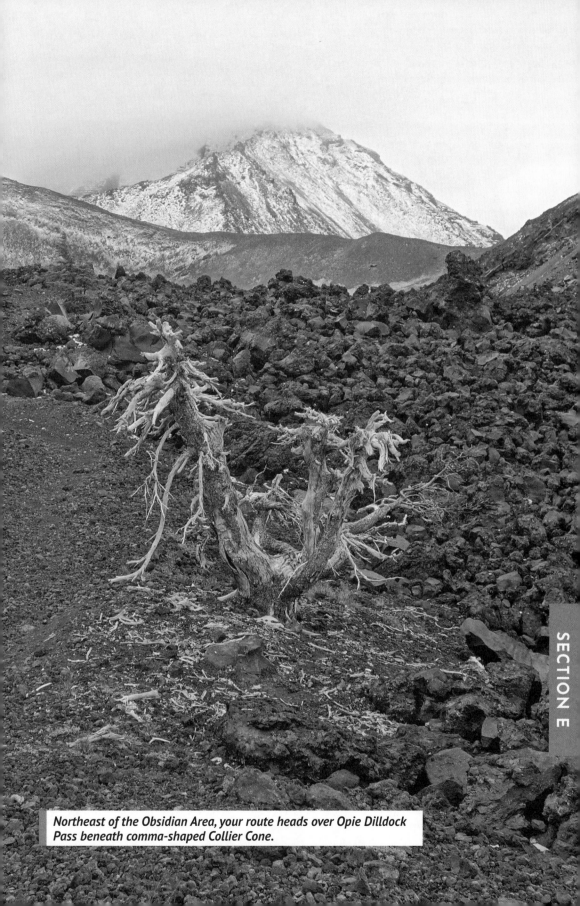

Northeast of the Obsidian Area, your route heads over Opie Dilldock Pass beneath comma-shaped Collier Cone.

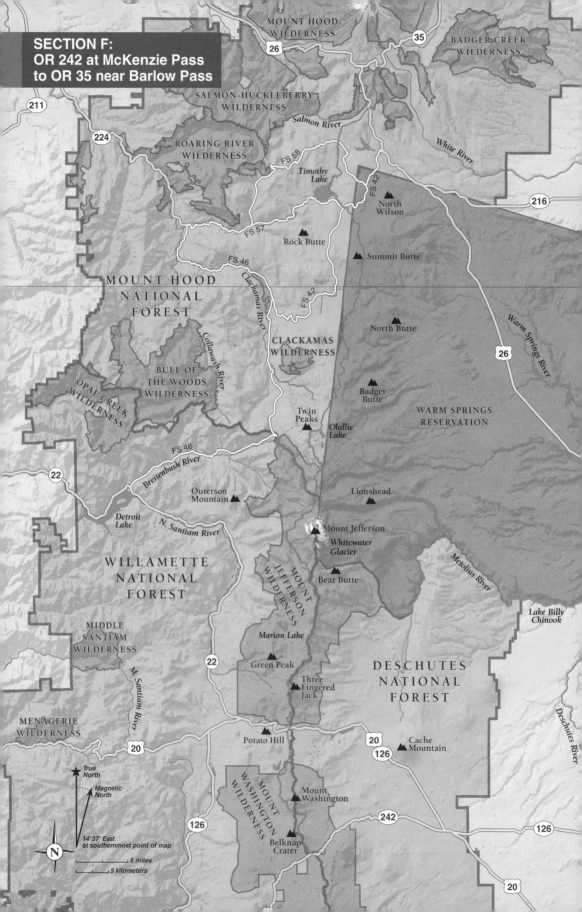

MOUNT HOOD
WILDERNESS

BADGER CREEK
WILDERNESS

35

26

211

224

SALMON-HUCKLEBERRY
WILDERNESS

Salmon River

White River

ROARING RIVER
WILDERNESS

FS 58

Timothy
Lake

216

FS 42

North
Wilson

FS 57

Rock Butte

Summit Butte

FS 46

N45°

Clackamas River

FS 42

MOUNT HOOD
NATIONAL
FOREST

CLACKAMAS
WILDERNESS

North Butte

Warm Springs River

26

Collawash River

BULL OF
THE WOODS
WILDERNESS

Badger
Butte

WARM SPRINGS
RESERVATION

OPAL CREEK
WILDERNESS

FS 46

Twin
Peaks

Olallie
Lake

Breitenbush River

22

Outerson
Mountain

Lionshead

Detroit
Lake

N. Santiam River

Mount Jefferson

Metolius River

Whitewater
Glacier

Lake Billy
Chinook

WILLAMETTE
NATIONAL
FOREST

MOUNT
JEFFERSON
WILDERNESS

Bear Butte

MIDDLE
SANTIAM
WILDERNESS

Marion Lake

DESCHUTES
NATIONAL
FOREST

M. Santiam River

22

Green Peak

Three
Fingered
Jack

MENAGERIE
WILDERNESS

20

Potato Hill

20

Cache
Mountain

126

Deschutes River

126

MOUNT
WASHINGTON
WILDERNESS

Mount
Washington

242

126

True
North

Magnetic
North

14°37' East
at southernmost point of map

N

Belknap
Crater

20

5 miles

5 kilometers

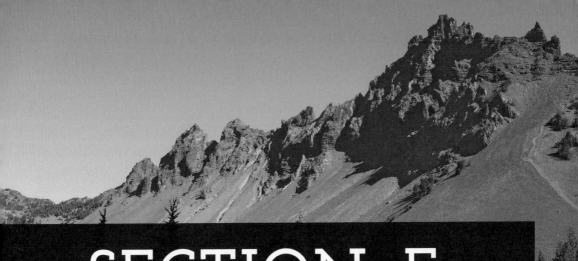

SECTION F

OR 242 at McKenzie Pass to OR 35 near Barlow Pass

THE TERRAIN CROSSED IN SECTION F is an approximate mirror image of that crossed in Section E. Starting from OR 242, you head north on the Pacific Crest Trail (PCT) across recent lava flows that also make up the last part of Section E. You then pass three major peaks—Mount Washington, Three Fingered Jack, and Mount Jefferson—just as you passed the Three Sisters. All six peaks are volcanoes in various stages of erosion. Mount Jefferson, the northernmost, and South Sister, the southernmost, are the two youngest.

North of Mount Jefferson, you hike through the lake-studded Breitenbush Lake–Olallie Lake area, which is a smaller version of the southern Three Sisters Wilderness. Finally, you hike a lengthy stretch across slopes that offer few views or lakes, just as you did in the first third of Section E. Both sections, on average, are fairly scenic, and it is difficult to say which is better. For many, Jefferson Park is the scenic high point of the Oregon PCT.

Above: Three Fingered Jack, the highest volcanic peak between the Three Sisters and Mount Jefferson, is the ruins of a small stratovolcano.

But on this spectacular plain, you'll find a backpacking crowd to match or exceed that on any other part of the tristate PCT.

DECLINATION 14°37'E

USGS MAPS

Boulder Lake, OR	Olallie Butte, OR
Fort Butte, OR	Pinhead Buttes, OR
Marion Lake, OR	Three Fingered Jack, OR
Mount Hood South, OR	Timothy Lake, OR
Mount Jefferson, OR	Wapinitia Pass, OR
Mount Washington, OR	Wolf Peak, OR
Mount Wilson, OR	

POINTS ON THE TRAIL, SOUTH TO NORTH

	Mile	Elevation in feet	Latitude/Longitude
OR 242 at McKenzie Pass	1,983.8	5,309	N44° 15' 35.4103" W121° 48' 18.7279"
Trail to Big Lake Youth Camp	1,995.1	4,775	N44° 21' 41.1012" W121° 52' 16.6800"
WA 20 at Santiam Pass	2,000.9	4,804	N44° 25' 25.6306" W121° 50' 58.9852"
Minto Pass	2,011.2	5,350	N44° 30' 48.9844" W121° 48' 42.9502"
Start of Pamelia Lake alternate routes	2,021.0	5,890	N44° 36' 58.7413" W121° 49' 01.5977"
Shale Lake	2,022.7	5,884	N44° 38' 10.1044" W121° 49' 01.4643"
Southern boundary of Jefferson Park	2,033.3	5,889	N44° 42' 23.1790" W121° 48' 39.1345"
FS 4220 near Breitenbush Lake	2,039.4	5,515	N44° 45' 55.1374" W121° 47' 13.5863"
Trail to Olallie Lake Resort	2,045.6	4,963	N44° 48' 51.8300" W121° 47' 32.2900"
Miller Trail junction to Clackamas Lake Campground	2,072.6	3,427	N45° 05' 43.2729" W121° 44' 18.8485"
US 26 at Wapinitia Pass	2,086.5	3,914	N45° 13' 44.3754" W121° 42' 03.2047"
Start of Twin Lakes alternate route	2,087.9	4,397	N45° 14' 13.1388" W121° 41' 11.2812"
OR 35 near Barlow Pass	2,091.7	4,164	N45° 17' 04.2880" W121° 40' 52.7708"

CAMPSITES AND BIVY SITES

Mile	Elevation in feet	Latitude/ Longitude	Number of tents	Feature	Notes
1,991.6	5,759	N44° 19' 33.0313" W121° 51' 17.6216"	>4	Mount Washington	
1,993.7	5,214	N44° 20' 43.0049" W121° 52' 03.0502"	2	Ephemeral spring nearby	
2,014.8	6,274	N44° 33' 10.4137" W121° 48' 14.4647"	>4	Rockpile Lake	
2,021.0 (alt. 2)	3,954	N44° 39' 21.3900" W121° 51' 04.3900"	>4	Pamelia Lake	

CAMPSITES AND BIVY SITES *(continued)*

Mile	Elevation in feet	Latitude/ Longitude	Number of tents	Feature	Notes
2,039.4	5,524	N44° 46' 04.0800" W121° 46' 57.0000"	2	Breitenbush Lake Campground	0.3 mile off-trail; vault toilet; no fee
2,041.1	5,200	N44° 46' 47.3484" W121° 47' 07.3716"	6	Horseshoe Lake Campground	0.75 mile east of PCT; vault toilet
2,043.2	5,384	N44° 47' 49.5877" W121° 48' 44.6334"	3	Upper Lake	
2,043.6	5,333	N44° 48' 08.6501" W121° 48' 42.1483"	2	Cigar Lake	
2,045.6	4,966	N44° 48' 54.1137" W121° 47' 27.5925"	>4	Head Lake	East shore
2,045.6	4,941	N44° 48' 01.2600" W121° 47' 08.5812"	35	Peninsula Campground	About 1 mile east of PCT at Olallie Lake; vault toilet
2,045.6	5,000	N44° 48' 10.4400" W121° 47' 22.2000"	10	Camp Ten	About 0.75 mile east of PCT at Olallie Lake; vault toilet
2,049.1	4,500	N44° 51' 36.7200" W121° 46' 22.4400"	7	Olallie Meadow Campground	0.75 mile northwest of PCT
2,049.3	4,623	N44° 51' 17.6828" W121° 45' 47.9532"	2	Jude Lake	
2,054.6	4,362	N44° 54' 22.5447" W121° 44' 55.2421"	>4	Lemiti Creek	Flat spot near trail on left
2,064.6	3,347	N45° 00' 02.4248" W121° 43' 00.7822"	>4	Warm Springs River	Flat spot near trail on left, north and south of river
2,072.6	3,400	N45° 05' 41.6040" W121° 44' 57.9840"	46	Clackamas Lake Campground	0.7 mile off-trail; vault toilet, potable water; 11 equestrian sites
2,077.8	3,246	N45° 08' 30.8067" W121° 45' 53.0990"	2	Timothy Lake	Fire ring
2,078.8	3,300	N45° 08' 54.0744" W121° 44' 43.9800"	16	Little Crater Lake Campground	0.3 mile off-trail; vault toilet, drinking water, picnic table, fire ring with grill
2,082.7	3,928	N45° 11' 50.9744" W121° 45' 13.9357"	3	Spring nearby	Flat spot near trail on right
2,086.6	3,800	N45° 13' 26.9976" W121° 41' 39.6996"	31	Frog Lake Campground	0.6 mile off-trail; vault toilet, well water, picnic table, fire ring with grill
2,091.5 (alt.)	5,400	N45° 19' 12.9396" W121° 42' 19.6992"	16	Alpine Campground	Toilets, drinking water

SUPPLIES

Just 11.3 miles north into this section, at a junction 1.4 miles north of Coldwater Spring, you can descend a broad trail 0.7 mile to the grounds of the Seventh-Day Adventists' Big Lake Youth Camp. This camp not only offers showers, a laundry, and meals (for a donation), but it also accepts PCT trekkers' packages at no charge. Mail them to Big Lake Youth Camp, 26435 Big Lake Road, Sisters, OR 97759.

Not far beyond this section's halfway point, you reach the Olallie Lake Guard Station and, just east of it, Olallie Lake Resort. The resort has a fair selection of food and cold, hopped beverages, but there's not really enough food for more than a couple of days' resupply.

At the end of this section, you could hike—or hitch—4.8 miles west to the village of Government Camp, which has a post office and a moderately well-stocked store, plus hotels, restaurants, and brewpubs. See page 194 for more details.

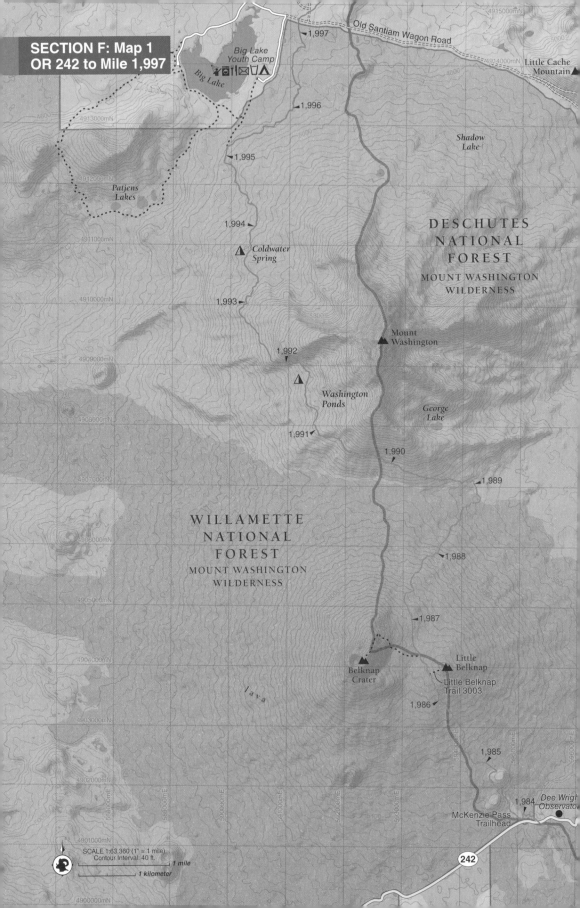

Old Santiam Wagon Road

Little Cache Mountain

1,997

Big Lake Youth Camp

Big Lake

1,996

1,995

Shadow Lake

Patjens Lakes

1,994

Coldwater Spring

DESCHUTES NATIONAL FOREST

MOUNT WASHINGTON WILDERNESS

1,993

1,992

Washington Ponds

Mount Washington

George Lake

1,991

1,990

1,989

WILLAMETTE NATIONAL FOREST

MOUNT WASHINGTON WILDERNESS

1,988

1,987

Belknap Crater

Little Belknap

Little Belknap Trail 3003

lava

1,986

1,985

1,984

Dee Wright Observato

McKenzie Pass Trailhead

242

SCALE 1:63,360 (1" = 1 mile)
Contour Interval: 40 ft.

1 mile

1 kilometer

PERMITS

If you're section hiking, you will need to obtain a Central Cascades Wilderness Permit to enter the Mount Washington and Mount Jefferson Wilderness areas from the Friday before Memorial Day through the last Friday in September. For more information, visit fs.usda.gov/detail/willamette /passes-permits/recreation/?cid=fseprd688355.

OR 242 AT MCKENZIE PASS TO OR 35 NEAR BARLOW PASS

>>>THE ROUTE

This section's PCT begins at a small trailhead parking area just west of ill-defined McKenzie Pass. This trailhead is easy to find because it is at a bend in OR 242 (1983.8–5,309'), where the road to the east is very curvy but the road to the southwest is as straight as an arrow.

From this trailhead, at the southern boundary of Mount Washington Wilderness, ascend the Belknap Crater basalt flows northwest, and pass between two forested islands of older, glaciated basalt that stand in a sea of younger basalt. **GEOLOGY** The desolate young basalt flows look as if they cooled only a few years ago, yet those emanating from Little Belknap (6,305') are 2,900 years old. The flows seen today on Belknap Crater (6,872') and its flanks are mostly 1,500–3,000 years old. All the flows between North Sister and Mount Washington compose a 65-square-mile field that represents the Cascades' greatest post-Pleistocene outpouring of lava. Belknap Crater is an excellent example of a shield volcano and is quite similar to the shields on which the Three Sisters and Mount Thielsen grew. **WILDLIFE** The route now takes you up to a junction with Little Belknap Trail 3003 (1,986.3–6,112') that leads east-northeast up to the summit of Little Belknap. This area you're in looks quite lifeless, yet up here among the rocks you might spot a whistling marmot scurrying for its hole or, even more astounding, a western toad. Mountain chickadees sing out their name as you enter a strip of forest near Belknap Crater and descend through it to the eastern edge of a fresh-looking flow.

First head north and then west, up along its edge, which borders the south slope of Mount Washington. The trail switchbacks northeast and in a couple of minutes switchbacks west-northwest.

From the point where the trail switchbacks west-northwest (1,989.0–5,310'), you climb steadily to the Cascade divide, where the PCT levels off. Now travel northwest about 0.7 mile before curving north 0.3 mile to a ravine just 0.1 mile southwest of the easily missed Washington Ponds (1,991.3–5,719').

From here, you climb slightly higher through a meadow that affords an excellent view of the basalt plug that makes up the steep-walled summit block of Mount Washington (7,794'). **CAMPING** Your route arcs west, descends moderately alongside the west spur, and then descends north around it to an

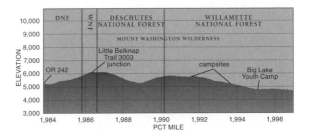

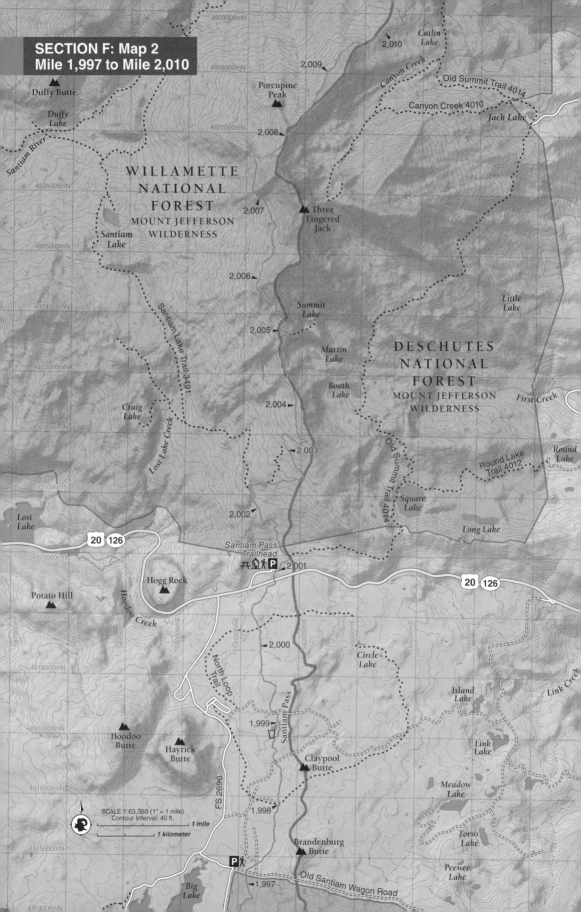

Duffy Butte

Duffy Lake

Santiam River

Porcupine Peak

2,009

2,010

Catlin Lake

Canyon Creek

Old Summit Trail 4014

Canyon Creek 4010

Jack Lake

WILLAMETTE
NATIONAL
FOREST
MOUNT JEFFERSON
WILDERNESS

Santiam Lake

2,008

2,007

Three Fingered Jack

2,006

Summit Lake

Little Lake

Santiam Lake Trail 3491

2,005

Martin Lake

DESCHUTES
NATIONAL
FOREST
MOUNT JEFFERSON
WILDERNESS

First Creek

Craig Lake

Lost Lake Creek

Booth Lake

2,004

2,003

Old Summit Trail 4014

Round Lake Trail 4012

Round Lake

Square Lake

Lost Lake

2,002

Long Lake

20 **126**

Santiam Pass Trailhead

2,001

Hogg Rock

Potato Hill

Hoodoo Creek

20 **126**

2,000

Circle Lake

Island Lake

Link Creek

North Loop Trail

Santiam Pass

1,999

Link Lake

Hoodoo Butte

Hayrick Butte

Claypool Butte

Meadow Lake

FS 2690

1,998

SCALE 1:63,360 (1" = 1 mile)
Contour Interval: 40 ft.

1 mile

1 kilometer

Brandenburg Butte

Torso Lake

1,997

Old Santiam Wagon Road

Peewee Lake

Big Lake

overused meadow with a hole that's euphemistically referred to as Coldwater Spring (1,993.7–5,200'). If the spring isn't dry, it may be the last fresh water on-route until Rockpile Lake, about 21 miles farther. Less desirable ponds and lakes also exist near the trail, and snow patches linger through mid-August on the northwest slope of Three Fingered Jack. Because this meadow is the only trailside PCT campsite in Mount Washington Wilderness that has fresh water, it has been overused, so much so that the spring sometimes dries up. Be prepared. If you are lucky enough to find water here, be sure to treat it.

On weekends, many mountaineers will make this their base camp and then climb the north spur to the 300-foot-high north arête of the summit block—the easiest summit route, but one that still requires ropes and other equipment.

RESUPPLY ACCESS

The PCT continues its northward descent through a hemlock forest, which burned in 2011. You pass an unmarked climbers' trail that ascends east–southeast toward the peak's north spur, and then descend north to a fork with a broad trail (1,995.1–4,775') that turns left (north) and heads to Big Lake Youth Camp. See "Supplies" on page 173 for more information.

The PCT veers right (northeast) and traverses slopes that are waterless once the snow patches disappear. Leave Mount Washington Wilderness just before reaching Old Santiam Wagon Road (1,997.1–4,686').

WATER ACCESS

From the Old Santiam Wagon Road, the PCT heads northeast past abandoned logging roads on a route that gradually turns north and reaches a 100-yard-long pond (1,999.0–4,796') just west of the trail. The next northbound water possibility is in 11.6 miles near Koko Lake, so use this opportunity to gather and treat water.

This stretch you have just passed through is easy to follow, despite old roads. Southbound along it, you'll have views of Mount Washington. Just north of the pond, you climb over a low saddle and into a mature forest once again, and about 0.7 mile through it, you intersect the North Loop Trail, a cross-country ski route. Next the route heads into the burn scar of the massive B&B Complex wildfire of 2003, which affects the trail on and off for the next 15 miles. The forest regeneration is inspiring to witness. However, be aware of standing snags, and don't put up your tent where they or their limbs may fall. Your route heads quite steadily north, then turns northeast, quickly crosses a minor road, and reaches Santiam Highway (US 20/OR 126) (2,000.9–4,804') about 200 yards west of the national forest boundary at Santiam Pass.

HISTORY This pass was first crossed in 1859 by Andrew Wiley. He

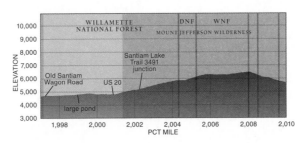

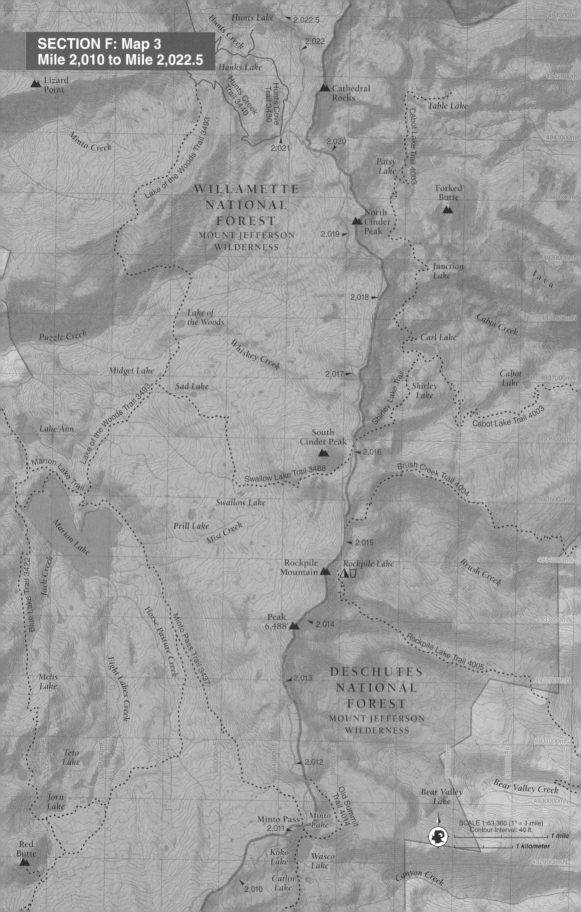

Hunts Lake
2,022.5
Hunts Creek
2,022
Hanks Lake
Lizard Point
Cathedral Rocks
Table Lake
Hunts Cove Trail 3430
Minto Creek
2,021
2,020
Cabot Lake Trail 4003
Patsy Lake
Forked Butte
Lake of the Woods Trail 3493
WILLAMETTE NATIONAL FOREST
MOUNT JEFFERSON WILDERNESS
North Cinder Peak
2,019
Junction Lake
lava
2,018
Lake of the Woods
Puzzle Creek
Whiskey Creek
Carl Lake
Cabot Creek
2,017
Midget Lake
Shirley Lake
Cabot Lake
Sad Lake
Lake of the Woods Trail 3493
Shirley Lake Trail
Cabot Lake Trail 4003
Lake Ann
South Cinder Peak
2,016
Marion Lake Trail
Swallow Lake Trail 3488
Brush Creek Trail 4004
Swallow Lake
Prill Lake
Mist Creek
2,015
Marion Lake
Blue Lake Trail 3422
Jack Creek
Rockpile Mountain
Rockpile Lake
Brush Creek
4931000mN
Minto Pass Trail 3437
Horse Pasture Creek
Peak 6,488'
2,014
Rockpile Lake Trail 4005
Eight Lakes Creek
2,013
DESCHUTES NATIONAL FOREST
MOUNT JEFFERSON WILDERNESS
Melis Lake
Teto Lake
2,012
Bear Valley Lake
Bear Valley Creek
Jorn Lake
Old Summit Trail 4014
Minto Pass
2,011
Minto Lake
SCALE 1:63,360 (1" = 1 mile)
Contour Interval: 40 ft.
1 mile
Red Butte
Koko Lake
Wasco Lake
1 kilometer
Catlin Lake
2,010
Canyon Creek

explored an old American Indian trail up the Santiam River and worked his way farther east each year on his hunting expeditions from the Willamette Valley.

Just 240 yards west of the highway crossing is a PCT access road that curves 0.2 mile northeast to a parking area with a vault toilet and picnic tables at the popular Santiam Pass Trailhead. Cross the highway and, after 200 yards, you'll see the parking area immediately to the west. Your trail bears north, curves northwest, enters Mount Jefferson Wilderness (2,001.3–4,959'), and then climbs increasingly steep slopes, passing a few stagnant ponds just before a junction with the Santiam Lake Trail 3491 (2,002.3–5,200'), which curves northwest around a prominent boulder pile. *Note:* You will need a Central Cascades Wilderness Permit to enter the wilderness area if you're section hiking (see page 175).

From the junction, you head slightly northeast for about 0.5 mile, and then turn northwest for another 0.5 mile before a final switchback to the ridge, which you follow north-northwest toward Three Fingered Jack. The trail eventually leaves the ridge, curves northeast across a prominent cliff above Martin Lake, then heads up a small ravine and promptly curves north–northwest (2,004.8–6,000').

Follow the trail as it switchbacks up to the ridge again, crosses it, and traverses up the lower west slope of Three Fingered Jack (7,841'). Up close, this peak has a totally different appearance from the one you saw from a distance. Here, he seems to have considerably more than three fingers.

GEOLOGY	The PCT rounds the peak's northwest spur, turns east

toward a snow patch that lasts through mid-August, and then curves northeast up to a saddle (2,008.0–6,500') along the Cascade divide. From this vantage point, you can observe Three Fingered Jack, the remaining structure of an ancient volcano.

Now the PCT descends four switchbacks, soon recrosses the divide, and then descends northeast along forested slopes to a smattering of stagnant ponds just southwest of an intersection with Minto Pass Trail 3437 (2,011.2–5,350') at Minto Pass. This trail heads about 4.5 miles northwest to Marion Lake.

The PCT turns north, climbs to a saddle, and reaches the Wasco Lake loop trail (2,011.7–5,430'), which descends southeast 0.5 mile to an unnamed lake before curving west to Wasco Lake. You continue north up the divide, switchback as it steepens, and then traverse to the southeast spur (2,013.7–6,210') of Peak 6,488, from which you can look south and see how Three Fingered Jack got its name.

WATER ACCESS

CAMPING Continuing north, contour to a saddle; then traverse the east slope of Rockpile Mountain (6,559') and pass Rockpile Lake Trail 4005, which descends southeast to Bear Valley, just before reaching a pond and beautiful Rockpile Lake (2,014.8–6,274'). This shallow but clear lake has an excellent campsite above

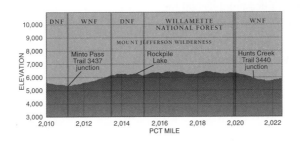

its southwest shore and a very good one at its north end. Help keep the forests green. Campfires are strictly forbidden at this lake.

Your trail heads north on the rocky slope along the lake's west shore and then descends the divide to a saddle where Brush Creek Trail 4004 (2,015.2–6,140') forks right and drops generally east toward roads near Abbot Butte.

WILDLIFE Your route stays west of the divide and climbs to a level, open area just east of a breached post-Pleistocene cinder cone. Although there are no lakes or ponds nearby, you may find that in midsummer this flat is crawling with 1-inch toads.

Continuing north, you pass a second cone, South Cinder Peak (6,746'), also of post-Pleistocene age. Soon the PCT reaches a saddle and trail junction (2,016.1–6,300'). Here, unmaintained Swallow Lake Trail 3488 descends 2 miles southwest to Swallow Lake, while Shirley Lake Trail 4003.1 heads 2 miles northeast to Carl Lake.

The PCT continues north along the west slope of the divide and reaches a saddle on a northwest ridge (2018.0–6,382'), from which a spur trail climbs west-northwest to a small knoll with a good view of Mount Jefferson to the north. Now the trail crosses a snow patch that lingers through late July, arcs east to the divide, and descends it to a level section that passes beside a small freshwater pond 50 yards east of the crest.

Hike once again up the ridge route, and then contour across the forested west slopes of North Cinder Peak (6,722') to a small, grassy meadow. A hidden, rock-lined pond lies on the other side of a low pile of rocks that borders the meadow. This might be a good water hole if you are passing through late in the summer.

HISTORY After a brief ascent north, you arrive at an escarpment where Mount Jefferson (10,497') towers above in all its presidential glory. On March 30, 1806, Lewis and Clark saw this snowy peak from the lower Willamette River and named it after their president.

GEOLOGY At the base of its south slope, below you, lies a bizarre glacio-volcanic landscape. During the last major glacial advance, glaciers cut a deep canyon on each side of the resistant Sugar Pine Ridge, seen in the east. After these glaciers disappeared, volcanic eruptions burst forth and constructed Forked Butte (6,483') east of North Cinder Peak. This butte was subsequently breached by outpourings of fluid basaltic andesite that flowed east down the glaciated Jefferson Creek and Cabot Creek canyons. A smaller cone with a crater lake, north of here, also erupted about this time, but it was aborted by nature before any flows poured forth. To its north stands the flat Table, and between it and the ridge of Cathedral Rocks is a large, deep, enigmatic depression that may represent a collapsed flow.

Time, which allowed nature to sculpt this surrealistic artwork, now forces you to press onward. Descend northwest, still marveling at the configurations below; leave the ridge; and switchback down to reach a saddle (2,021.0–5,890'), from where you have a choice of three routes: the PCT and two alternate routes. We recommend one of the alternates.

ALTERNATE ROUTE 1 This older route follows Hunts Cove Trail 3430 down the glaciated valley and curves west to shimmering, pure Hanks Lake. Along its north shore, you can take a spur trail north to another gem, Hunts Lake. Back at Hanks Lake, take Hunts Cove Trail west to meet Hunts Creek Trail 3440, described below in "Alternate Route 2."

ALTERNATE ROUTE 2 This second, newer alternate route follows Hunts

Creek Trail 3440 to a junction with Lake of the Woods Trail 3493, near a saddle, before it switchbacks down to Hunts Cove Trail 3430, where the older alternate route joins this newer one. You continue to descend into the glaciated valley on Hunts Creek Trail, and finally arrive at the southeast shore of shallow Pamelia Lake (3,884').

CAMPING Paralleling the shore, the route curves west to a junction with Pamelia Lake Trail 3439, which takes you down to many campsites near the lake's deeper end. Early in the season, the lake is high and attractive, but by August, Pamelia is reduced to a puddle dotted with hikers who climb the easy 2.3-mile trail to this lake. Back at the junction with Pamelia Lake Trail, ascend north and then northeast 0.6 mile on Hunts Creek Trail, toward Milk Creek, to regain the PCT route.

At mile 2,021.0, the PCT begins a gentle descent north-northeast from the saddle and traverses the lower slopes of the inspiring Cathedral Rocks. The route curves northwest to the crest of a lateral moraine well above sparkling Hunts Lake and enters the Pamelia Lake Area.

CAMPING Beginning at mile 2,022.0 and ending at mile 2,023.4, no camping is permitted without a special permit. This is a no-camping zone for long-distance hikers.

WATER ACCESS

The trail leaves this escarpment and winds north to the west shore of placid Shale Lake (2,022.7–5,884'), where Leave No Trace camping is permitted—and appreciated (but see above note for thru-hikers).

GEOLOGY The shale implied by the lake's name is actually basaltic andesite that has become highly fractured along many parallel planes.

Just north of this popular lake, you reach a shallow, seasonally larger lake that in late summer dwindles to a mudhole. Beyond it, the trail drops west to the glaciated escarpment and then gently descends it before entering a Douglas-fir forest and reaching a junction with Hunts Creek Trail 3440 (2,027.5–4,315') just south of Milk Creek. (If you took one of the alternate routes to Pamelia Lake, this is where you rejoin the PCT.)

Ascend the gravelly, bouldery outwash deposits of Milk Creek canyon and pass a lavish display of wildflowers and shrubs before hiking north to a crossing of aptly named Milk Creek. If you are running low on water, be sure to gather it along your descent because the water in Milk Creek is nonfilterable: disappointment will set in if you try to filter this or any of the other many silty water sources that you'll encounter along your journey north.

Beyond this minor torrent, you now enter an area that burned in 2017, affecting the next 5 miles of trail. Be aware there may not be many campsites free of the hazard of dead falling trees.

WATER ACCESS

Make tracks northwest across many small, deceptive ridges before reaching the real Woodpecker Ridge and a junction with lightly used Woodpecker Ridge Trail 3442 (2,029.3–5,051'), which

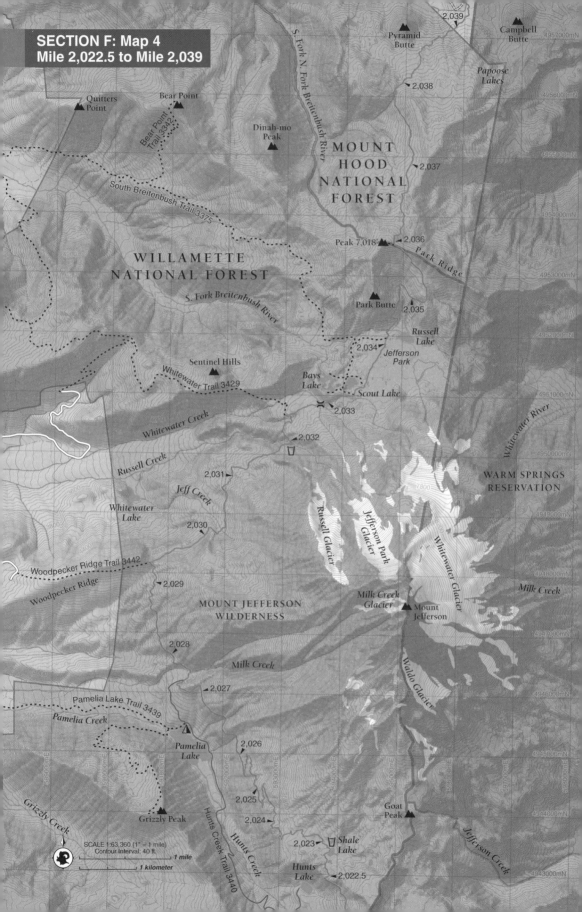

Quitters Point

Bear Point

Bear Point Trail 3342

Dinah-mo Peak

Pyramid Butte

Campbell Butte

2,039

2,038

Papoose Lakes

S. Fork N. Fork Breitenbush River

MOUNT HOOD NATIONAL FOREST

2,037

South Breitenbush Trail 3375

WILLAMETTE NATIONAL FOREST

2,036

Peak 7,018'

Park Ridge

S. Fork Breitenbush River

Park Butte

2,035

Russell Lake

2,034

Jefferson Park

Sentinel Hills

Whitewater Trail 3429

Bays Lake

Scout Lake

2,033

Whitewater Creek

2,032

Whitewater River

Russell Creek

2,031

Jeff Creek

WARM SPRINGS RESERVATION

Whitewater Lake

2,030

7,800

Russell Glacier

Jefferson Park Glacier

Whitewater Glacier

Woodpecker Ridge Trail 3442

2,029

Woodpecker Ridge

Milk Creek

MOUNT JEFFERSON WILDERNESS

Milk Creek Glacier

Mount Jefferson

Milk Creek

2,028

Milk Creek

Waldo Glacier

2,027

Pamelia Lake Trail 3439

Pamelia Creek

2,026

Pamelia Lake

Grizzly Creek

2,025

2,024

Goat Peak

Grizzly Peak

Hunts Creek Trail 3440

2,023

Shale Lake

Jefferson Creek

Hunts Creek

Hunts Lake

2,022.5

SCALE 1:63,360 (1" = 1 mile)
Contour Interval: 40 ft.

1 mile

1 kilometer

descends west to its trailhead. Head east on the PCT easily down from the ridge, soon passing a tranquil pond where you may be able to gather water.

PLANTS The open forest here is successfully regenerating with an understory of spirea, corn lily, gooseberry, rhododendron, and the ubiquitous huckleberry. You'll easily identify Whitewater Lake, way below you, by its milky color.

Not much farther along, you pass a small spring and then cross a creeklet whose ravine is a channel for periodic avalanches. Two minutes past it, you cross seasonal Jeff Creek (2,030.3–4,956') and see more evidence of avalanches.

WATER ACCESS

After 0.5 mile of gently ascending north, the trail ascends east, sometimes moderately, and then quickly drops to a ford of Russell Creek (2,031.9–5,447').

This can be a dangerous stream to cross, so plan to ford it *before 11 a.m.* The afternoon's warmer temperatures greatly increase the snowmelt from the Russell and Jefferson Park Glaciers, and that increased flow can take unwary hikers on a one-way trip down the gorge immediately below the ford. If the creek looks too brisk for safe crossing, look for a better spot about 70–100 yards upstream.

The trail now curves around a minor, westward-descending ridge; soon makes a loop around a small, boggy area; and then briefly descends to cross the headwaters of a Whitewater Creek tributary. From its north bank, you make a minute's walk west to a junction with heavily traveled Whitewater Trail 3429 (2,032.5–5,581'). Starting from the end of Whitewater Road, this trail—the shortest one into popular Jefferson Park—climbs 3.7 miles to the main branch of Whitewater Creek and then climbs an additional 0.4 mile to your junction.

From this point, the PCT/Whitewater Trail makes an easy climb east-northeast to cross that branch (2,032.9–5,700'). A sturdy wooden bridge makes this creek crossing safe, unlike the ford of Russell Creek. Continue this easy ascent in the same general direction, and then curve north for a momentary climb to the south rim of beautiful but overpopulated Jefferson Park (2,033.3–5,889').

CAMPING As a response to the popularity of the lakes in Jefferson Park, the U.S. Forest Service has designated specific sites around the lakes with posts embedded trailside to mark where campers can enjoy their stay without pressure on the area or on other hikers. Campfires are prohibited, but backpacking stoves are permitted. As always, try to leave your tent area in better shape than you found it. Contact the Willamette National Forest for information on permit reservations. *Note:* Long-distance hikers are not permitted to camp here, so plan to camp before or after Jefferson Park's boundaries.

VIEWS Beneath hemlocks on the north shore of Scout Lake, you get beautifully framed views across the reflective

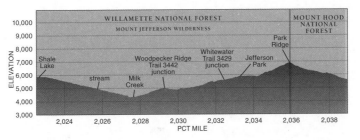

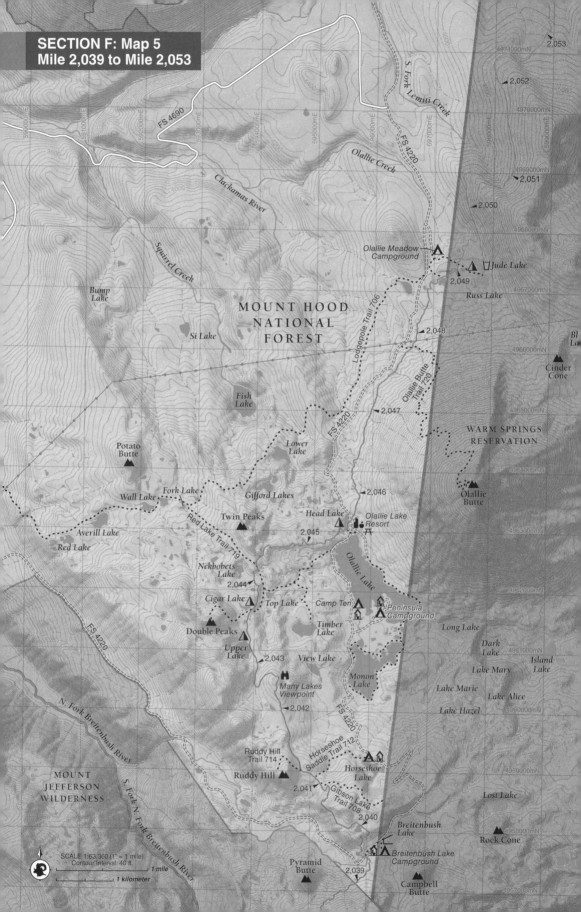

2,053

2,052

S. Fork Lemiti Creek

FS 4220

Olallie Creek

2,051

FS 4690

Clackamas River

2,050

Olallie Meadow Campground

Jude Lake

2,049

Russ Lake

Squirrel Creek

Bl La

Bump Lake

MOUNT HOOD NATIONAL FOREST

Cinder Cone

Si Lake

2,048

Lodgepole Trail 706

Fish Lake

Olallie Butte Trail 720

2,047

FS 4220

WARM SPRINGS RESERVATION

Lower Lake

2,046

Potato Butte

Olallie Butte

Fork Lake

Wall Lake

Gifford Lakes

Head Lake

Olallie Lake Resort

Averill Lake

Twin Peaks

Red Lake Trail 719

2,045

Red Lake

Nekhobets Lake

2,044

Olallie Lake

Long Lake

Cigar Lake

Top Lake

Camp Ten

Peninsula Campground

Dark Lake

Double Peaks

Timber Lake

Island Lake

FS 4220

Upper Lake

2,043

View Lake

Lake Mary

Lake Alice

N. Fork Breitenbush River

Many Lakes Viewpoint

Monon Lake

Lake Marie

2,042

Lake Hazel

MOUNT JEFFERSON WILDERNESS

Ruddy Hill Trail 714

Horseshoe Saddle Trail 712

FS 4220

Ruddy Hill

Horseshoe Lake

Lost Lake

2,041

S. Fork N. Fork Breitenbush River

Gibson Lake Trail 708

2,040

Breitenbush Lake

Rock Cone

Breitenbush Lake Campground

Pyramid Butte

2,039

Campbell Butte

SCALE 1:63,360 (1" = 1 mile)
Contour Interval: 40 ft.

1 mile

1 kilometer

lake of stately Mount Jefferson (10,497') with its ermine robe of glaciers. At this lake and the adjacent lakes of Jefferson Park, you might make a strange catch while fishing for trout: Pacific giant salamanders that inhabit the shady waters.

The PCT turns right (northeast) at the first spur-trail junction; follows blazes past radiating, narrow spur trails; curves north past a seasonal pond; and reaches a spur trail that heads west to Scout and Bays Lakes. Now you hike north-northeast across the open flat of Jefferson Park, with impressive views back at the peak all the way to a junction with South Breitenbush Trail 3375 (2,034.1–5,886'), which starts west-southwest before descending northwest. Just 30 yards farther, a prominent spur trail branches northeast 250 yards to shallow Russell Lake (5,856'). By late season, the lake may be fairly depleted, and the others in the basin may be completely dry.

The PCT turns abruptly northwest at this junction with South Breitenbush Trail and then quickly descends northeast to a step-across ford of South Fork Breitenbush River. The trail now climbs steeply up a slope and into a glacial cirque, which it explores via two undulating turns, and then climbs moderately southeast to a spur on the Cascade divide. Climb this in an arc to Park Ridge, and then traverse 70 yards west to a viewpoint (2,036.0–6,880'), where you get a last look down at justifiably popular Jefferson Park.

VIEWS SIDE TRIP A short trail climbs 200 yards west to Peak 7,018 for an even better view. In the distance, just east of north, towers magnificent Mount Hood (11,235'), and just west

of north stands southern Washington's decapitated Mount St. Helens (8,364').

Now you descend the trail—or, rather, the semipermanent snowfield—toward small, shallow lakes and ponds. As the gradient eases, the trail becomes obvious as it selects a pond-dotted route north out of the alpine realm and into the hemlock forest. The path momentarily takes you over a low saddle and then meanders northeast, giving views of locally dominant Pyramid Butte (6,095') as it crosses many minor gullies and ridges. Views disappear, and soon the trail starts through a small flat with a low hill on your left. Here you leave Mount Jefferson Wilderness (2,039.0–5,591'). *Note:* Southbound hikers who are section hiking will need a Central Cascades Wilderness Permit to enter the wilderness (see page 175).

CAMPING Your trail rambles onward 0.3 mile, passing a small, volcanic butte of shalelike rocks before it meets Breitenbush Lake's outlet creek. Beside it is a spur road, which goes east to a large, nearby trailhead parking area. Immediately east of it is the Warm Springs Reservation boundary, and squeezed between that boundary and the southwest shore of Breitenbush Lake is the Breitenbush Lake Campground, which is administered by the U.S. Forest Service. It is located on the Warm Springs Reservation and governed by its rules and regulations.

On the PCT, walk a few paces past the spur road to FS 4220 (2,039.4–5,515'), crossing it just 30 yards northeast of the start of the spur road. Keeping within Mount Hood National Forest, you climb a winding trail to the east shore of a shallow lake (2,040.0–5,750'), curve

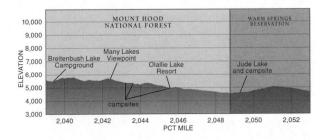

around to its north shore, and then pass near a smaller, triangular lake. The trail then traverses the bouldery southwest slope of summit 5,975 before winding down to a junction with the old OST route (2,041.0–5,552'), now Gibson Lake Trail 708. Starting northwest, you shortly reach Horseshoe Saddle Trail 712 (2,041.1–5,520')— logically atop a saddle above Horseshoe Lake.

CAMPING You can follow this trail 0.75 mile down to its trailhead by FS 4220's Horseshoe Lake Campground.

VIEWS A short distance northwest along this ridge route, you encounter Ruddy Hill Trail 714 (2,041.4–5,600'), which climbs steeply west to the summit of Ruddy Hill for great views of Mount Jefferson to the south and Mount Hood to the north.

Now you contour north through a thick forest and then climb to a low knoll before descending slightly to Many Lakes Viewpoint (2,042.4–5,667'), which, due to wonderful tree growth, barely lives up to its description. Mile-long Olallie Lake is the focal point of the basin,

and andesitic Olallie Butte (7,215') rules above it. (*Olallie* is what the American Indians called the huckleberries.) This volcano has been active in both glacial and postglacial times.

CAMPING After hiking counterclockwise down the knoll's northern slopes, you reach a dry flat from which southbound hikers see the lofty crown of Mount Jefferson beckoning. Here the trail crosses a seasonal creek, descends north steeply alongside it, and veers northwest to a very good campsite at restful Upper Lake (2,043.2–5,384'). As always, set your tent no closer than 200 feet to the shore.

Continuing north, you pass several seasonal ponds and shallow, linear Cigar Lake (2,043.6–5,333'), from which a 0.6-mile trail first winds northeast down to Top Lake (5,170') and then climbs back to a mile-high crest junction with the PCT. Leaving Cigar Lake, the PCT takes an easier, more direct route to that crest junction (2,044.1–5,294'), from which Red Lake Trail 719 goes 1.25 miles northwest to Fork Lake.

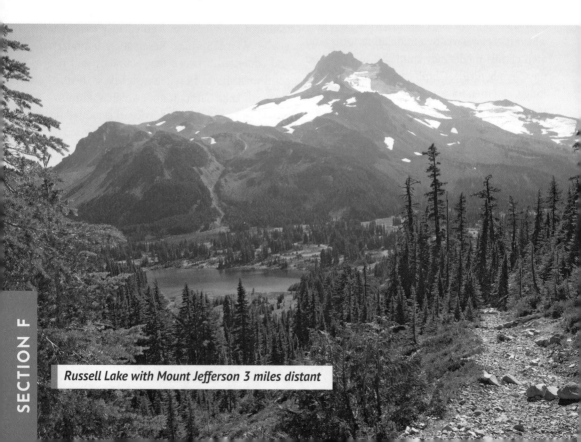

Russell Lake with Mount Jefferson 3 miles distant

RESUPPLY ACCESS

The PCT contours north along the divide, curves northeast and crosses it, and follows it east down past a small triangular, semiclear lake. About 0.5 mile past this lake, a spur trail to the east (2045.6–4,963') leads to Olallie Lake Resort. See "Supplies" on page 173 for more information.
CAMPING Also at Olallie Lake, you'll find the Camp Ten and Peninsula Campgrounds.

From the spur trail, the PCT climbs above the southeast shore of Head Lake to reach FS 4220 (2,045.7–4,969') at a point 20 yards north of its signed 4,991-foot divide.

From the FS 4220 crossing, the PCT starts northeast and then makes a long, gentle descent north along the lower slopes of Olallie Butte (7,215') to an intersection with Olallie Butte Trail 720 (2,047.8–4,680'), which descends 220 yards west alongside the southern power line to FS 4220. Cross under the three sets of power lines, and parallel the unseen road, going north-northeast, until you observe a flat, bushy, open depression on the right (east). Then the trail veers northeast, and a trail continues north. The latter trail (2,048.7–4,570') is a 230-yard link between the PCT and the old OST (now Lodgepole Trail 706). The PCT now enters Warm Springs Reservation land and will remain on it almost to Clackamas Lake. While traveling the PCT through the Warm Springs Reservation, you must stay within the trail's 200-foot-wide right-of-way.

TRAIL INFO *Note:* There is ongoing logging on the reservation, and the PCT crosses logging roads in various states

of use. Not all of these are shown on the maps or mentioned in the text.

CAMPING Continue northeast on a low ridge, angle north, and intersect Russ Lake Trail 716 (2,049.1–4,606'), ascending southeast from Olallie Meadow Campground. This trail continues 0.3 mile southeast past an adequate campsite at Jude Lake to another one at deeper Russ Lake (4,600'). If camping at Jude Lake, choose a site on the southwestern side at least 200 feet from the shore.

WATER ACCESS

On the PCT, start north and then ramble northeast to shallow Jude Lake (2,049.3–4,623'). Refill your water bottles here, for you have a long, dry (though shady) walk around the lower ends of two ridges before you descend to trickling Lemiti Creek (2,054.6–4,362') at the lower end of Lemiti Meadow. You can also gather water ahead at Trooper Spring (2,055.0–4,394').

The PCT continues southeast 0.1 mile and then turns north to climb over the low Cascade divide. It more or less follows the divide north through a continuous forest canopy until South Pinhead Butte (5,348'), where you reach the trailside Chinquapin Viewpoint (2,057.5–5,000')—rather disappointing, but at least it permits you to see over the forest. Better views are just ahead. Contour the butte's slopes to the north; cross Pinhead Saddle, which has an abandoned spur road going west; and then reach the southeast slope of North Pinhead Butte (5,450'), which is the youngest of the three andesite buttes. Looking south, you see Mount Jefferson once again and are reminded of the beauties of Jefferson Park.

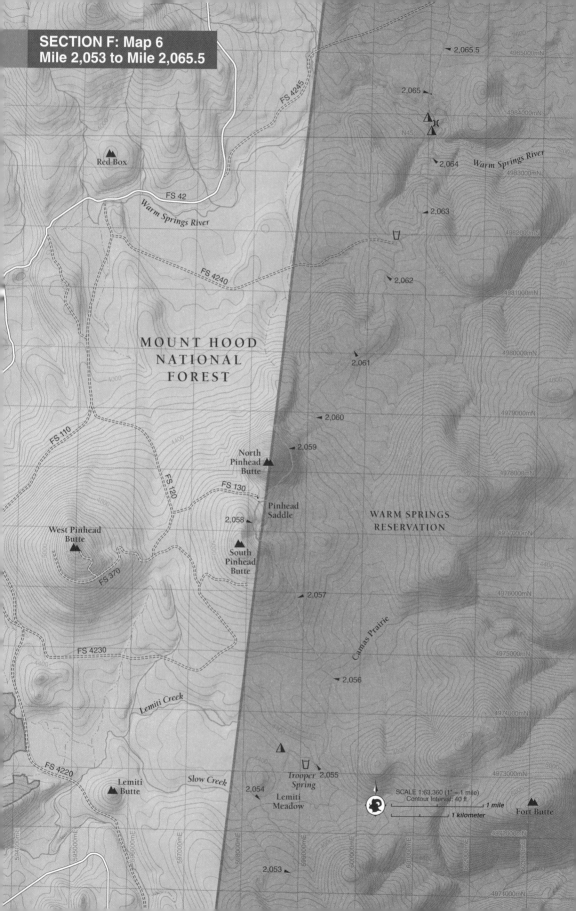

2,065.5

2,065

N45

Warm Springs River

2,064

Red Box

2,063

FS 42

Warm Springs River

2,062

FS 4240

2,061

MOUNT HOOD
NATIONAL
FOREST

2,060

FS 110

2,059

North
Pinhead
Butte

FS 120

FS 130

Pinhead
Saddle

WARM SPRINGS
RESERVATION

2,058

West Pinhead
Butte

South
Pinhead
Butte

FS 370

2,057

FS 4230

Camas Prairie

2,056

Lemiti Creek

FS 4220

Trooper
Spring

2,055

Lemiti
Butte

Slow Creek

2,054

Lemiti
Meadow

SCALE 1:63,360 (1" = 1 mile)
Contour Interval: 40 ft.

1 mile

1 kilometer

Fort Butte

2,053

WATER ACCESS

Now you descend north to a lava flow, make a switchback, descend back into the depths of the forest, and generally follow a gentle ridge route down to a junction with a spur trail (2,062.5–3,950') that descends west–southwest 70 yards to a seeping spring.

CAMPING The slopes steepen, and so does the route, which switchbacks down to a dry creek, contours north, then turns west, where a two-log crossing with handrails spans Warm Springs River (2,064.6–3,347'), with campsites on both sides.

TRAIL INFO You've also just crossed the N45° latitude line and are midway between the equator and the North Pole. If you hike the entire PCT, about 2,650 miles long, you'll cover only 16.5° of latitude, going from about 32.5° at the Mexican border to about 49° in Manning Park.

Climb north above a tributary ravine and reach a flat, where you meet a signed spur trail (2,064.9–3,450'), which heads 70 yards east–southeast to a spring.

CAMPING While traversing the Warm Springs Reservation, heed the warning signs, which caution hikers not to trespass or stray or camp outside of the legal 200-foot corridor. Violations are considered serious and are handled as such. Camp can be made only within the 200-foot right-of-way corridor even in this open-forest area.

Beyond the spring, you cross a linear meadow that is being invaded by lodgepole pines and then climb gradually increasing slopes to a junction with FS 4245 (2,066.1–3,807'); traveling southwest along this road, you would reach FS42 in 3.4 miles. Walk 17 yards northeast up FS 4245 to a resumption of the trail, and follow it north up to the east slope of andesitic Summit Butte (4,790'). Next make a gentle descent north, pass under a high-voltage power line (2,068.1–4,210'), cross northwest past unseen Red Wolf Pass (2,069.0–4,099'), and then reach a jeep road (2,069.4–3,990') that diagonals northeast across the route.

The trail continues its descent north and parallels a seasonal creek on the right (east) shortly before intersecting closed Mount Wilson Road/FS S549 (2,070.7–3,580'), which, like the PCT, heads toward the Clackamas Lake area, reentering Mount Hood National Forest. Cross this road and roughly parallel it northwest, leaving the Warm Springs Reservation before reaching a junction with Miller Trail 534 (2,072.6–3,427').

WATER ACCESS

CAMPING Miller Trail makes a moderate descent northwest before contouring west to large, well-maintained Clackamas Lake Campground, 0.7 mile distant. Why it is so popular is a mystery, for the nearby lake appears to be little more than a polluted cattle pond, and campground vistas are virtually nonexistent. Could it be the

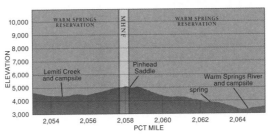

> campground's two old-fashioned, muscle-powered water pumps? Actually, the lake's water is better than you'd guess at first, for it is spring-fed.

The PCT turns north; proceeds through the forest bordering the meadow's edge to a usually dry crossing of Oak Grove Fork Clackamas River; and, after 40 yards west, reaches a spur trail that goes 280 yards southwest to Joe Graham Horse Camp. On the PCT, you go 300 yards west; meet Headwaters Trail 522, starting northeast toward the upper Oak Grove Fork Clackamas River; and then in a few yards reach paved FS 42 (2,073.4–3,370'). The PCT crosses this road just 90 yards northeast of the entrance to Joe Graham Horse Camp, which in turn is 200 yards northeast of a junction with FS 57. Start west on the trail and soon see Oak Grove Fork Clackamas River below on the left (southwest). Shortly you descend to this creek, climb a little, and then pass a spring 0.3 mile before reaching Timothy Lake Trail 528 (2,074.7–3,286'), which makes an 8-mile traverse around Timothy Lake (3,232'), passing campgrounds, picnic areas, and creeks before rejoining the PCT near the lake's northeast end.

You can see the lake from this junction, from which the PCT winds gradually down to the lake's unappealing east shore. The shoreline improves as you head north, and the trail contours northeast around it, passing several trailside springs, some of them seasonal, a few minutes before you reach a bridge over wide, clear Crater Creek (2,078.5–3,234'). Just north of this crossing, Timothy Lake Trail 528 rejoins the PCT from the west.

CAMPING About 450 yards beyond that junction, you reach Little Crater Lake Trail 500 (2,078.8–3,245'). This trail strikes east 220 yards to 45-foot-deep, extremely clear Little Crater Lake, which is an oversize artesian spring. Its

purity is maintained by a fence that keeps out the cattle. You can camp at pleasant Little Crater Lake Campground, which is just 200 yards east of the lake. Little Crater looks like the ideal swimming hole, but stick your arm down into it—brrrr! As with most springs, its water stays an almost constant year-round 40°F.

PLANTS Back on the PCT, the path north to Mount Hood is now deficient in views, lakes, creeks, and weekday hikers, but it is great if you like the solitude of a shady forest such as this one. This forest has Douglas-fir; western and mountain hemlocks; western red and Alaska cedars; silver, noble, grand, and subalpine firs; and western white and lodgepole pines.

The trail starts northwest and then gradually curves north up to FS 5890 (2,080.3–3,355'), which gently descends northeast to a crossing of Crater Creek. Bear north 30 yards on a diagonal across the road, and then continue north up to FS 58 (2,081.9–3,879'), which would lead you back to Little Crater Lake Campground and FS 42. Traversing through a forest of mountain hemlock and lodgepole, you next reach FS 240 (2,082.4–3,878').

WATER ACCESS

CAMPING Not far beyond it, you pass through a small campsite (2,082.7–3,928') that has a seeping spring. If you make camp here, set it up 75 feet away from, and tread lightly around, the spring. This could be your last on-trail

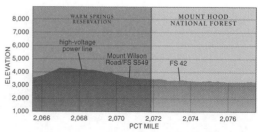

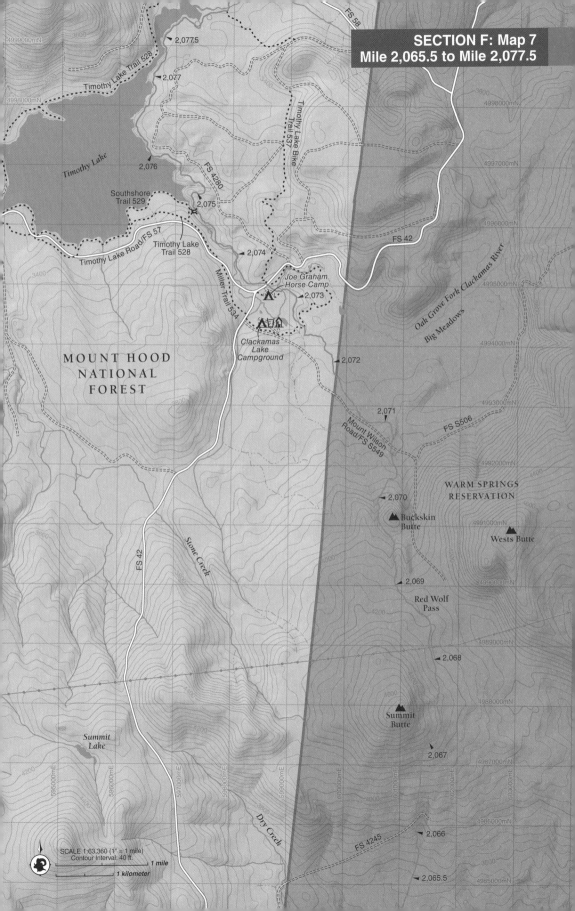

4999000mN

2,077.5

2,077

Timothy Lake Trail 528

FS 58

4998000mN

Timothy Lake Bike Trail 537

4997000mN

Timothy Lake

2,076

FS 4280

Southshore Trail 529

2,075

4996000mN

FS 42

Oak Grove Fork Clackamas River

Timothy Lake Road/FS 57

Timothy Lake Trail 528

2,074

Miller Trail 534

Joe Graham Horse Camp

2,073

Big Meadows

4995000mN

Clackamas Lake Campground

2,072

4994000mN

MOUNT HOOD NATIONAL FOREST

2,071

Mount Wilson Road/FS S549

FS S506

4993000mN

4992000mN

WARM SPRINGS RESERVATION

2,070

4400

3600

Buckskin Butte

Wests Butte

4991000mN

FS 42

Stone Creek

2,069

Red Wolf Pass

4990000mN

4200

2,068

4989000mN

Summit Butte

Summit Lake

2,067

4988000mN

595000mE

596000mE

597000mE

598000mE

599000mE

600000mE

601000mE

602000mE

603000mE

4987000mN

Dry Creek

2,066

FS 4245

4986000mN

2,065.5

4985000mN

SCALE 1:63,360 (1" = 1 mile)
Contour Interval: 40 ft.

1 mile

1 kilometer

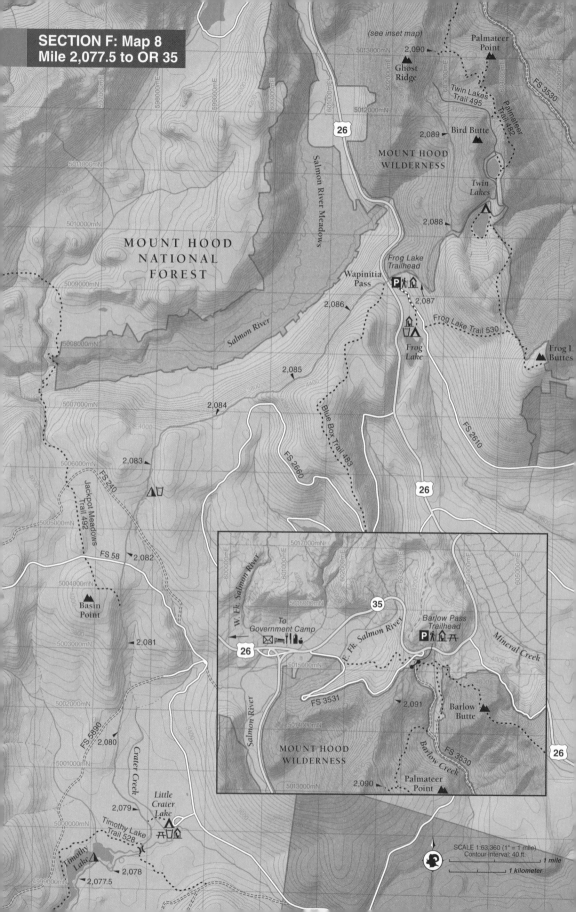

Palmateer Point

2,090

Ghost Ridge

5013000mN

FS 3530

Twin Lakes Trail 495

2,089 ► Bird Butte

Palmateer Trail 482

5012000mN

MOUNT HOOD WILDERNESS

Salmon River Meadows

26

Twin Lakes

5011000mN

2,088 ►

Frog Lake Trailhead

Wapinitia Pass

5010000mN

2,086 ►

2,087

Frog Lake Trail 530

Frog Lake

MOUNT HOOD NATIONAL FOREST

5009000mN

FS 2610

Frog L. Buttes

2,085

Salmon River

5008000mN

3800

2,084 ►

Blue Box Trail 483

5007000mN

FS 2660

26

2,083 ►

FS 240

5006000mN

Jackpot Meadows Trail 492

5005000mN

FS 58   2,082 ►

5004000mN

Basin Point

2,081 ►

5003000mN

5017000mN

W. Fk. Salmon River

601000mE

35

Barlow Pass Trailhead

Mineral Creek

5016000mN

To Government Camp

E. Fk. Salmon River

FS 5890

2,080 ►

26

5015000mN

Crater Creek

FS 3531

2,091 ►

Barlow Butte

5002000mN

5014000mN

Salmon River

26

5001000mN

Barlow Creek

FS 3530

Little Crater Lake

5013000mN

2,090 ► Palmateer Point

MOUNT HOOD WILDERNESS

5000000mN

2,079 ►

Timothy Lake Trail 528

4999000mN

Timothy Lake

2,078 ►

SCALE 1:63,360 (1" = 1 mile)
Contour Interval: 40 ft.

1 mile

1 kilometer

► 2,077.5

water until the upper Salmon River, 14 miles farther. However, water can be obtained 0.6 mile off the PCT at Frog Lake Campground, about 4 miles away.

The PCT now climbs north to a saddle, and then makes a long traverse northeast through a beautiful forest filled with rhododendron and occasional glimpses of Mount Hood through the trees to a junction with Blue Box Trail 483, which strikes south to Clear Lake (3,500').

RESUPPLY ACCESS

In 50 yards you reach US 26 (2,086.5–3,914') near Wapinitia Pass. Hikers can follow this highway 6.7 miles north to the post office and village store at Government Camp. Or walk across where the highway widens and traffic coming uphill in either direction naturally slows at the wide pullout, from where you can hitch a ride. Oregon has a strong understanding about hitchhiking, especially here. A quicker route to Government Camp that starts from Barlow Pass is described at the end of this chapter.

Walk another 70 yards and you'll reach a spur trail that goes 40 yards to the Frog Lake PCT trailhead parking lot beside the busy highway.

CAMPING From the parking lot, FS 2610 curves southeast and after 0.3 mile gives rise to Frog Lake Road 230, branching southwest. Starting on it, you'll come to the entrance to Frog Lake Campground. You might plan to camp here or at least get water.

Only 120 yards past the parking-lot trail, the PCT meets southbound Frog Lake Trail 530, which quickly crosses FS 2610, soon crosses FS 230, and then parallels FS 230 to the northwest lobe of Frog Lake.

Leaving Trail 530, the PCT continues northeast through a solemn forest of western hemlock, curves southeast upward, and then switchbacks north to a near-crest junction with Twin Lakes Trail 495 (2,087.9–4,397').

From this point, you can either stay on the PCT or take an alternate route. On the PCT, there is no reliable water from here until off-route sources about 4 miles ahead near Barlow Pass.

ALTERNATE ROUTE From here, the Twin Lakes Trail immediately crosses a crest saddle, visits the two glistening orbs, and then, after a total length of 2.75 miles, rejoins the PCT. This lake loop used to be a part of the PCT, but the easily accessible Twin Lakes became overused, and the PCT was rerouted in the mid-1970s. Still, many PCT hikers prefer this longer route, if not for its aesthetics then at least for its water.

Beyond the near-crest junction, the PCT makes a shady, viewless traverse north to a

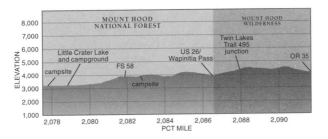

broad saddle, and then continues northwest to a reunion with the alternate-route loop trail (2,089.5–4,356').

From this junction the PCT heads north, passes southeast-descending Palmateer Trail 482 (2,090.0–4,450'), and then soon hugs the crest for a 1.5-mile descent to an old section of OR 35 at Barlow Pass (2,091.5–4,157'). You'll find a PCT trailhead parking area immediately west of here.

RESUPPLY ACCESS

Most hikers will continue along Section G's PCT to Timberline Lodge, which serves good but expensive food and which also holds parcels for hikers—for a fee (see Section G, "Supplies"). Long-distance PCT hikers on a shoestring budget may want to have their parcels mailed to Government Camp Post Office rather than to Timberline Lodge.

To reach Government Camp, descend west along the old section of OR 35, now FS 3531. Starting at Barlow Pass, this takes you down past an obvious roadside spring to a scenic hairpin turn and then down to a pioneer woman's grave, on your left, about 100 yards before crossing the East Fork Salmon River. Just 0.3 mile west of the crossing, FS 3531 ends at OR 35, 2.5 miles from Barlow Pass.

Continuing west, you soon pass through the large, high-speed interchange of US 26 and OR 35 and then follow traffic over to the start of Timberline Highway, opposite the Summit Ranger Station. Just 0.25 mile past it, you fork right and take the Government Camp road through town, reaching Government Camp Post Office just 250 yards past the moderately well-stocked village store.

Now backtrack 0.8 mile to Timberline Highway, follow it 4.5 miles up past the entrance to Alpine Campground, and then go up to the road's end at giant Timberline Lodge. At the north end of the large hikers' parking lot, below the lodge, register at a small hut. You'll find the PCT making an obvious slice across the slopes just above the lodge. Although you've bypassed part of the PCT by taking this route, you can see from a distance the best part of what you've missed by scanning along the PCT for a long 0.5 mile east to the White River buried forest overlook, described in Section G.

As you start to parallel the old section of OR 35 northeast, you immediately cross FS 3530, descending south. Past it, the PCT soon becomes an abandoned road that takes you on a minute's walk to this section's end, a crossing of OR 35 (2,091.7–4,164'). You should be able to find water in a small ravine about 130 yards east of this crossing. If not, and if you're desperate, start down the resupply access to Government Camp that begins 0.2 mile back, at Barlow Pass.

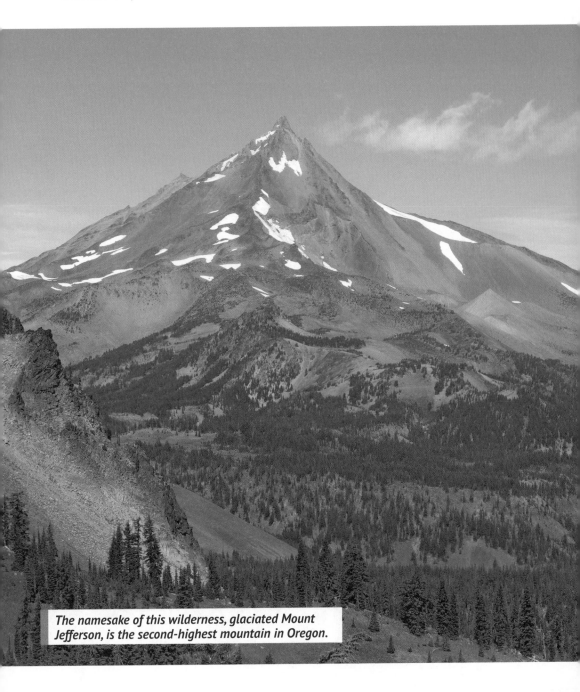

The namesake of this wilderness, glaciated Mount Jefferson, is the second-highest mountain in Oregon.

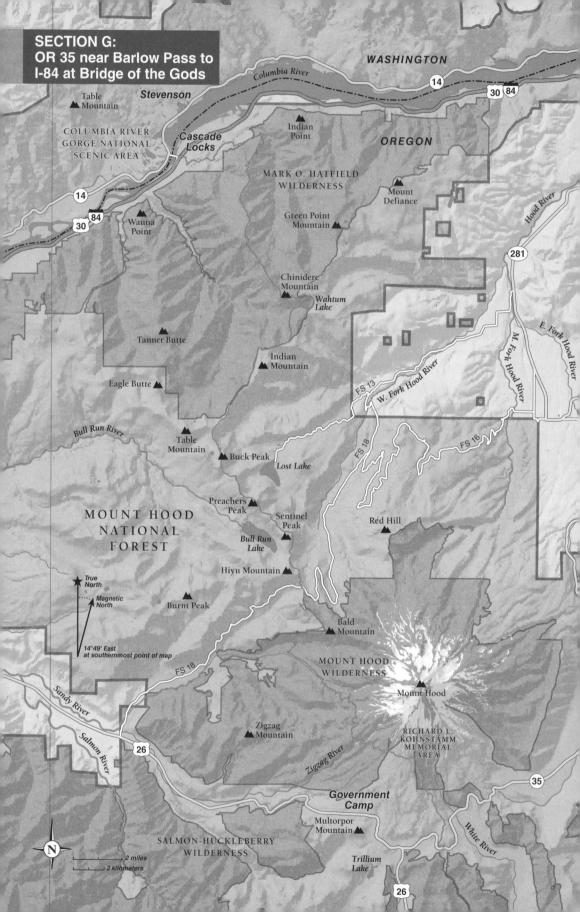

SECTION G:
OR 35 near Barlow Pass to
I-84 at Bridge of the Gods

WASHINGTON

Columbia River

14

30 84

Stevenson

Table
Mountain

COLUMBIA RIVER
GORGE NATIONAL
SCENIC AREA

Cascade
Locks

Indian
Point

OREGON

MARK O. HATFIELD
WILDERNESS

Mount
Defiance

Hood River

14

84

30

Wauna
Point

Green Point
Mountain

281

Chinidere
Mountain

Wahtum
Lake

E. Fork Hood River

Tanner Butte

Indian
Mountain

FS 13

W. Fork Hood River

M. Fork Hood River

Eagle Butte

FS 18

FS 16

Bull Run River

Table
Mountain

Buck Peak

Lost Lake

MOUNT HOOD
NATIONAL
FOREST

Preachers
Peak

Sentinel
Peak

Red Hill

Bull Run
Lake

Hiyu Mountain

★ True
   North

Magnetic
North

Burnt Peak

Bald
Mountain

14°49' East
at southernmost point of map

MOUNT HOOD
WILDERNESS

FS 18

Sandy River

Mount Hood

Salmon River

RICHARD L.
KOHNSTAMM
MEMORIAL
AREA

26

Zigzag
Mountain

Zigzag River

35

White River

Government
Camp

Multorpor
Mountain

N

SALMON-HUCKLEBERRY
WILDERNESS

Trillium
Lake

2 miles

2 kilometers

26

26

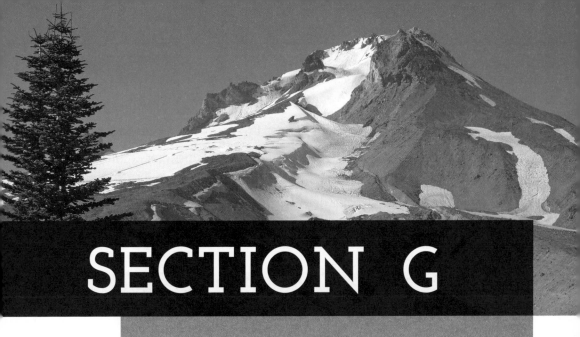

SECTION G

OR 35 near Barlow Pass to I-84 at Bridge of the Gods

IN THIS SHORT SECTION, you traverse around Oregon's highest and most popular peak: glacier-robed Mount Hood. If you start your hike at Timberline Lodge, you can make it around the peak in one long (about 19 miles), though relatively easy, day. Hiking in the opposite direction, however, requires considerable effort, for in that direction you have a *net* (not total) gain of 2,520 feet instead of a net loss.

From Bald Mountain north past Lolo Pass to Wahtum Lake, the scenery is subdued—a typical, forested Oregon Cascades crest. North of Wahtum Lake, the Pacific Crest Trail (PCT) travels through a quiet plateau blanketed by a majestic forest, partly burned in a 2017 fire, then makes a relentless descent into the Columbia River Gorge. Many hikers prefer the unusually dramatic Eagle Creek Trail as an alternate route, with its abundant waterfalls within a steep-walled canyon. However, this canyon is also

Above: From the Barlow Pass trailhead, Mount Hood rises over 7,000 feet. Fortunately, hikers don't have to climb that high to reach Timberline Lodge.

regenerating from the fire of 2017, and as we went to press, Eagle Creek Trail was closed to the public. Crews are hard at work restoring the footpath and bridges, and the trail is expected to reopen. To check its status, visit pcta.org/discover-the-trail/closures/oregon/eagle-creek-columbia -river. Note that Eagle Creek Trail is a foot trail only; it is impassable and prohibited for stock.

DECLINATION 14°49'E

USGS MAPS

Mount Hood South, OR	Carson, WA
Wahtum Lake, OR	Bull Run Lake, OR
Government Camp, OR	Bonneville Dam, WA

POINTS ON THE TRAIL, SOUTH TO NORTH

	Mile	Elevation in feet	Latitude/Longitude
OR 35 near Barlow Pass	2,091.7	4,164	N45° 17' 04.2880" W121° 40' 52.7708"
Join the Timberline Trail	2,095.6	5,345	N45° 19' 19.0545" W121° 41' 45.7769"
Trail junction to Timberline Lodge	2,097.0	6,048	N45° 19' 49.9452" W121° 42' 37.9006"
Paradise Park Loop Trail first junction	2,100.7	5,020	N45° 20' 35.1672" W121° 45' 08.4276"
Paradise Park Loop Trail second junction	2,103.2	5,447	N45° 21' 39.8448" W121° 45' 07.4376"
Ramona Falls Trail first junction	2,106.9	3,323	N45° 22' 47.6150" W121° 47' 03.1763"
Ramona Falls Trail second junction	2,108.9	2,810	N45° 23' 44.0105" W121° 48' 02.8736"
Leave the Timberline Trail	2,111.4	4,341	N45° 24' 19.0351" W121° 46' 42.4926"
Lolo Pass	2,114.2	3,437	N45° 25' 37.5717" W121° 47' 48.4938"
Huckleberry Mountain Trail junction	2,118.4	4,020	N45° 28' 04.2503" W121° 49' 45.3876"
Wahtum Lake at Eagle Creek Trail junction	2,130.3	3,751	N45° 34' 48.7344" W121° 47' 57.7312"
Teakettle Spring	2,139.0	3,403	N45° 39' 26.2471" W121° 50' 32.3763"
Junction with lateral trail to Herman Creek	2,142.5	978	N45° 40' 18.2328" W121° 50' 20.6740"
Bridge of the Gods (east end)	2,146.9	219	N45° 39' 42.4383" W121° 53' 51.1225"

CAMPSITES AND BIVY SITES

Mile	Elevation in feet	Latitude/ Longitude	Number of tents	Feature	Notes
2,100.7 (alt.)	5,699	N45° 21' 06.4249" W121° 44' 50.2775"	3		1.2 miles off PCT; former site of Paradise Park Shelter; shade
2,106.9 (alt.)	3,536	N45° 22' 47.8200" W121° 46' 34.0800"	2	Ramona Falls	Camp at least 500 feet from falls
2,106.9 (alt.)	4,176	N45° 23' 22.3837" W121° 44' 53.4618"	>4	Muddy Fork tributary	

CAMPSITES AND BIVY SITES *(continued)*

Mile	Elevation in feet	Latitude/ Longitude	Number of tents	Feature	Notes
2,108.9	2,797	N45° 23' 41.8545" W121° 48' 05.6826"	3		Horse camp
2,114.2	3,435	N45° 25' 36.6099" W121° 47' 46.3973"	3	Road nearby	
2,118.6	4,085	N45° 28' 14.5552" W121° 49' 48.5824"	2	Salvation Spring Camp	Shaded bivy
2,121.3	4,230	N45° 29' 20.2447" W121° 51' 31.6635"	2		Flat spot near trail on right; no fires
2,130.2 (alt.)	1,440	N45° 34' 15.2868" W121° 51' 11.6172"	>4	7.5 Mile Camp	Campfires discouraged
2,130.2 (alt.)	908	N45° 35' 20.3568" W121° 51' 39.2760"	4	Blue Grouse Camp	No campfires June 1–September 15; access to Eagle Creek
2,130.2 (alt.)	836	N45° 35' 40.8480" W121° 52' 05.2320"	8	Wy'East Camp	No campfires
2,130.2 (alt.)	200	N45° 38' 32.0784" W121° 55' 31.0224"	17	Eagle Creek Campground	14 of the sites must be reserved; vault toilet, fire ring
2,127.6	4,260	N45° 33' 25.3447" W121° 49' 36.0950"	4	Indian Springs	Spring nearby
2,130.6	3,900	N45° 34' 38.3160" W121° 47' 32.8920"	5	Wahtum Lake Campground	Just east of trail; vault toilet, picnic table, fire pit
2,130.6	3,774	N45° 34' 45.5644" W121° 47' 39.8027"	>4	Wahtum Lake	
2,136.6	3,966	N45° 37' 53.1104" W121° 51' 07.7012"	2	Along Ruckel Creek Trail	0.6 mile off PCT; near spring
2,146.9 (alt.)	105	N45° 40' 03.2880" W121° 53' 44.2752"	>15	Cascade Locks Marine Park	PCT campsites; restrooms, showers, water, Wi-Fi

SUPPLIES

This section is short enough that most hikers don't worry about supplies. However, long-distance hikers will certainly want to pick up packages they've mailed to Timberline Lodge, which lies only 5.3 miles into this section's route. Packages are held at Guest Services at the Wy'East Day Lodge, which has a $10 charge for each package. Send your packages to: Guest Services, Timberline Lodge, 27500 E. Timberline Road, Government Camp, OR 97028. Timberline Lodge, like other premier mountain lodges, is expensive. Those who can afford it can get rooms, meals, and showers, plus the use of a heated pool and a sauna. There is also a shower for PCT hikers in the Salmon River parking lot.

You can avoid a charge by mailing packages to the Government Camp post office (also 97028), a few miles off-route. Government Camp also has a small market, a motel and a hotel, breweries, restaurants, and a gas station. See page 194 at the end of Section F for directions on reaching this small settlement.

Halfway through your trek, you can take the Huckleberry Mountain Trail down to a small store at the north end of Lost Lake. However, few hikers do so. Finally, at trail's end in Cascade Locks (post office 97014), you can find almost anything you need. If you can't, take the bus west into Portland or east to much-closer Hood River.

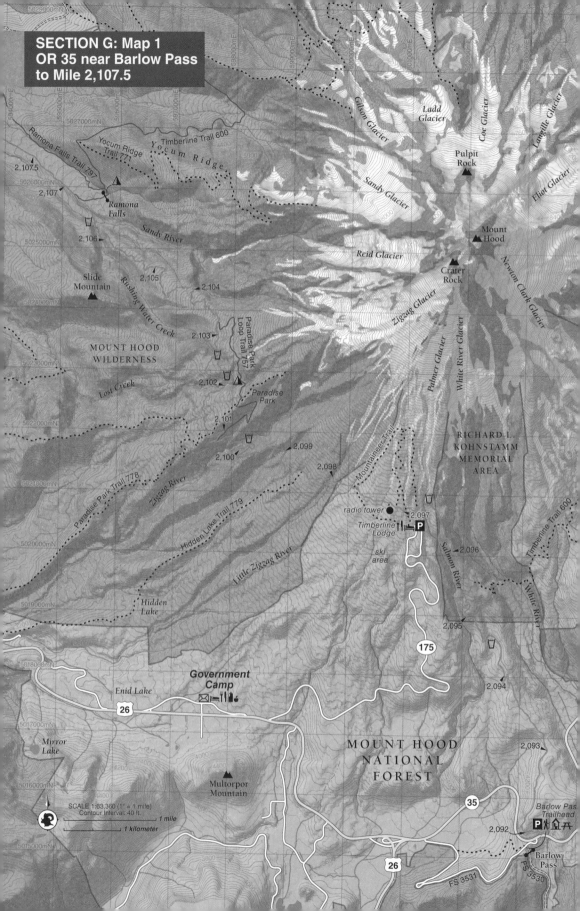

Gilson Glacier

Ladd Glacier

Coe Glacier

Langille Glacier

Pulpit Rock ▲

Sandy Glacier

Eliot Glacier

Ramona Falls Trail 797

Yocum Ridge Trail 771

Timberline Trail 600

Yocum Ridge

2,107.5

⚑

2,107

● Ramona Falls

Mount Hood ▲

Reid Glacier

Sandy River

Crater Rock ▲

Newton Clark Glacier

2,106 ⎕

Rushing Water Creek

Slide Mountain ▲

2,105

2,104

Zigzag Glacier

Palmer Glacier

White River Glacier

MOUNT HOOD WILDERNESS

Lost Creek

Paradise Park Loop Trail 757

2,103 ⎕

2,102 ⎕ ⚑

Paradise Park

RICHARD L. KOHNSTAMM MEMORIAL AREA

2,101

Paradise Park Trail 778

Zigzag River

2,100

2,099

2,098

Mountaineer Trail

Timberline Trail 600

Hidden Lake Trail 779

radio tower ●

⎕

2,097

Timberline Lodge

P

Salmon River

2,096

Little Zigzag River

ski area

2,095

White River

Hidden Lake

175

2,094

Government Camp

✉ 🏕 ⛽

Enid Lake

26

2,093

MOUNT HOOD NATIONAL FOREST

Mirror Lake

⎕

Multorpor Mountain

35

Barlow Pass Trailhead

P 🏕 ⛺

2,092

SCALE 1:63,360 (1" = 1 mile)
Contour Interval: 40 ft.

1 mile

1 kilometer

26

Barlow Pass

FS 3531

FS 3530

OR 35 NEAR BARLOW PASS TO I-84 AT BRIDGE OF THE GODS
>>>THE ROUTE

Section G begins where the PCT heads diagonally across OR 35 (2,091.7–4,164') just east of Barlow Pass. This crossing is 90 yards northeast of a junction with the northeast end of Barlow Road 3530. Drive 0.25 mile southwest down this road to find a PCT trailhead parking area—the start of Section F's alternate route that goes to Government Camp. If you must stock up on water, get it at an obvious roadside spring 0.5 mile southwest past the parking area or in a small ravine about 130 yards east of where the PCT crosses OR 35.

From OR 35, the PCT starts northeast, but it immediately angles west for a climb to the Cascade divide. Ascending north, it stays close to the crest of the divide, and you may see one or more cross-country ski routes, marked by blue diamonds nailed to trees. For a short stretch, the PCT is part of a ski route when under snow.

WATER ACCESS

Eventually, the PCT curves northwest over to a ravine (2,094.5–4,822') with *usually* flowing water.

From this cool forest retreat, your trail methodically climbs over to the slopes of the Salmon River canyon, where you can look west toward Alpine Campground (not accessible from the trail) and see a cliff below it. The trail then climbs northeast to a junction with

Timberline Trail 600 (2,095.6–5,345'), which starts a descent east to the White River. This trail, which stays near timberline as it circles Mount Hood (11,249'), offers an alternative 25.7-mile route if you take it counterclockwise to a reunion with the PCT near Bald Mountain. Clockwise, it coincides with the PCT, which starts northwest up a ridge of loose, gravelly debris.

GEOLOGY If you look east at the cliff composed of unsorted volcanic debris that is above the White River, you'll get an idea of the type of sediments you're walking on. These deposits, which are on the south and southwest slopes of Mount Hood, are remnants of a huge debris fan of hornblende andesite formed 1,800–1,400 years ago when a crater was blasted out near the mountain's summit and a plug dome of viscous lava welled up, melting the surrounding ice field. The sudden release of water created devastating mudflows that carried the volcanic debris down to these slopes that the PCT crosses today. Due north, you can identify Crater Rock (10,564'), which is a remnant of that plug dome. Just north of it, numerous fissures still emit steam and hydrogen sulfide gas. On clear, windless days, the gas emissions from these fumaroles are visible from as far away as Portland. Mount Hood had minor eruptions in the mid-1800s, and you can be sure that it is still alive today.

Not too far ahead, you reach the White River buried forest overlook (2,096.3–5,799'). If you scrutinize the lower mudflow sediments

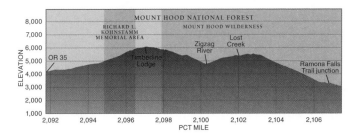

in the canyon's wall, you should be able to recognize a few buried snags. Radiocarbon dating was used on these snags to date the eruptions mentioned above.

Leaving the overlook, the trail soon curves northwest away from the canyon views, crosses a dry creekbed, and then crosses the upper Salmon River (2,096.7–5,982'), which derives its flow from an arm of the Palmer Glacier.

WATER ACCESS

This flow is the first reliable on-route water since a seeping spring just past Linney Creek Road 240, 14 trail miles south.

The trail now contours southwest past an ascending dirt road and then quickly reaches a spur trail (2,097.0–6,048')—one of many—that descends to the east side of Timberline Lodge. Stock are not allowed on the PCT between the lodge and Paradise Park Loop Trail 757.

RESUPPLY ACCESS

No hiker should pass up the opportunity to inspect this grand structure, built by the Works Progress Administration in the late 1930s. See "Supplies" on page 199 for more information. Timberline Lodge serves a breakfast buffet at 7:30 a.m. Lunch and dinner buffets are also available for latecomers.

SIDE TRIP Just east of and below the lodge's parking lot is an even larger lot for backpackers and mountaineers; at its north end is a small hut

where you should register if you plan to hike any farther or if you plan to climb Mount Hood. Mountaineers who climb it often try to reach the summit by sunrise to avoid avalanche hazards due to warming snow and ice. By early July rockfalls can also become a real danger along south-slope routes. Don't attempt to climb the peak unless you are an experienced mountaineer and are familiar with Hood's routes and hazards.

After ascending one of the spur trails or roads from the lodge back to the PCT, hike west 0.1 mile under the ski lift and past a radio tower below, and then gradually descend west with views south across a rolling topography to lofty Mount Jefferson (10,497'). You enter Mount Hood Wilderness (2,097.7–5,959') and cross several seasonal creeks before making a 3-yard boulder-hop across silty Little Zigzag River (2,098.0–5,832') and continuing your descent to a junction with Hidden Lake Trail 779 (2,098.4–5,715'), which goes southwest down a morainal ridge to Hidden Lake. The PCT continues its rambling descent and then climbs to a narrow ridge from which you get a great view of Mount Hood and glaciated Zigzag Canyon.

WATER ACCESS

Now switchback down the steep slope, jump across the silty Zigzag River (2,100.3–4,776'), and climb moderately into and out of a tributary canyon, up to a point where you have a choice of two routes: the official PCT and the older, also scenic former PCT route, given as an alternate.

ALTERNATE ROUTE Those on foot can take the older PCT route, a stretch of the old Oregon Skyline Trail (OST) that is more scenic. The Paradise Park Loop Trail 757 (2,100.7–5,020') starts northeast up the tributary canyon of Zigzag Canyon. The ascent finally eases just after gaining access to a ridge and, after a full mile, meeting Paradise Park Trail 778, which descends west-southwest through an alpine meadow. Continuing straight (north) on the Paradise Park Loop Trail, you now hike 0.2 mile to Lost Creek.

PLANTS The banks of this creek are ablaze with common and Lewis monkeyflowers, lupine, bistort, corn lily, mariposa lily, yarrow, paintbrush, pasqueflower, aster, and eriogonum.

CAMPING Push onward to reach the site of the former Paradise Park Shelter 500 feet ahead in an open forest of dwarf hemlock. Though the shelter is gone, the site is still good for camping. Campsites must be at least 200 feet from any creek or body of water. From here, the trail makes a slight climb and then contours across more alpine meadows before it switchbacks down to a reunion with the PCT in another mile.

The official PCT, which equestrians *must* take, starts west-southwest and switchbacks up to a broad ridge where Paradise Park Trail 778 (2,101.2–5,247') crosses the trail.

WATER ACCESS

Your route ascends north across the ridge and turns northeast to descend to splashing Lost Creek (2,102.0–5,375'), which cascades down a cliff just to the east. Cross it and its more reserved tributary, and then climb west to a ridge, top the ridge, and descend once again—this time to a crossing of Rushing Water Creek (2,102.6–5,480') just below its narrow waterfall.

After climbing steeply north out of this cliff-bound canyon, you follow a rather direct trail down to rejoin the alternate route through Paradise Park (2,103.2–5,447').

VIEWS Now you make a switchbacking descent along the PCT and obtain two fantastic views: up toward the glacier-mantled summit above and down on the mountain below. There's one more view, from a vertical-sided ridge at the end of a 50-yard spur trail, and it is the most revealing of all. The cliffs of the Sandy River canyon and its tributary canyon are composed of andesite flows and interbedded pyroclastic deposits. As if this flood of magnificent scenery were not enough to satisfy, the trail takes you down to the west side of the ridge, where your view is saturated with the impressive, naked cliffs of Slide Mountain (4,872') and of Rushing Water Creek canyon.

WATER ACCESS

If you are low on water, get some from Rushing Water Creek (2,106.3–3,388') at the bottom of the switchbacks from the

SECTION G

> viewpoint because Sandy River is just that—a sandy river.

Beyond the creek, the PCT quickly reaches the bouldery, bushy bottom of the Sandy River canyon. During floods, the river can be wall-to-wall, up to 100 yards wide, and when it is, it can obliterate the trail. Generally, however, the river is only a few yards wide, and depending on what a past flood did to the trail, you'll hike down either one side of the river or the other, or perhaps even between two parallel streams.

After about a 300-yard ramble downstream among boulders and brush, you reach a low cliff of unsorted, poorly bedded sediments. The PCT makes a short climb up it and reaches a flat bench (2,106.7–3,258'). From it, a steep path climbs about 50 yards east to Upper Sandy River Guard Station, which is locked and unmanned. From the bench, the PCT climbs north to reach a junction with Ramona Falls Trail 797–Timberline Trail 600 (2,106.9–3,323').

Here, hikers have a choice of three routes: the official PCT route and two alternates. The author highly recommends either of the alternate routes; the preferred route is the Ramona Falls Trail–Timberline Trail alternate. Equestrians are restricted to the official PCT, although they can ride west to a stock fence near Ramona Falls and catch a glimpse of it.

ALTERNATE ROUTES Ramona Falls Trail–Timberline Trail: This combination of trails is 1.2 miles longer than the PCT and the other alternate route. From the junction just north of the Upper Sandy River Guard Station, the route starts southeast on Ramona Falls Trail 797 and follows it east across a broad terrace that sprouts a dry, open forest. Within earshot of the falls, you

reach a stock fence. Equestrians must leave their animals here.

CAMPING East beyond the fence is a backpackers' camping area, and you can find sites above and below the trail; you must camp at least 500 feet from the falls.

About 0.4 mile from the trail junction, descend to the base of Ramona Falls, which splashes down moss-draped rocks. A few yards after the trail crosses the falls' creek, there is a junction. From here, go north-northwest on Timberline Trail 600. This leg starts with a serious 0.6-mile climb to a ridge junction with Yocum Ridge Trail 771, which climbs to alpine slopes near the south edge of Sandy Glacier.

CAMPING The Timberline Trail climbs more easily as it leaves this ridge trail, and then it levels and travels in and out of ravines before dropping to a cluster of small campsites about 70 yards before the first glacier-fed tributary of Muddy Fork.

You may have to wade across the first two tributaries, particularly if you are crossing them on a hot afternoon. Between the first and second fords, you get impressive views upcanyon of a serrated, pinnacle-studded ridge that separates cascading creeks from spreading Sandy Glacier. Beyond the second ford, you make a minute's stroll over to the jump-across third ford, which, unlike the others, is clear and flows beneath forest cover. Another minute down it, you come to

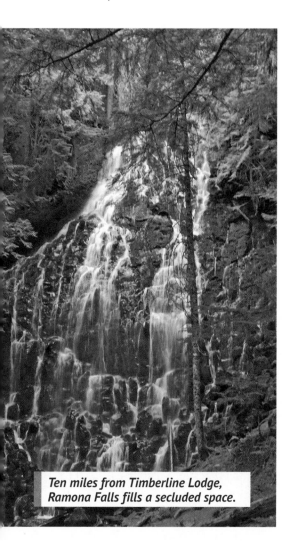

Ten miles from Timberline Lodge, Ramona Falls fills a secluded space.

Views disappear as you curve north out of Mount Hood Wilderness, enter forest cover, and make a 0.25-mile easy descent to a shady crest junction with the official PCT (2,111.4–4,341'), climbing from the west. Here you leave Timberline Trail 600 to rejoin the official PCT route, while Timberline Trail 600 strikes east to continue the loop of Mount Hood's slopes.

Ramona Falls Trail: In terms of scenery, this trail is the middle choice. From the junction just north of the Upper River Sandy Guard Station, this alternate route follows the Ramona Falls Trail–Timberline Trail, described above, as far as the junction just beyond the crossing of Ramona Falls' creek. From here, go northwest on the north arm of Ramona Falls Trail 797, descend 1 mile northwest along Ramona Falls' creek, and then go another 0.7 mile north to a junction with the official PCT (2,108.9–2,810'). Continue in accordance with the official PCT description, on the next page, from the paragraph beginning, "Here, the Ramona Falls Trail alternate route ..."

a spur trail that immediately crosses the creek.

Just past the spur, Timberline Trail 600 leaves the canyon floor and, over the next 0.5 mile, makes a gentle ascent west. Ascend past several creeklets before traversing Bald Mountain's south slopes. From these, there are unrestricted views—weather permitting—of towering Mount Hood as well as of forested Muddy Fork Canyon and the upper canyon's glacier-fed cascades.

From the intersection of the Ramona Falls Trail–Timberline Trail and the PCT, the PCT heads northwest, descending on a usually gentle grade as it parallels Sandy River at a distance. By the time you reach a junction with the Sandy River Trail 770 (2,108.4–2,767'), the lodgepole forest has become quite open.

CAMPING SIDE TRIP Should you need to reach civilization, you can take the Sandy River Trail 770 1.25 miles west from this junction to a popular trailhead and perhaps hitch a ride out. Also, from it, Forest Service Road 1825-100 goes about 0.5 mile west down to a junction, where you can head 0.3 mile south to Lost Creek Campground.

CAMPING The PCT continues 250 yards northeast to the Ramona Falls branch of the Sandy River before going 0.3 mile farther to a junction (2,108.9–2,810'); there's a nearby horse camp. Here, the Ramona Falls Trail alternate route rejoins the official PCT.

WATER ACCESS

From this point, you take the PCT north 70 yards to aptly named Muddy Fork. Be prepared for a difficult crossing and choose your crossing point carefully. The U.S. Forest Service has no plans to replace the previous bridge, as the banks are not stable enough to support it.

Now you make a moderate to steep, major switchbacking ascent to a ridge (2,110.6–3,876'), where you briefly leave the Mount Hood Wilderness. Ahead you have a moderate climb east to a junction just north of Bald Mountain (2,111.4–4,341'), where the Ramona

Falls Trail–Timberline Trail alternate route rejoins the official PCT. With all three routes finally back together at this junction north of Bald Mountain, you begin the next leg of the PCT, whose route from here to the Columbia River is more down than up.

Descending northwest just 50 yards, you reach a junction with the Top Spur Trail 785, which descends 0.4 mile west to FS 1828-118. Continue your forested route northwest to the crest's end, as you parallel the Mount Hood Wilderness boundary, and then start north down a series of switchbacks. Here, you briefly enter and then exit the wilderness. The thorny gooseberries, thimbleberries, and giant devil's clubs attest to the cool, moist slope of this forest, which you leave behind as you descend a drier north ridge to a clearing just south of Lolo Pass Road 18 (2,114.2–3,437') at Lolo Pass.

WATER ACCESS

A quarter mile west of here, you can find water running down to the road. Immediately east of the PCT, FS 1810 branches southeast from FS 18, going 0.4 mile to spring-fed water.

The northbound trailhead is about 20 yards southwest along paved FS 18 and 30 yards before this road's junction with paved FS 1828.

Start northwest from Lolo Pass, cross north under four sets of buzzing power lines, and then glance back northeast at Mount Hood's north

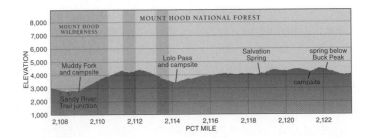

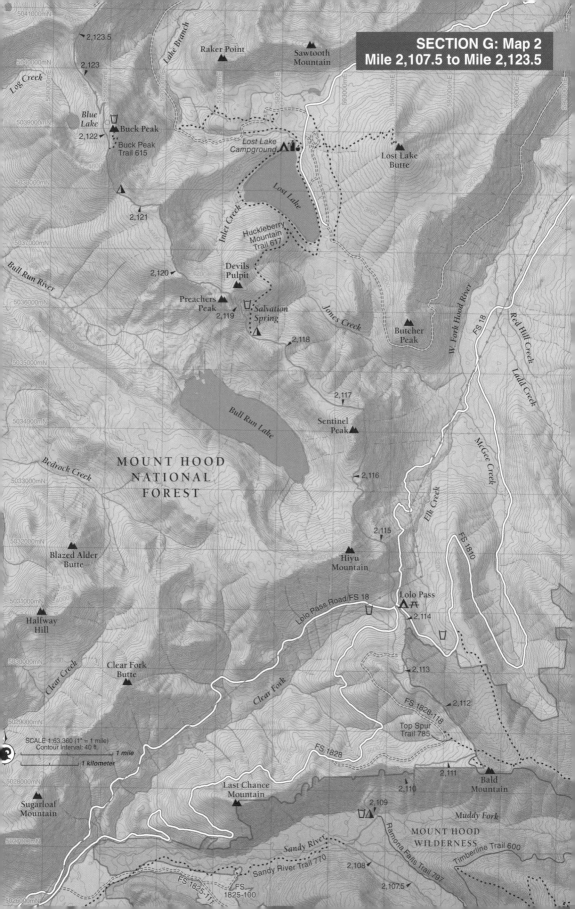

5041000mN

2,123.5

Log Creek

2,123

Lake Branch

Raker Point

Sawtooth
Mountain

5040000mN

Blue
Lake

Buck Peak

2,122

Buck Peak
Trail 615

Lost Lake
Campground

Lost Lake
Butte

5039000mN

5038000mN

2,121

Inlet Creek

Lost Lake

5037000mN

Huckleberry
Mountain
Trail 617

Bull Run River

Devils
Pulpit

2,120

W. Fork Hood River

FS 18

Red Hill Creek

5036000mN

Preachers
Peak

2,119

Salvation
Spring

Jones Creek

Butcher
Peak

Ladd Creek

5035000mN

2,118

2,117

McGee Creek

Bull Run Lake

Sentinel
Peak

5034000mN

2,116

Elk Creek

5033000mN

Bedrock Creek

MOUNT HOOD
NATIONAL
FOREST

2,115

FS 1810

5032000mN

Blazed Alder
Butte

Hiyu
Mountain

5031000mN

Halfway
Hill

Lolo Pass

2,114

Lolo Pass Road/FS 18

5030000mN

Clear Fork
Butte

Clear Creek

2,113

2,112

5029000mN

Clear Fork

FS 1828-118

Top Spur
Trail 785

SCALE 1:63,360 (1" = 1 mile)
Contour Interval: 40 ft.

FS 1828

1 mile

2,111

1 kilometer

Bald
Mountain

5028000mN

Last Chance
Mountain

2,110

Sugarloaf
Mountain

2,109

Muddy Fork

MOUNT HOOD
WILDERNESS

5027000mN

Sandy River

Ramona Falls Trail 797

Timberline Trail 600

5026000mN

Sandy River Trail 770

2,108

FS 1825-117

FS
1825-100

2,107.5

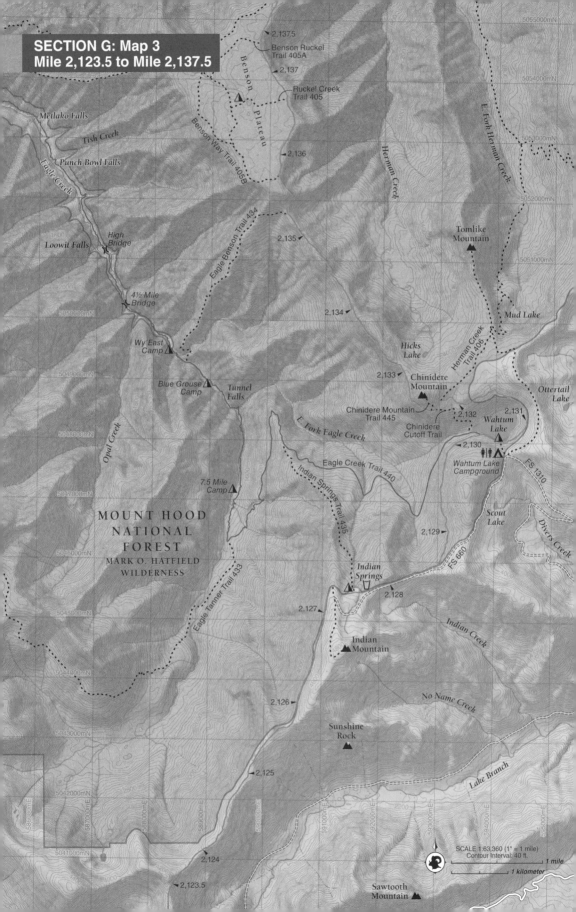

Metlako Falls

Tish Creek

Punch Bowl Falls

Eagle Creek

Loowit Falls

High Bridge

4½ Mile Bridge

Wy'East Camp

Blue Grouse Camp

Tunnel Falls

Opal Creek

7.5 Mile Camp

MOUNT HOOD
NATIONAL
FOREST

MARK O. HATFIELD
WILDERNESS

Eagle Tanner Trail 433

Eagle Benson Trail 434

Benson Way Trail 405B

2,137.5

Benson Ruckel Trail 405A

2,137

Ruckel Creek Trail 405

Benson Plateau

2,136

2,135

2,134

Herman Creek

E. Fork Herman Creek

Tomlike Mountain

Mud Lake

Hicks Lake

2,133

Chinidere Mountain

Herman Creek Trail 406

Ottertail Lake

Chinidere Mountain Trail 445

E. Fork Eagle Creek

2,132

Chinidere Cutoff Trail

2,131

Wahtum Lake

2,130

Wahtum Lake Campground

FS 1310

Eagle Creek Trail 440

Indian Springs Trail 435

2,129

Scout Lake

FS 660

Divers Creek

Indian Springs

2,128

2,127

Indian Creek

Indian Mountain

No Name Creek

2,126

Sunshine Rock

2,125

Lake Branch

2,124

2,123.5

Sawtooth Mountain

SCALE 1:63,360 (1" = 1 mile)
Contour Interval: 40 ft.

1 mile

1 kilometer

face. You soon reach a gully with a trickling creek (2,114.6–3,609') and then climb gradually north to the divide and circle the east slope of Sentinel Peak (4,565'). Rejoining the divide, the trail contours northwest past two low summits before arriving at a junction with Huckleberry Mountain Trail 617 (2,118.4–4,020').

CAMPING **SIDE TRIP** Huckleberry Mountain Trail 617 descends slightly 0.3 mile to a trickling creek in the gully below the Preachers Peak–Devils Pulpit saddle. If you descend this trail farther, you reach Lost Lake after another 1.9 miles; follow its east shore north to Lost Lake Campground, 0.8 mile along, and soon reach a small store by the lake's north end.

WATER ACCESS

CAMPING From the junction, contour 0.2 mile to a sharp bend in the trail, where a spur trail descends 50 yards to a trickling creek and the small, flat Salvation Spring Camp (2,118.6–4,085').

Back on route, continue north to a ravine, then switchback up to the Preachers Peak–Devils Pulpit saddle. From its two summits, you follow a huckleberry-lined path in a forest of hemlock and fir, descend to a saddle, climb

north up the ridge above Lost Lake, and then descend west to a notch.

Now a short, stiff climb north takes you to a saddle and a junction with Buck Peak Trail 615 (2,121.8–4,491'), which continues along the ridge up to Buck Peak (4,751').

WATER ACCESS

Descend north across the west slope of this peak to discover a small spring (2,122.1–4,426') a couple of feet below the west edge of the trail.

A little farther down the trail, you reach the ridge again and then switchback down to a long saddle from which you glimpse Blue Lake (3,770') below to the southwest. As the trail arcs northeast, you leave Portland's Bull Run Watershed behind for good, and with it the posted NO CAMPING signs you may have seen since Lolo Pass. Camping is prohibited to prevent forest fires.

Ahead the PCT flirts with the southeast boundary of the Mark O. Hatfield Wilderness for about 4.5 miles, as both the PCT and the wilderness boundary parallel an old crest-line road northeast.

TRAIL INFO The Mark O. Hatfield Wilderness, about 61 square miles with about 125 miles of trail, was created in 1984. Before then, the area had long been a de facto wilderness, spared the logger's ax. You won't see any clear-cutting once you reach Wahtum Lake,

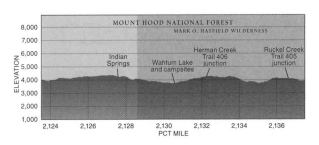

but you'll certainly see enough of it to the east on the upcoming crest-line traverse.

This next stretch follows a fairly level crest northeast; contours across the southeast slope of a low, triangular summit; and then finally climbs gently northeast to quickly reach abandoned FS 660 (2,125.8–4,279'), which is momentarily atop the ridge. Locate the trail on the northwest side of the road, parallel it north-northeast, and then round the north spur of Indian Mountain (4,920'), from which you see Mounts St. Helens (8,363'), Rainier (14,410'), and Adams (12,276').

WATER ACCESS

CAMPING   Descend east to Indian Springs (2,127.6–4,212'). Unfortunately, this area had to be logged over to remove snags left by a devastating 1920 fire. Make sure to camp at least 200 feet away from water sources.

Just beyond the spring, Indian Springs Trail 435 starts northwest toward Indian Mountain's north spur, follows it, and then steeply descends it 1.9 miles into the area burned in 2017. The PCT continues east past the spring and parallels the abandoned road, first below it and then above it, to a saddle, where it leaves the roadside to enter the Mark O. Hatfield Wilderness (2,128.6–4,099'). The trail then winds gently down a forested slope and then northeast down to a junction with Eagle Creek Trail 440 (2,130.3–3,751') just above the southwest shore of Wahtum Lake (3,723').

Here, you have a choice of the official PCT or an alternate route. Eagle Creek Trail 440, described below, was a popular alternate trail on the way to the Columbia River Gorge before it was closed due to fire damage in 2017. When it reopens, the author highly recommends this alternate route to nonacrophobic hikers only.

However, the trail can be crowded, especially in the last few miles, and sections are merely notches blasted into cliff walls to make passages suitable for nonacrophobic hikers but too low for riders. Therefore, equestrians must, and acrophobic hikers should, take the official PCT.

ALTERNATE ROUTE   The hike from Wahtum Lake down to the Columbia River is far more scenic, but also more crowded, along the Eagle Creek Trail than along the PCT. We describe it here as a highly recommended alternate route when it becomes available for hikers. Unfortunately, the terrain surrounding this trail was burned in a massive wildfire, started by humans, in 2017. The burn is a patchy mosaic. Many of the trees closer to the creek itself were spared, but high-intensity heat at the top of the canyon walls dislodged tons of rock that's still falling. Pacific Crest Trail Association volunteer and U.S. Forest Service crews are hard at work repairing the trail. We hope to join you on this trail in the future.

From the Wahtum Lake outlet, which is the East Fork Eagle Creek, Eagle Creek Trail 440 heads west then southwest. You then arc west down to a ford of the Indian Springs fork of East Fork Eagle Creek, which could be tricky to cross in early summer.

PLANTS   Begin a descent northwest that takes you past a regenerating understory of rhododendron, gooseberry, red elderberry, thimbleberry, huckleberry, devil's club, and Oregon grape.

Along this descent, 3 miles from the lake, you may see Indian Springs Trail 435, which climbs south 1.9 steep miles back to the PCT. After reaching a viewpoint at the tip of a north spur, your trail turns south and, in 1 mile, descends past a shallow ravine, crosses seasonal creeklets, turns north, and then makes a switchback in 0.7 mile. From here, Eagle Tanner Trail 433 heads upcanyon (southwest).

You continue on the Eagle Creek Trail. The slope is now much gentler, and in the near distance you can hear Eagle Creek splashing merrily down its course. In 0.5 mile you reach a rockbound creek.

WILDLIFE Don't be too surprised if a red-spotted garter snake is climbing a rock behind you; it needs water too. It is not uncommon to encounter half a dozen of these beneficial snakes in a day's hike along this verdant route.

CAMPING Just beyond the pleasant creek, you meet several trails that descend about 50 yards west to 7.5 Mile Camp. If you intend to camp before reaching the trailhead, this is a good place to stop if you set your tent away from overhead widowmakers. Before you lies a string of impressive waterfalls.

The trail gradually descends to the bank of Eagle Creek, and you see a 50-foot cascade—not too impressive, but a sample of what's to come. In 0.3 mile, the creek enters a safe,

very deep, crystal-clear pool that is extremely tempting for an afternoon swim, but the cool water will ensure that you won't stay in for long. Immediately beyond it is a two-stage, 100-foot-high waterfall, sliced into a narrow gorge, which you don't see until you round a vertical cliff where this exposed trail, blasted from the cliff, heads another 0.3 mile toward 150-foot-high Tunnel Falls.

This trail is definitely not for the faint-hearted; neither is its ceiling sufficient for those on horseback. The fall, in its grotto of vertical-walled basalt, is spectacular enough to make it the climax of this route, but your sensations of it are heightened even more as you head through a wet tunnel blasted behind the fall about midway up it. Leave this grotto of the East Fork in expectation of more high adventure. Below you, Eagle Creek cascades 30 feet down to another layer of this Miocene Columbia River basalt.

CAMPING The trail's exposure decreases considerably as you leave the falls' narrow gorge. In another 0.3 mile, you reach pleasant Blue Grouse Camp.

You then continue 0.5 mile farther to a junction with Eagle Benson Trail 434, which climbs steeply to the PCT. *Warning:* We do not recommend this footpath; it is too narrow to be safely climbed or descended with a heavy pack. In places it is quite easy to slip on loose gravel and then fall over a 100-foot cliff.

Just around the corner from this junction, the trail enters another side canyon and bridges a murmuring tributary 100 yards downstream from its slender, 80-foot-high fall.

CAMPING Continuing 0.5 mile northwest, you soon enter another side canyon, and this one provides you with Wy'East Camp, which is just above the trail. Downstream 0.6 mile, you reach a bridge across Eagle Creek, 20 feet below.

Now above the creek's west bank, you follow the singing creek 0.3 mile down to the once-popular 4 Mile Camp, also known as Tenas Camp. Since the 2017 fire, two trees have fallen across the most desirable campsite, and there is now limited space here; camping is no longer recommended here. However, be sure to check out the nearby two-step, 40-foot waterfall.

WILDLIFE Near it you'll find the dipper, or water ouzel, a gray, chunky, water-loving bird that tenaciously clings to the bottoms of swift streams in search of aquatic animal life. The name *dipper* refers to the bird's bobbing motions while standing on land.

After a quick, invigorating frolic in the pools below the lower fall, you can stretch out in the afternoon sunlight to thaw out before you begin hiking once again.

Back on the trail, you walk spiritedly 0.3 mile north to a bridge across

a 90-foot-deep gorge that is only 30 feet wide. A hundred yards downstream from this crossing, the swirling creek has cut deep potholes that would make superb swimming holes were it not for the cool temperature. The 6-inch trout don't seem to mind it, though. Above the potholes, wispy Loowit Falls emerges from the vegetation to flow silently down the polished rock and into one of the pools.

Continuing downstream, you soon enter another side canyon, bridge a creek 50 feet above it, and then pass massive, vertical-walled flows of Columbia River basalt. In just 1.4 miles, you cross Tish Creek and arrive at an overlook above Punch Bowl Falls, which drops 40 feet into a churning cauldron below.

Here the trail starts to climb high above the now-impassable gorge, and you soon see more reasons that horses aren't allowed on the trail. At times the overhanging walls seem to press you terribly close to the brink of the dead-vertical cliff below, and you are thankful that the trail crew installed cables along these stretches. You now reach another overlook after 0.6 mile where you can gaze 200 yards upstream to Metlako Falls, whose silvery course plummets another step down into the inaccessible gorge.

The route gradually descends toward the trailhead, and you leave the threatening, moss-covered cliffs behind. All too soon, another 1.5 miles has passed and the verdant route reaches the trailhead, which is by a bridge that spans Eagle Creek.

CAMPING To reach Bridge of the Gods, take Gorge Trail 400, which starts from the parking area. This trail climbs through a picnic area, crosses the short road 0.1 mile up to Eagle Creek Campground, passes between the campground and I-84, and then quickly reaches a part of the abandoned, narrow Columbia River "highway." On this, you curve 0.7 mile over to Ruckel Creek, on the east bank of which Ruckel Creek Trail 405 makes a 5.3-mile climb to the PCT.

Your shady gorge trail continues 1.9 miles northeast, and at times it almost touches I-84. After traversing a few hundred yards across grassy slopes—absolutely miserable in the rain—the trail ends at Moody Avenue opposite the PCT.

The official PCT route, which is 0.7 mile shorter than the Eagle Creek route, starts a traverse east along Wahtum Lake's southwest shore and then meets a lateral trail (2,130.6–3,778'), where hikers keep left.

CAMPING This lateral trail climbs 0.3 mile to Wahtum Lake Campground, atop a saddle. From that saddle, FS 1310 descends southeast toward other roads that lead out to the city of Hood River.

From the lateral-trail junction, the PCT circles Wahtum Lake, leaving its popular south-shore campsites behind. The trail's gentle, long, counterclockwise climb ends high above the lake at a junction with the Herman Creek Trail. In 200 yards, the now-level trail reaches another junction, this time with the Chinidere Mountain Trail (2,132.4–4,302').

VIEWS SIDE TRIP If you're having good weather, don't pass up this 0.3-mile-long, 400-foot ascent to Chinidere Mountain's superb panoramic summit. From the summit, you can see Mount St. Helens rising skyward above the north-northwest horizon, massive Mount Adams lording over the north-northeast horizon, and graceful Mount Hood dominating the south-southeast horizon. You can also see the Columbia River and Wind River Canyons, due north, while closer by, you're surrounded by deep canyons.

Leaving the Chinidere Mountain Trail junction, the PCT curves northwest around this miniature mountain to a saddle and then contours across southwest slopes to a crest viewpoint. It then drops to a second saddle, and then a third saddle (2,135.3–3,798'), this one signed CAMP SMOKEY, perhaps because these two saddles and the southwest-facing slopes between them were part of an area burned by a large forest fire. And it burned again in 2017, leaving lots of charred snags with too many limbs that are no match for gravity, so camping is not recommended here.

Pushing toward the deep Columbia River Gorge, you leave the Camp Smokey saddle and climb to spreading Benson Plateau. In a gully on the plateau's southeast edge, you meet the *first*—and lightly used—Benson Way Trail 405B (2,135.7–4,070'), which starts west but eventually curves north over to Ruckel Creek Trail 405. Staying near the plateau's east edge, the PCT winds north to meet Ruckel Creek Trail 405 (2,136.6–4,097').

CAMPING Follow Ruckel Creek Trail 405 west 0.8 mile to a campsite that escaped the 2017 fire unburned and in good condition. This site is the only one between

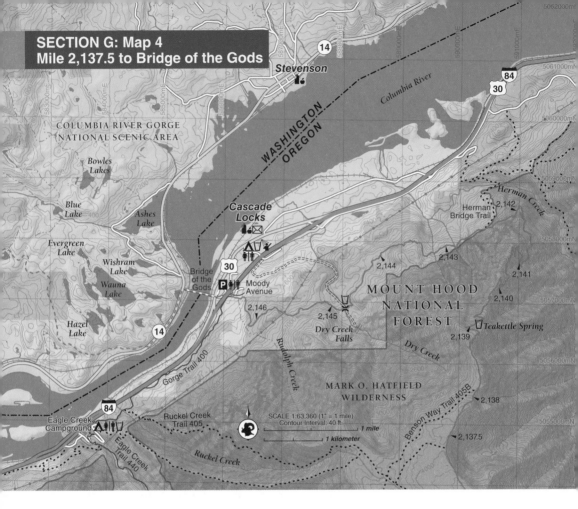

Wahtum Lake and Dry Creek that is suitable for equestrians. Forty yards south of this campsite, you'll find a spring in a small meadow. From this campsite, you could continue 4.9 miles down the trail to Gorge Trail 400, mentioned at the end of the alternate Eagle Creek Trail route, described beginning on page 210.

Beyond the Ruckel Creek Trail junction, the PCT descends gently northwest along the plateau's east edge and soon meets the Benson Ruckel Trail 405A (2,137.4–3,930'), which heads west-southwest 0.8 mile to Ruckel Creek Trail 405. Past this junction, the PCT curves northeast and leaves Benson Plateau by the time it arrives at a junction with the *second* Benson Way Trail 405B (2,138.1–3,764').

Now you hike north along a forested crest just before the trail curves east to begin a descent into the Columbia River Gorge.

Your moderately to steeply dropping trail briefly descends the crest, then heads west to a switchback.

WATER ACCESS

Immediately past this turn, which you could easily miss without its sign, is Teakettle Spring (2,139.0–3,403').

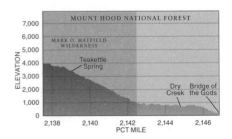

VIEWS Past the spring, the trail switchbacks once again down to the crest, on which it reaches a barren area that gives you revealing views of the giant Columbia River Gorge. From here, you can identify the towns of Cascade Locks, Stevenson, and Carson. To the west you see an impressive set of cliffs composed of pyroclastic rocks, the same kind of volcanic rocks that compose this barren area.

From the barren area atop the crest, the trail starts west, turns north, soon crosses the crest, and then makes a fairly steep descent into the Columbia River Gorge, recrossing the crest—now a ridge—near its lower end. In another mile, you enter the Columbia River Gorge National Scenic Area (2,141.4–1,753') while overlooking Herman Creek's canyon far below.

The PCT heads north then west to a junction (2,142.5–978') with the Herman Bridge Trail that provides a fast way out to the highway, crossing Herman Creek and ending at the Columbia Gorge Work Center. This trail junction is also where you leave the Mark O. Hatfield Wilderness.

If you intend to cross into Washington, continue along the westbound PCT. Departing from the Herman Bridge Trail junction, the PCT continues across open talus slopes and then enters an area of Douglas-fir and maple where the fire burned at low intensity, so the canopy is intact, but the moss and understory are regenerating. You soon cross a creek (2,142.9–966'), with an ethereal wisp of a waterfall high overhead called Pacific Crest Falls. Just beyond the creek you pass through a shallow saddle and then round a steep bowl. As the trail reaches a ridge and turns west to leave the bowl, notice an interesting set of pinnacle rock formations on the downhill side.

WATER ACCESS

The PCT heads southwest about a mile, dropping slowly; turns south; and quickly descends to a bridge across perennial, misnamed Dry Creek (2,144.8–705'). Immediately beyond it, you reach a dirt road.

SIDE TRIP You can follow this dirt road 0.2 mile south to its end, where you'll see an ideal shower: 50-foot-high Dry Creek Falls. Beautiful and mossy, this waterfall offers a taste of what hikers would see along the Eagle Creek Trail.

From this junction, the PCT starts west, contours over toward a saddle, and joins a power line road (2,145.6–698') that climbs up and over that saddle. Head northwest down this road 70 yards, and then branch left on the trail. This segment undulates southwest 0.5 mile around the north slopes of a low summit, turns north, and descends to Moody Avenue in the town of Cascade Locks. The Eagle Creek Trail alternate route ends here, opposite the PCT.

With the PCT and Eagle Creek Trail now rejoined, the PCT follows dirt Moody Avenue 70 yards to its junction with Southwest Undine Street (2,146.6–229'), where the road becomes paved. Moody Avenue immediately passes under the freeway. Five yards west of the freeway's largest pillar, the PCT resumes. It curves 200 yards northwest over to the paved loop road that leads up to Bridge of the Gods (2,146.9–219') and a toll booth.

Near the toll booth is a trailhead parking area with toilets, covered picnic tables, and a lawn. Section G ends here in Oregon, and Section H crosses the Columbia River into Washington. Hikers and bikers can cross Bridge of the Gods toll-free.

RESUPPLY ACCESS

If you're a long-distance hiker, you'll want to resupply in Cascade Locks. Walk down to the town's nearby thoroughfare, Wa Na Pa Street. On it, you walk 0.3 mile northeast to the Cascade Locks Post Office, which is conveniently located opposite a general store, a restaurant, and other stores.

CAMPING In another 0.3 mile, you reach a road that heads north to Cascade Locks Marine Park. It has a campground and, in the nearby visitor center, showers. One great feature of the campground is its roofed cooking area with tables, under which you can keep dry on rainy days.

HISTORY In this park, you can visit the shipping locks, built in 1896, which allowed ships to travel upriver beyond the Columbia River's Cascade Rapids. The park also has a historical museum.

If you are waiting for the weather to improve, you might spend some time at Cascade Locks Ale House, which has a great hiker box and register. Thunder Island Brewing Co.'s relaxed atmosphere is also friendly to PCT hikers.

Across the river and a 3-mile walk upstream brings you to Stevenson, Washington, which has a grocery store, pharmacy, bank, and Walking Man Brewing. You can reach Stevenson via a pedestrian-friendly route that follows Ash Lake Road and Rock Creek Drive instead of the parallel WA 14.

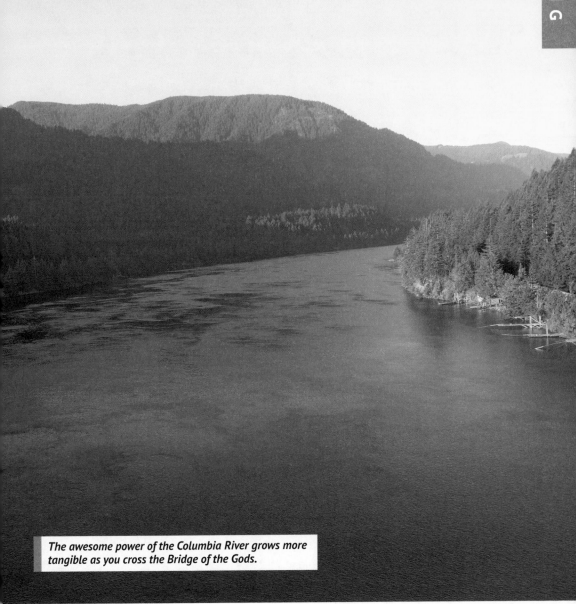

The awesome power of the Columbia River grows more tangible as you cross the Bridge of the Gods.

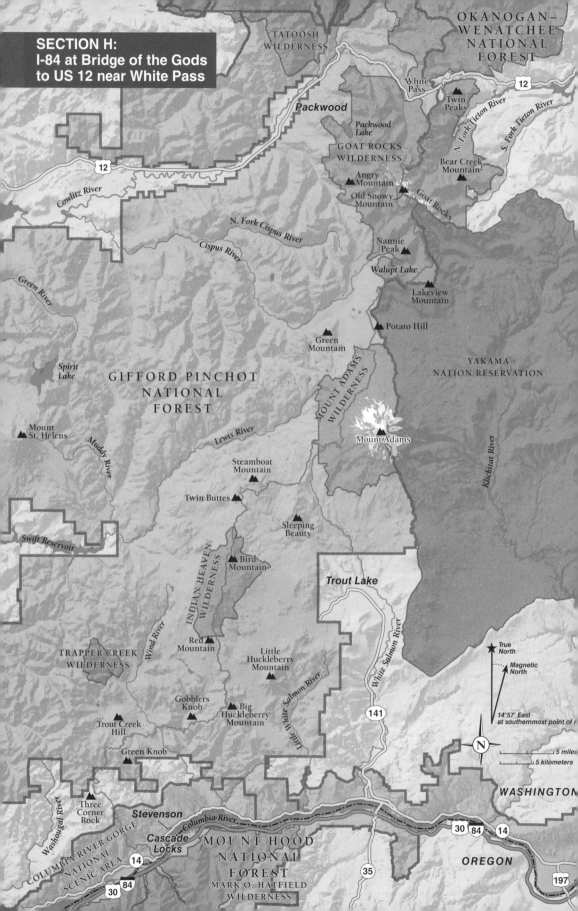

SECTION H:
I-84 at Bridge of the Gods
to US 12 near White Pass

OKANOGAN–
WENATCHEE
NATIONAL
FOREST

TATOOSH
WILDERNESS

White
Pass

12

Twin
Peaks

Packwood

Packwood
Lake

GOAT ROCKS
WILDERNESS

N. Fork Tieton River

S. Fork Tieton River

12

Angry
Mountain

Bear Creek
Mountain

Cowlitz River

Old Snowy
Mountain

Goat Rocks

N. Fork Cispus River

Cispus River

Nannie
Peak

Walupt Lake

Lakeview
Mountain

Green River

Potato Hill

Green
Mountain

YAKAMA
NATION RESERVATION

Spirit
Lake

GIFFORD PINCHOT
NATIONAL
FOREST

MOUNT ADAMS WILDERNESS

Mount
St. Helens

Lewis River

Mount Adams

Klickitat River

Muddy River

Steamboat
Mountain

Twin Buttes

Sleeping
Beauty

Swift Reservoir

Bird
Mountain

Trout Lake

INDIAN HEAVEN WILDERNESS

White Salmon River

TRAPPER CREEK
WILDERNESS

Wind River

Red
Mountain

Little
Huckleberry
Mountain

Little White Salmon River

True
North

Magnetic
North

Gobblers
Knob

Big
Huckleberry
Mountain

141

14°57' East
at southernmost point of r

Trout Creek
Hill

N

Green Knob

5 miles

5 kilometers

Three
Corner
Rock

Stevenson

Columbia River

WASHINGTON

Washougal River

30

84

14

COLUMBIA RIVER GORGE
NATIONAL
SCENIC AREA

14

*Cascade
Locks*

MOUNT HOOD
NATIONAL
FOREST

35

OREGON

197

30

84

MARK O. HATFIELD
WILDERNESS

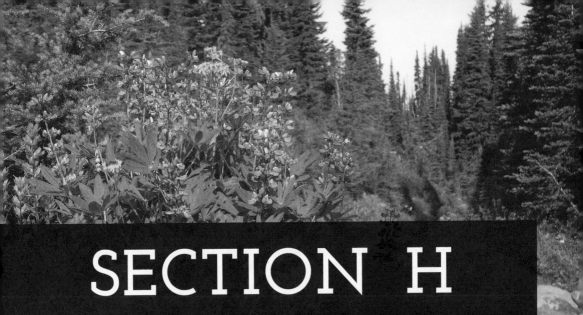

SECTION H

I-84 at Bridge of the Gods to US 12 near White Pass

BECAUSE THIS IS THE LONGEST SECTION of the Pacific Crest Trail (PCT) and because it has the greatest elevation change, it is the most diverse. It starts at Bridge of the Gods, which, at 188 feet elevation at its west end, is one of the lowest points on the official PCT (the lowest point— 99 feet—is just 1 mile southwest of the start of this section). Near this section's end, the trail climbs to 7,095 feet—its second-highest elevation in Washington—before traversing the upper part of Packwood Glacier.

Between these two extremes, you pass through several environments. After starting in a lush, damp Columbia River forest, you climb usually viewless slopes; wind past an extensive, recent lava flow; navigate a lake-speckled, glaciated lava plateau; and climb to a subalpine forest. The trail then circles a major, periodically active volcano, Mount Adams; traverses

Above: In Washington, it's not all tall trees and glaciers. The PCT boasts refreshing displays of small-flowered paintbrush, big-leaved lupine, and arrowleaf groundsel.

high on the walls of deep, glaciated canyons; and finally climbs to an alpine landscape at Packwood Glacier. Along this section, then, you pass through all of the landforms and vegetation belts that you see along the PCT from central Oregon to trail's end in southern British Columbia.

DECLINATION 14°57'E

USGS MAPS

Sleeping Beauty, WA	Big Huckleberry Mountain, WA
Bonneville Dam, WA	Walupt Lake, WA
Steamboat Mountain, WA	Gifford Peak, WA
Beacon Rock, WA	Old Snowy Mountain, WA
Mount Adams West, WA	Lone Butte, WA
Lookout Mountain, WA	White Pass, WA
Green Mountain, WA	Little Huckleberry Mountain, WA
Stabler, WA	Spiral Butte, WA (PCT barely enters map)
Hamilton Buttes, WA	

POINTS ON THE TRAIL, SOUTH TO NORTH

	Mile	Elevation in feet	Latitude/Longitude
Bridge of the Gods (east end)	2,146.9	219	N45° 39' 42.4383" W121° 53' 51.1225"
Bridge of the Gods (west end) and WA 14	2,147.2	192	N45° 39' 46.4918" W121° 54' 18.4007"
Spur trail junction to Three Corner Rock water trough	2,162.1	3,255	N45° 44' 10.6628" W122° 02' 35.0721"
FS 43 alongside Trout Creek	2,176.6	1,195	N45° 48' 41.0828" W121° 57' 22.7777"
Big Huckleberry Mountain spur trail junction	2,191.1	3,975	N45° 50' 48.0363" W121° 47' 12.6571"
Alternate route to Crest Horse Camp	2,194.6	3,246	N45° 52' 49.0624" W121° 47' 18.5118"
Sawtooth Trail junction	2,212.1	4,852	N46° 03' 40.0824" W121° 46' 26.8109"
FS 24	2,214.7	4,269	N46° 05' 30.4683" W121° 45' 57.5100"
FS 88 at Grand Meadows Trailhead	2,223.4	3,482	N46° 08' 05.7027" W121° 41' 24.0079"
FS 23 to Trout Lake	2,228.9	3,849	N46° 09' 42.4897" W121° 37' 54.3526"
Round the Mountain Trail junction	2,235.5	5,901	N46° 10' 47.2062" W121° 34' 07.8296"
Lava Spring	2,249.5	4,522	N46° 18' 18.5378" W121° 31' 04.4101"
Walupt Lake Trail junction	2,264.6	4,964	N46° 24' 37.1356" W121° 24' 08.7577"
Bypass Trail junction	2,274.0	5,964	N46° 29' 15.5312" W121° 27' 35.3406"
Old Snowy Alternate junction	2,276.6	7,095	N46° 30' 51.7705" W121° 27' 39.1234"
Junction with North Fork Tieton and Clear Fork Trails	2,283.3	4,807	N46° 33' 11.5535" W121° 25' 10.6030"
US 12 near White Pass	2,294.9	4,409	N46° 38' 37.1687" W121° 22' 45.4575"

CAMPSITES AND BIVY SITES

Mile	Elevation in feet	Latitude/ Longitude	Number of tents	Feature	Notes
2,159.9	3,025	N45° 43' 33.5052" W122° 00' 38.1485"	3		In shade
2,166.1	1,487	N45° 46' 00.8946" W122° 02' 19.3444"	>4	Wide Rock Creek	Bivy on both sides of creek in shade
2,176.6	1,186	N45° 48' 40.4859" W121° 57' 24.8276"	2	Trout Creek	
2,182.1	902	N45° 49' 04.3251" W121° 52' 43.3728"	>4	Panther Creek Campground	Vault toilets, drinking water, picnic table, grill
2,193.0	3,529	N45° 52' 00.1477" W121° 47' 14.1961"	4	Nearby spring	Shaded bivy on left and right
2,197.9	3,495	N45° 54' 33.0753" W121° 48' 08.5159"	4	Crest Horse Camp	PCT trailhead; pit toilet, picnic table
2,205.2	4,659	N45° 59' 01.6688" W121° 47' 42.2298"	>4	Blue Lake	Some protected areas
2,205.2	4,720	N45° 59' 13.9800" W121° 47' 45.9600"	3	Lake Sahalee Tyee	0.25 mile off-trail
2,208.2	4,791	N46° 01' 04.6200" W121° 47' 16.0800"	2	Bear Lake	Just off-trail
2,208.9	4,944	N46° 01' 25.0200" W121° 46' 55.8000"	3	Clear Lake	0.3 mile off-trail
2,218.7	3,940	N46° 07' 34.0011" W121° 44' 59.7656"	4	Mosquito Creek nearby	Flat spot near trail on right in shade
2,221.3	3,700	N46° 07' 56.4204" W121° 42' 55.2996"	2	Steamboat Lake Campground	0.75 mile off-trail
2,229.0	3,849	N46° 09' 47.3517" W121° 37' 51.8073"	2	Nearby stream	Fire ring; popular with car campers
2,229.9	4,095	N46° 10' 23.9475" W121° 37' 31.4975"	>4		On left; fire ring
2,234.5	5,638	N46° 11' 12.1577" W121° 34' 36.6181"	4		Flat spot near trail
2,235.5	5,519	N46° 10' 52.9800" W121° 33' 59.7000"	5	Dry Lake Camp	0.25 mile off-trail
2,240.4	5,852	N46° 13' 35.1475" W121° 33' 45.3527"	2	Mutton Creek	Flat spot near trail in shade
2,249.2	4,613	N46° 18' 15.7515" W121° 30' 46.9541"	2	Streams nearby	Fire ring
2,253.7	4,699	N46° 21' 21.1167" W121° 31' 04.8564"	2	Midway Creek	South of creek on right
2,258.2	5,254	N46° 23' 42.0603" W121° 28' 51.9385"	4		Fire ring
2,258.8	5,468	N46° 23' 50.3993" W121° 28' 16.3978"	2		Flat spot near trail on left; fire ring
2,260.4	5,272	N46° 23' 33.4658" W121° 27' 12.2050"	3		Flat spot near trail on left
2,273.6	5,983	N46° 29' 08.3431" W121° 27' 04.8771"	3	Vista	Flat spot near trail on left
2,274.0	5,571	N46° 29' 18.6000" W121° 28' 20.2800"	2	Bypass Camp	0.6 mile off-trail; protected
2,279.9	5,994	N46° 32' 22.4923" W121° 26' 34.9435"	2	Nearby stream	Flat spot near trail on left
2,281.1	5,558	N46° 32' 20.9968" W121° 25' 40.1003"	2		Flat spot near trail in shade
2,282.3	5,081	N46° 32' 39.6600" W121° 25' 05.5200"	2	Lutz Lake	

SUPPLIES

At almost 148 miles, this section is the longest on the entire PCT, so many hikers will want to resupply twice. This is easy to do with a fill-up at Cascade Locks, Oregon, or Stevenson, Washington, along with another stop for more chow in pleasant Trout Lake. (See the end of Section G for directions to Cascade Locks or Stevenson.) Hikers will be able to resupply again at White Pass at the end of this section.

Trout Lake is one of the many near-trail towns that take extra efforts to make hikers feel welcome—and properly fed. It's a 13-mile hitch to Trout Lake on Forest Service Road 23; however, several residents routinely assist hikers to and from this trailhead. (Remember to reimburse the driver with some fuel money.) The Trout Lake General Store accepts and holds hiker packages at no charge. The store is also well stocked with hiker-approved foods. Trout Lake Country Inn and the Station Cafe will serve their fine food and cold, hopped beverages to you at your table. There are several nice motels and inns, but not all are centrally located.

At White Pass, you can pick up mailed parcels (USPS or UPS) at the Kracker Barrel Store (48851 US 12, Naches, WA 98937). The store has a gas station; some hiker staples, such as tortillas, cheese, hazelnut spread, beer, and chips; and some quick, hunger-eliminating items, such as pizza, sandwiches, and snacks. And it surprisingly provides an espresso bar, showers, and a laundromat. Hikers may also opt to stay at White Pass Campground and take a quick, chilly dip in adjacent Leech Lake.

SPECIAL RESTRICTIONS

The U.S. Forest Service would like to see you camp at least 200 feet from the PCT when you are in an official wilderness area. Unfortunately, topographic and/or vegetative constraints often make this rather challenging. Nevertheless, choose a site that will not negatively impact the environment or other trail users. Camp on durable surfaces such as mineral soil and practice Leave No Trace principles, respecting your fellow, and future, campers. Packers mustn't let their animals graze within 200 feet of lakes, and, if they pack in feed, it must be processed so as to prevent seed germination. All of these rules apply to *all* of Washington's wilderness areas.

BRIDGE OF THE GODS TO US 12 NEAR WHITE PASS

>>>THE ROUTE

RESUPPLY ACCESS

Stevenson is 4.5 miles from Cascade Locks, where it is pretty easy to find a ride across the river. The town has a nice market, convenience store, and motels, plus diners, java shops, and brewpubs, making this a worthwhile stop.

This section of the PCT begins by exploring hilly hummocks and small lakes that were deposited by a huge landslide hundreds of years ago. This is the same landslide that temporarily dammed the Columbia River, creating the original legendary Bridge of the Gods, a natural bridge. It then climbs a short series of ridges offering scenic vistas. Between these ridges, descend into forests of mossy creeks and occasional old-growth giants.

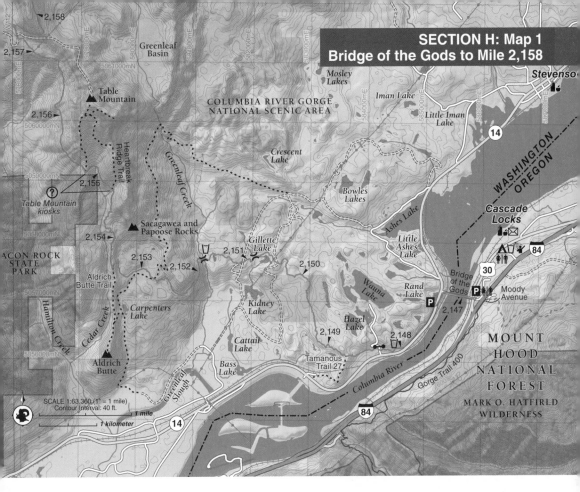

Cross the Columbia River via the Bridge of the Gods (2,146.9–219'), which is toll-free for pedestrians, and enter Washington. From the west end of the Bridge of the Gods toll road (2,147.2–192'), head south on WA 14 past an oversize pond, and just 80 yards beyond it reach the PCT trailhead (2,147.4–155'). You'll find limited parking nearby, plus access for equestrians. The "trail" at first is along an old power line road that parallels WA 14, just below you. The roadbed is rather overgrown, and in some places the trail sticks to the road's outer edge, which can leave the trail somewhat exposed, so caution is highly advised here.

WATER ACCESS

The short clifftop stretch soon gives way to safer slopes, and presently you reach a spring, which is your first source of reliable water (2,148.1–156').

In 0.2 mile cross a gated, paved road, which climbs from WA 14 to private Wauna Lake. Leaving civilization, you first climb to a ridge (2,148.7–372') from where Tamanous Trail 27 starts southwest, meandering 0.6 mile to a large parking area opposite the Bonneville Lock and Dam. Ahead, the forested, often

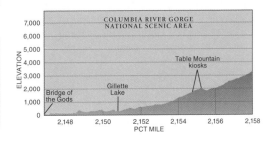

fern-bordered PCT takes a convoluted, rolling route across a giant landslide.

GEOLOGY Large and small landslides have descended from both walls of the Columbia River Gorge. This is due in part to the steepness of the gorge's walls but is also a result of their composition: the volcanic flows and associated volcanic sediments composing the walls belong to two distinct time periods. The lower layers are about 25 million years old, while the upper ones are about 15 million years old. The surface of the lower layers thus had about 10 million years to deeply weather to clay in this area's warm, humid, preglacial climate before the clay was buried under a sea of younger deposits. This clay layer is the structurally weak element that causes overlying layers to give way, as in the landslides from Table Mountain and the Red Bluffs. The landslides can temporarily dam the Columbia River, and such temporary dams perhaps provided a basis for the American Indian legend about Bridge of the Gods.

After about an hour of meandering through recent timber harvests in various stages of regeneration (the PCT is on easements through private land here), you emerge from forest cover at a utility road (2,150.5–420'), which serves three sets of Bonneville Dam power lines.

TRAIL INFO Across this major road, the PCT follows an abandoned road down toward Gillette Lake (2,150.8–311'). This lake was, until recently, on private land, but the Pacific Crest Trail Association (PCTA) and the U.S. Forest Service joined forces to acquire it in 2016, in the interest of protecting it in a more natural state for the future. Swimmers will find the water relatively warm.

Now the trail reenters forest, in a couple of minutes passes the lake's seasonal inlet creek,

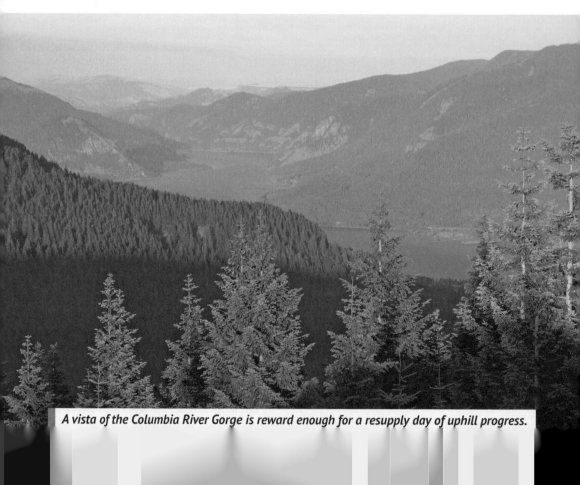

A vista of the Columbia River Gorge is reward enough for a resupply day of uphill progress.

and then climbs 0.25 mile to a mowed pipeline corridor. From the pipeline corridor you follow an old road 70 yards west before leaving it. Eastbound trekkers could be led astray if they miss the PCT tread starting from the east side of the pipeline corridor.

WATER ACCESS

On trail tread, westbound trekkers make an easy climb to a lily-pad pond before momentarily dropping to a horse bridge across Greenleaf Creek (2,151.7–482'). This is your last totally reliable, on-trail water source until Rock Creek, 14.4 miles farther. Fortunately, some near-trail water sources are available.

Switchback upward from the creek and get your only views of sprawling Bonneville Dam as you make a short trek southwest. Then angle northwest to a ravine with a seasonal creeklet, ramble west to a second creeklet, and then climb north along a third before switchbacking up to a low ridgecrest (2,153.6–1,107'). Here you turn north and parallel an abandoned road up Cedar Creek canyon.

After a crest walk north, you cross the road (2,154.1–1,411') and then recross it in less than 0.2 mile. Shortly, the climb north takes you to a creeklet (2,154.7–1,707'), just beyond which you meet a junction with Heartbreak Ridge Trail, which climbs very steeply up a minor ridge to Table Mountain. On a moderate grade, you climb northwest then southwest up to a larger ridge (2,155.2–2,015'), where you meet a junction with West Table Mountain Trail.

Now you exchange the Cedar Creek drainage for the larger Hamilton Creek drainage. The trail drops a bit, quickly emerges from forest cover, and then drops some more to avoid steep slopes on the west side of towering Table Mountain. Enjoy the panoramic views as you tackle the 1,500 feet of climbing ahead. Try not to obsess about every ounce in your pack just now. The earlier in the morning you make this protracted climb out of the Columbia River Gorge, the better.

On a shady bench due west of Table Mountain, the PCT latches onto an abandoned roadbed that, fortunately, is alder-shaded along its first 0.5 mile. You'll need the shade, for the gradient averages a stiff 17%. Just before the gradient abates, you get a view. Stop and listen for music to your ears—a never-failing creek.

Onward, in about 140 yards, the trail reenters forest cover and bends west. Soon you leave the old roadbed, pass under a buzzing power line, travel along a short stretch of bear grass turf, and then ramble over to a nearby road (2,157.2–2,761'). You climb briefly north and then head east on a rather steep, very rocky tread across a rubbly open slope that offers fine views south down Hamilton Creek canyon. Mount Hood, poking over the shoulder of multilayered Table Mountain, also comes into view. With a final burst of effort, you reach a ridge above a power line saddle.

Having put most of the elevation gain behind, you can enjoy the next stretch, which has views east past Greenleaf Basin and Peak to the Columbia River Gorge and south past Table Mountain to Mount Hood. Typical of a crest route, the PCT climbs to a saddle and crosses it, giving you your first view of Three Corner Rock, a conspicuous knob to the northwest. Here, the PCT leaves the Columbia River Gorge National Scenic Area and enters private land (2,158.7–3,462'). The trail climbs briefly, topping out at just over 3,500 feet, and then makes a minimal descent over to flowery, bushy slopes.

Next you wind around a ridge, absorbing panoramic views to the south, west, and northwest; enter a regenerating, young forest; and cross three dirt roads on your 0.4-mile descent

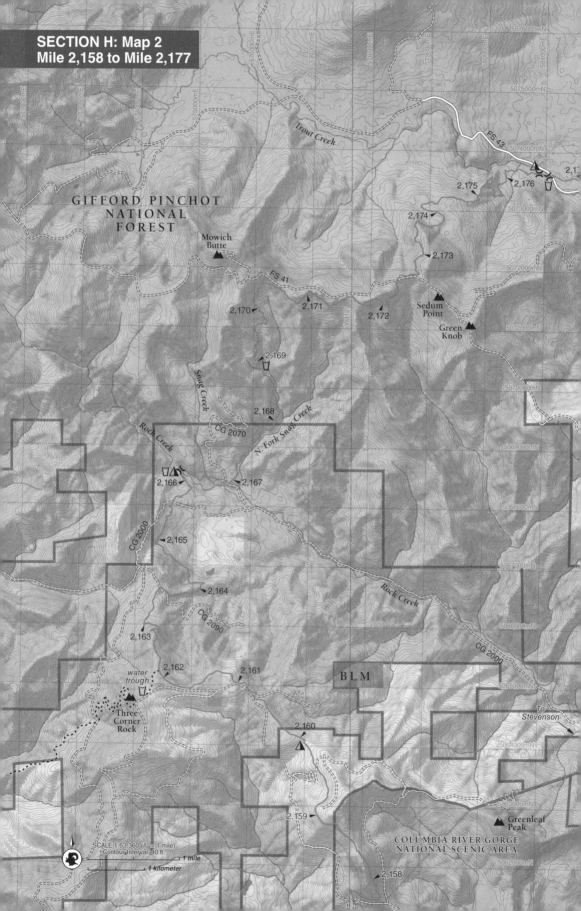

Trout Creek

FS 43

2,1

2,175

2,176

GIFFORD PINCHOT
NATIONAL
FOREST

2,174

Mowich
Butte

2,173

FS 41

Sedum
Point

2,170

2,171

2,172

Green
Knob

2,169

Snag Creek

2,168

N. Fork Snag Creek

CG 2070

Rock Creek

2,166

2,167

CG 2000

2,165

2,164

Rock Creek

CG 2090

2,163

CG 2000

2,162

2,161

B L M

water
trough

Three
Corner
Rock

To
Stevenson

2,160

Greenleaf
Peak

2,159

COLUMBIA RIVER GORGE
NATIONAL SCENIC AREA

SCALE 1:63,360 (1" = 1 mile)
Contour Interval: 40 ft.

1 mile

1 kilometer

2,158

to a forested saddle with a crest-line road (2,159.9–3,025'). This jeep road heads over to Three Corner Rock, and the PCT parallels it in the same direction. Along this stretch, a newer road crosses the PCT and quickly meets the jeep road. Traversing along the PCT, you get sporadic views to the north and east, with Mount Adams and clear-cuts catching your attention. Views disappear about 0.25 mile before the trail touches the jeep road, and ahead you climb, first viewlessly southwest and then viewfully west, up to a spur trail (2,162.1–3,255'). If you'd like to take in the impressive 360-degree panorama offered atop Three Corner Rock, this is the spur that leads to it.

> ## WATER ACCESS
>
> Also, there's sometimes water in an old trough along the way to the rock. The next on-trail water is way down at Rock Creek, a hefty 4 miles away.

From the junction, you get a few views of recent timber harvest on state and private lands as the trail winds and switchbacks north down to a viewless saddle (2,163.5–2,343'), which is crossed by CG 2090. Next you skirt east just below a ridgecrest and soon duck through a crest gap. After immediately switchbacking west below the gap, you quickly plunge into a deep forest and wander in and out of numerous, usually dry ravines before crossing CG 2000 (2,165.6–1,737'). This is found after a

0.5-mile hike through a former clear-cut, now a young single-species forest. *Note:* If you need to abort your trip, take this well-maintained road 11 miles east down to Stevenson.

> ## WATER ACCESS
>
> Follow the PCT down and across ravines ultimately to a bridging of Rock Creek (2,166.1–1,487').

This 4-mile stretch from the spur trail to Three Corner Rock is a well-graded, very steady descent across intricately complex terrain.

Water availability now is less of a problem, at least until you leave Panther Creek Campground, some 16 miles ahead. You quickly climb above Rock Creek and travel southeast to Snag Creek (2,166.6–1,500'). You soon emerge from forest cover and then reach CG 2070 (2,166.9–1,465'). Prepare for a challenging ascent.

At first, you have a pleasant stroll through a forest of Douglas-firs, alders, and vine maples. You soon enter Gifford Pinchot National Forest (2,167.3–1,464'); since leaving the Columbia River Gorge National Scenic Area, you've been traveling through a mix of state forest and private land. The North Fork Snag Creek stays close by for the first 0.75 mile; then the trail enters and leaves a prominent ravine and climbs to a north-trending North Fork tributary. It is usually flowing but is a problem to reach because the PCT typically stays 200 feet above it on steep, densely vegetated slopes.

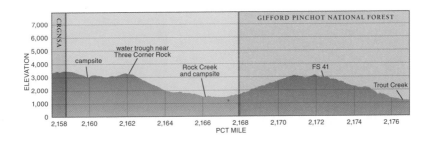

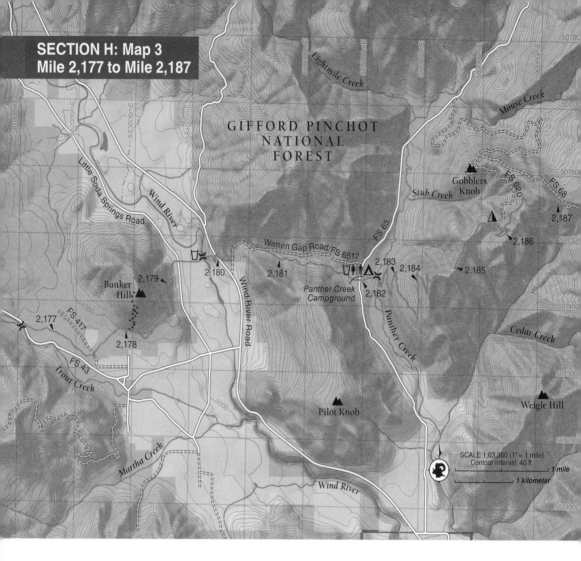

GIFFORD PINCHOT
NATIONAL
FOREST

Eightmile Creek

Mouse Creek

Little Soda Springs Road

Wind River

Gobblers
Knob

Stub Creek

FS 020

FS 68

2,187

2,186

Warren Gap Road/FS 6517

FS 65

2,183

2,180

2,181

2,184

2,185

Panther Creek
Campground

2,182

Bunker
Hill

2,179

FS 417

2,177

Wind River Road

Panther Creek

Cedar Creek

2,178

FS 43

Trout Creek

Pilot Knob

Weigle Hill

Martha Creek

Wind River

SCALE 1:63,360 (1" = 1 mile)
Contour Interval: 40 ft.

1 mile

1 kilometer

WATER ACCESS

Finally the trail crosses a seasonal creeklet (2,168.8–2,159'), your last hope for any water until a Trout Creek tributary 6.8 miles away.

Switchbacks carry you up to gentler slopes, across which you climb to a lushly vegetated, though dry, ravine. Ahead, the trail climbs east to a ridge and then north to the base of steep slopes below crest-hugging Sunset Hemlock Road 41. You climb southeast 0.5 mile, obtaining spotty views before reaching a south-trending ridge. Next you skirt over to an adjacent crest saddle and then, just beyond it, have your first good views as the trail skirts the base of a lava cliff. At a second saddle, the trail almost touches FS 41. The trail climbs once more, topping out at 3,124 feet near a scenic, south-trending ridge, and then descends to

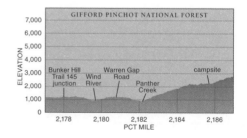

GIFFORD PINCHOT NATIONAL FOREST

ELEVATION

7,000
6,000
5,000
4,000
3,000
2,000
1,000
0

Bunker Hill
Trail 145
junction

Wind
River

Warren Gap
Road

Panther
Creek

campsite

2,178   2,180   2,182   2,184   2,186
PCT MILE

Sedum Ridge, where it finally crosses abandoned FS 41 (2,172.4–2,974').

The PCT reaches a gully, descends briefly north, turns east around a knife-blade ridge, and then drops north through a lush forest to the main ridge. Here you get the first good view north and see Bunker Hill to the east, standing alone in a flat-floored valley.

WILDLIFE The view disappears, and once again you disappear into a lush forest. If you are hiking the trail on one of those damp, misty days so common to this area, you may see a dozen or more rough-skinned newts.

The trail quickly reaches gentler slopes, angles northeast down to a viewless saddle, and then continues northeast down into several ravines that often, though not always, provide water.

WATER ACCESS

CAMPING The trail leaves these ravines and in 0.3 mile crosses a wide, splashing tributary (2,176.4–1,301') of Trout Creek. Now on nearly level ground, the trail curves east to Trout Creek and crosses it on a concrete span built to last as long as the PCT does. This is a good spot to camp.

Immediately past the bridge, the trail crosses FS 43 (2,176.6–1,195'), which gently descends 1.3 miles east to the Hemlock Picnic Area, with a good swimming hole. The PCT soon parallels unseen FS 43 southeast to FS 417 (2,177.4–1,156'). Walking east 30 yards on this road, you locate the PCT's tread, which follows the road's north edge 120 yards to another road junction; that road goes 0.5 mile southeast to the Wind River Work Center, near Hemlock

Picnic Area. FS 417 heads northwest along one edge of a private tree farm/campground, while the PCT heads east along the treed and fenced south edge.

Briefly parallel the tree farm's east edge, hiking north, and then in 40 yards angle northeast for a steepening walk up to a junction with the Bunker Hill Trail (2,178.0–1,216'), which switchbacks up to the summit. The PCT now winds, dips, and climbs east along the hill's viewless lower slopes; crosses a crest; and then descends gradually north down to a crossing of Little Soda Springs Road (2,179.4–966'). Here, the trail briefly leaves the national forest. East of the road, a row of trees bisects a large meadow, and the PCT stays along the row's north side as it heads east and reenters the national forest.

WATER ACCESS

The trail leaves this meadow just before crossing Wind River (2,179.7–942') on a major bridge built in 1978, one of the largest bridges to be found along the entire PCT.

From this river, climb 0.2 mile to busy Wind River Road, and cross it just 0.2 mile northwest of the road's junction with Warren Gap Road 6517. The PCT starts a climb southeast, almost touches FS 6517, eventually crosses it (2,180.8–1,191') just past Warren Gap, and then winds east down to FS 65 (2,182.0–939') near Panther Creek Campground.

CAMPING The entrance to Panther Creek Campground is 230 yards up the road, opposite the end of FS 6517. You should plan to camp there, for once you leave Panther Creek, you won't have a campsite with good water until Blue Lake, 23 miles farther.

WATER ACCESS

From FS 65, the PCT winds east 300 yards to Panther Creek (2,182.2–890'); just before the creek is a lateral trail that goes 150 yards north to the southeast corner of Panther Creek Campground. After bridging Panther Creek, you switchback upward, passing two trickling springs long before reaching the westernmost end of a ridge.

From the edge of the ridge, the trail starts by paralleling a slightly climbing ridgecrest northeast to a saddle (2,185.7–2,248'), from which a good dirt road starts a northeast descent and a vegetated one starts a southeast traverse. Follow the vegetated road 300 yards, curving around a brushy wash and then meeting a trail once again, just before the road curves south around a ridge. Hike east up this trail, recross the head of the wash, and wind around two minor ridges before coming to a saddle. This you cross; then, after a 0.5-mile climb across south slopes, the trail becomes an old road that quickly arrives at a junction with FS 68 (2,187.1–2,784'), on a saddle.

The trail continues east from the road, staying just south of the crest as it goes through a logged-out area; then, just before a saddle, it curves around the forested south slopes of the ridge, soon returning to the crest. Now you stay fairly close to the crest, which narrows to 5 feet in one spot and soon descends to a broad, open saddle. Next you climb and then head to a junction (2,190.1–3,577') with Cedar Creek Trail 149A.

WATER ACCESS

From here, a steep trail makes tight switchbacks south 0.3 mile down to Cedar Creek.

Onward, the PCT immediately switchbacks to climb up and around a small, open lava cap, from which there is a fine view of Mount Hood. Better views await at the summit of Big Huckleberry Mountain. From the lava cap, the PCT climbs 0.6 mile to a junction with southeast-descending Grassy Knoll Trail 146. In several paces, you reach a junction with the steep, 300-yard-long Big Huckleberry Mountain summit trail (2,191.1–3,975').

VIEWS **SIDE TRIP** Don't miss this opportunity to survey the lands of southern Washington and northern Oregon from Big Huckleberry's little summit. To the south is Mount Hood, rising prominently, and, just right of it, the summit of Mount Jefferson. To the northeast is your next major volcano, Mount Adams. All around are patches of clear-cuts in various stages of reforestation.

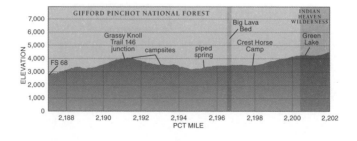

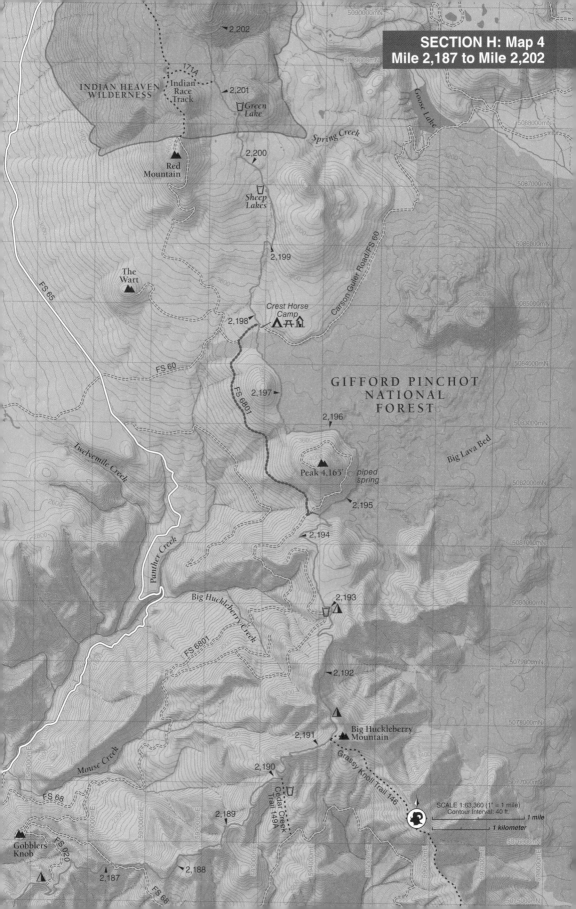

2,202

INDIAN HEAVEN
WILDERNESS

171A

Indian
Race
Track

2,201

Green
Lake

Goose Lake

Spring Creek

2,200

Red
Mountain

Sheep
Lakes

2,199

Carson Guler Road/FS 60

The Wart

Crest Horse
Camp

2,198

FS 65

FS 60

GIFFORD PINCHOT
NATIONAL
FOREST

FS 6801

2,197

2,196

Big Lava Bed

Twelvemile Creek

Peak 4,165'

piped
spring

2,195

Panther Creek

2,194

Big Huckleberry Creek

2,193

FS 6801

2,192

Mouse Creek

Big Huckleberry
Mountain

2,191

Grassy Knoll Trail 146

2,190

Cedar Creek
Trail 149A

SCALE 1:63,360 (1" = 1 mile)
Contour Interval: 40 ft.

1 mile

2,189

1 kilometer

FS 68

Gobblers
Knob

FS 020

2,187

2,188

FS 68

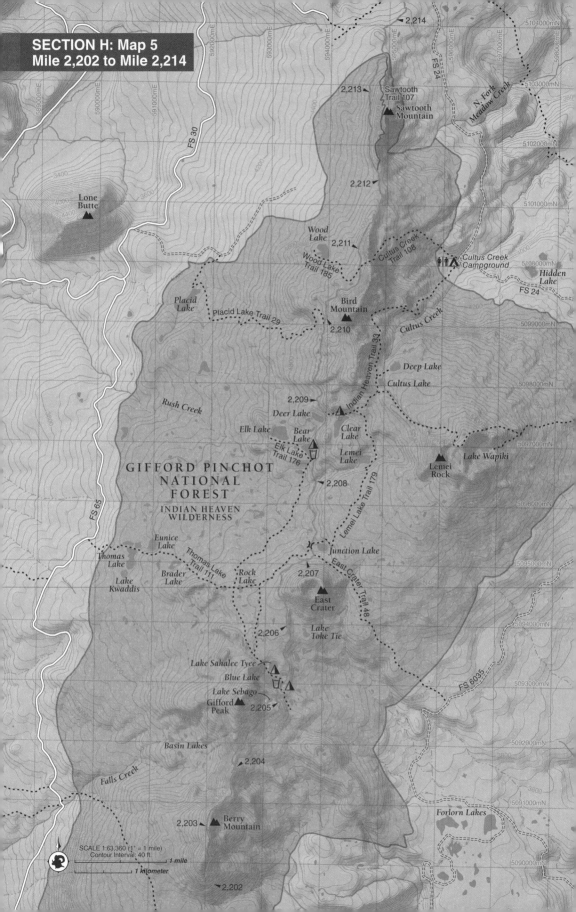

2,214

N. Fork Meadow Creek

FS 24

Sawtooth Trail 107

2,213 ◄ Sawtooth Mountain

2,212 ◄

Lone Butte ▲

Wood Lake

2,211 ◄ Wood Lake Trail 185

Cultus Creek Trail 108

Cultus Creek Campground

Hidden Lake

FS 24

FS 30

Placid Lake

Placid Lake Trail 29

Bird Mountain ▲

2,210 ◄

Cultus Creek

Deep Lake

Indian Heaven Trail 33

Cultus Lake

Rush Creek

2,209 ◄

Deer Lake

Elk Lake

Bear Lake

Elk Lake Trail 176

Clear Lake

Lemei Lake

Lake Wapiki

Lemei Rock ▲

2,208 ◄

Lemei Lake Trail 179

GIFFORD PINCHOT NATIONAL FOREST

INDIAN HEAVEN WILDERNESS

Eunice Lake

Thomas Lake Trail 111

Junction Lake

Thomas Lake

Brader Lake

Rock Lake

2,207 ◄

East Crater Trail 48

Lake Kwaddis

East Crater ▲

FS 65

2,206 ◄

Lake Toke Tie

FS 6035

Lake Sahalee Tyee

Blue Lake

Lake Sebago

Gifford Peak ▲ 2,205 ◄

Basin Lakes

2,204 ◄

Forlorn Lakes

Falls Creek

2,203 ◄ Berry Mountain ▲

2,202

The PCT now eases off and curves north to cross a saddle 0.4 mile from the last junction. Onward, the trail skirts across open slopes that provide excellent views of Mount Adams, and then it soon enters viewless forest.

WATER ACCESS

From a second saddle crossing, the trail descends to a ravine (2,193.0–3,556') that has a fairly reliable spring. This spring, 10.8 miles beyond Panther Creek, will be your last on-trail water until the Sheep Lakes, 6.6 miles farther.

CAMPING About 130 yards past the spring, a spur trail goes 50 yards southeast to a developed campsite. It certainly beats waterless, roadside Crest Horse Camp, which can have lumber-related traffic very early in the morning.

Onward, you contour north through a shady forest of Douglas-fir, western hemlock, and western white pine to reach a viewless, broad saddle and then wind down to the edge of Big Lava Bed, also by a broad saddle (2,194.6–3,246').

ALTERNATE ROUTE From this vicinity, a lateral trail winds 0.1 mile northwest to FS 6801. If you've been having snow problems, you might consider following this road 2.3 miles north to FS 60 and then 0.25 mile east to the PCT and Crest Horse Camp.

CAMPING Contouring counterclockwise around Peak 4,165, you may quickly encounter one or two springs, neither absolutely reliable. You follow the edge of geologically recent Big Lava Bed, cross one of its western overflow channels—which reveals the detailed intricacies of the flow—and then contour around another summit and cross another channel to the back of Crest Horse Camp (2,197.9–3,495'), which is on the south side of Carson Guler Road 60.

The campground has a picnic table but no water, so pick your pack off the table, put it on your back, and trudge north up the signed PCT. This moderate ascent up a fern-decked path is quite nice if you aren't running low on water.

WATER ACCESS

Climb to a flat and reach a duck pond (2,199.6–4,027'), which is no more than an oversize mud puddle after your arrival frightens the ducks away. Nevertheless, it boasts the name Sheep Lake. If absolutely necessary, you can gather water at this trailside pool or at the adjacent western or eastern Sheep Lakes.

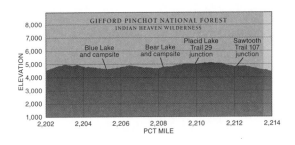

After climbing northwest through a more open forest, you enter Indian Heaven Wilderness and reach 35-yard-wide Green Lake (2,200.7–4,257'), which gets as deep as a foot in early summer and serves as a vital water supply.

If you find Green Lake too polluted to suit your standards, prepare for a dry march. Start northwest past a meadow, and then reach a junction with Indian Race Track Shortcut Trail 171A (2,201.1–4,238'), which strikes west-northwest 0.6 mile to a large, stagnant pond and to the Race Track, which was used by American Indian equestrians. On the PCT, hike north-northwest through a forest, and then climb several long switchbacks up the sunny south slope of Berry Mountain before reaching its crest.

VIEWS The PCT provides excellent views of Mount St. Helens (8,363') to the northwest, Mount Adams (12,276') to the northeast, and Mount Hood (11,249') to the south.

WATER ACCESS

Upon reaching the north end of linear Berry Mountain, you descend short switchbacks to a saddle, follow a rambling path down past the seasonal outlet creek of Lake Sebago, and come to an overlook of a 100-yard-wide stagnant pond, beyond which you finally reach the welcome, clear waters of Blue Lake (2,205.2–4,634'), nestled at the foot of Gifford Peak (5,368').

CAMPING Here you'll find the first good bivy sites since Panther Creek Campground, 23 miles back. Blue Lake is a popular destination for weekend backpackers and suffers from overuse. Please be careful to dispose of your human waste properly. You can learn the specifics at the PCTA website: pcta.org/discover-the-trail/backcountry-basics/leave-no-trace/honest-talk-toilet-paper-uncovered-feces.

CAMPING Starting along the lake's east shore, Thomas Lake Trail 111 heads 0.25 mile northwest over to an additional good campsite at shallow, circular Lake Sahalee Tyee. Camp at it if the Blue Lake campsites are full. Set up your tent at least 250 feet from either lake, and use only designated sites.

The PCT, which barely touches Blue Lake, starts northeast from the lake's southeast corner and then winds north up to a west arm of East Crater. The trail curves northeast around this youthful feature and then angles north for a short drop to a junction with East Crater Trail 48 (2,207.1–4,775'), which starts east along a skinny west finger of pleasant Junction Lake.

At the tip of the finger, you cross the lake's outlet and in 0.1 mile meet Lemei Lake Trail 179, which climbs east before swinging north past Lemei Lake to Indian Heaven Trail 33. The PCT stays on lower slopes just east of and above Indian Heaven's mosquito-populated ponds and lakes, avoiding bogs, but in early season, snow patches may be quite a problem.

WATER ACCESS

A quarter mile past the crossing of usually dry Lemei Lake creek, you meet a junction with Elk Lake Trail 176 (2,208.2–4,791') above the southeast corner of Bear Lake.

CAMPING From above the southeast corner of Bear Lake, Elk Lake Trail first skirts the southwest shore, offering you access to established campsites. Both Acker and Elk Lakes, which are nearby, are less desirable.

Along the PCT, you travel above Bear Lake and then over to a slope above the east end of Deer Lake. Rounding slopes above the lake, you meet Indian Heaven Trail 33 (2,208.9–4,897').

CAMPING This 3.1-mile trail takes the long way out to fairly large and often popular Cultus Creek Campground, which usually has a summertime host present, should you need help. By going just 0.3 mile on this trail, you can reach an adequate campsite by the northeast corner of Clear Lake. A couple of more-remote lake campsites can be reached with some cross-country effort.

With no more trailside lakes before FS 24, you continue north, pass two seasonal ponds, and then soon reach Placid Lake Trail 29 (2,209.9–5,000'), which offers neither nearby camps nor water. Still northbound, the trail crosses a saddle and then traverses northeast

to another one. Staying high, the PCT contours around Snow Lake and soon meets Wood Lake Trail 185 descending west to its namesake, which is not worth a visit. Also by Trail 185 is the west end of Cultus Creek Trail 108 (2,210.8–5,140').

CAMPING SIDE TRIP Cultus Creek Trail 108 climbs briefly northeast to a wooded saddle and then drops 1.5 miles at a hefty 15% gradient to the aforementioned Cultus Creek Campground, along FS 24.

The trail now stays close to a well-defined crest, which it eventually crosses, giving you views of massive Mount Adams and the terrain being logged around it. Just past the crest crossing, the trail heads briefly south, only to switchback north and descend to a crest saddle.

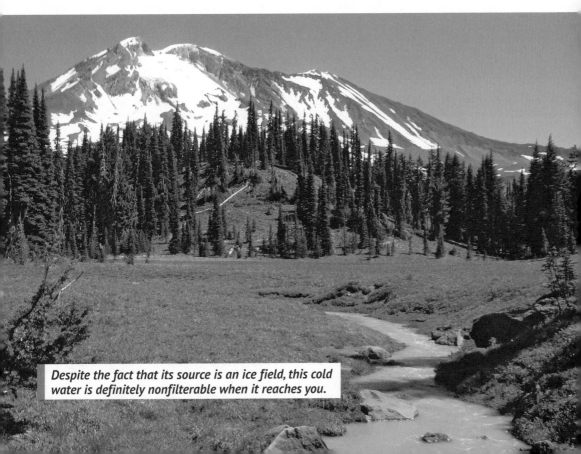

Despite the fact that its source is an ice field, this cold water is definitely nonfilterable when it reaches you.

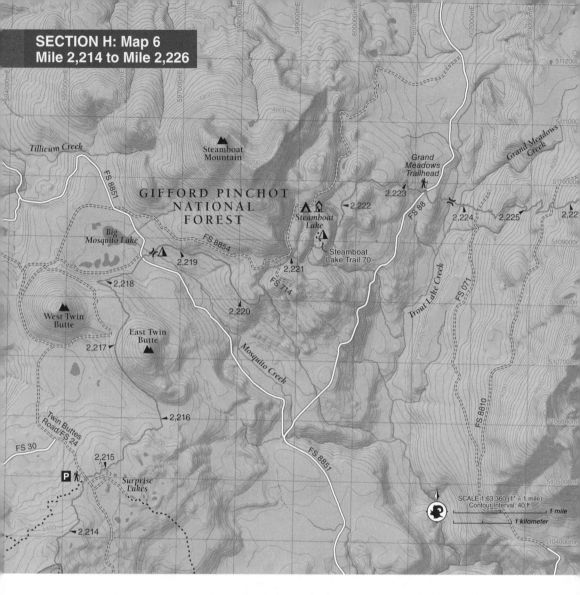

GIFFORD PINCHOT
NATIONAL
FOREST

Tillicum Creek

FS 8851

Steamboat
Mountain

Grand
Meadows
Trailhead

Grand Meadows Creek

2,223

FS 88

2,222

2,224

2,225

2,22

Big
Mosquito Lake

Steamboat
Lake

2,219

Steamboat
Lake Trail 70

Trout Lake Creek

FS 071

FS 8854

2,221

2,218

FS 714

2,220

West Twin
Butte

East Twin
Butte

2,217

Mosquito Creek

FS 8810

2,216

FS 8851

Twin Buttes
Road/FS 24

FS 30

2,215

P

Surprise
Lakes

SCALE 1:63,360 (1" = 1 mile)
Contour Interval: 40 ft.
1 mile
1 kilometer

2,214

At the switchback, you'll see a prominent huckleberry field just below, with berries in season from about mid-August until mid-September. You might sample these if you haven't already made a side trip to huckleberry fields back near Indian Heaven.

There is a junction here (2,212.1–4,852') where the Sawtooth Trail 107 veers northeast and to the western flanks of its namesake.

VIEWS **ALTERNATE ROUTE**

From the crest saddle, a 1.6-mile footpath switchbacks almost up to

the knife-edge crest of Sawtooth Mountain before switchbacking down to the PCT. Be sure to stay on the trail. From the serrated crest, you get an unobstructed view of

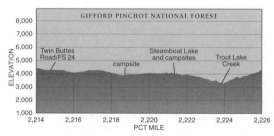

GIFFORD PINCHOT NATIONAL FOREST

8,000
7,000
6,000
5,000
4,000
3,000
2,000
1,000

ELEVATION

Twin Buttes
Road/FS 24

campsite

Steamboat Lake
and campsites

Trout Lake
Creek

2,214   2,216   2,218   2,220   2,222   2,224   2,226
PCT MILE

Mount Adams. On a clear day, you also see three other snowy peaks: distant Mount Hood in the south, bleak Mount St. Helens in the west-northwest, and distant Mount Rainier in the north.

If you keep to the official PCT route, the PCT stays low as it heads north gently down the west slopes of Sawtooth Mountain to a reunion with that summit's footpath, the boundary of the Indian Heaven Wilderness (2,213.5–4,591'), and the alternate route.

The PCT then descends into the Sawtooth Huckleberry Field, reaches a spur road, and parallels it 60 yards northeast to a signed PCT crossing of FS 24 (2,214.7–4,269').

HISTORY George B. McClellan's exploration party observed American Indians harvesting huckleberries here when the party passed through in 1854. Important treaties signed in 1854 and 1855 recognized the ancestral right to harvest the berries seen growing here, considered a spiritually endowed food crop for countless generations, exclusively by the American Indians whose descendants today comprise the Yakama Nation. After the turn of the 20th century, roads were built up to the berry fields. To stem the incursion of nontribal berry pickers, the original treaties were reinforced by the chief of the Yakama Nation and the supervisor of the Gifford Pinchot National Forest. This important agreement in 1932 was sealed with a handshake. Since then, the berry-picking rights of part of the Sawtooth berry fields east of FS 24 have been reserved exclusively for members of the Yakama Nation.

The trail now descends gently east-northeast, enters forest, and passes above the little-developed Surprise Lakes Campground, which, like Cold Spring and Meadow Creek Campgrounds south of it, is for American Indians only. Continuing northeast on the Surprise–Steamboat Lakes section of the PCT, you descend to a saddle, climb northwest up this well-graded trail, and then round the west slopes of East Twin Butte (4,651'). You reach a platform between the two Twin Buttes, which are obvious cinder cones. Descend northwest, switchback northeast, and descend to a crossing of a trickling creek immediately before reaching FS 8851 (2,218.5–3,921') at a junction 35 yards southeast of the west-trending Little Mosquito Lake road.

CAMPING The PCT bears northeast from FS 8851, and it quickly reaches the wide, refreshing outlet creek coming from Big Mosquito Lake (3,982'). Just northeast beyond this creek is a campsite. When conditions are boggy, you might prefer to follow FS 8851 north briefly down to where it bridges the creek. Just beyond it, on the left, is a parking area, which could serve as an early-season campsite.

The PCT leaves the creek and climbs gently east along the upper margin of a sheep-inhabited clearing, rounds a spur, and shortly crosses a dirt road (2,220.8–4,115') that snakes northwest 130 yards up to FS 8854. Continue northeast and descend to a small streambed with a seasonal creek (2,221.3–4,014') to meet a spur trail to Steamboat Lake.

CAMPING This spur trail to Steamboat Lake climbs north moderately 0.2 mile to Steamboat Lake (4,022'), and from it you can climb to waterless Steamboat Lake Campground, 0.75 mile from the PCT.

From the Steamboat Lake spur-trail junction, the PCT curves counterclockwise from the ravine; makes a gentle descent to an outlet creek 70 yards downstream from an unseen, unnamed lake; and then climbs briefly north to a saddle. Here the PCT descends northeast then east, weaving through a quiet forest down to a junction with FS 88 (2,223.4–3,482'). The swath cut by this road through the forest is oriented such that it affords an open view of Mount Adams.

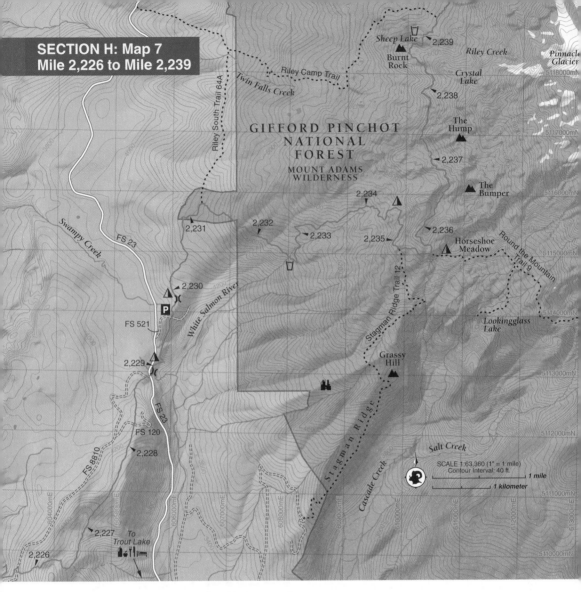

The PCT recommences 50 yards northeast up this road. You then top a minor ridge before descending to 3-yard-wide Trout Lake Creek (2,223.8–3,318'). About 100 yards later, cross the smaller Grand Meadows Creek. The trail now ascends east, crossing FS 071 one-third of the way up to a ridge. Soon your route momentarily descends to a tributary before making a final, stiff climb to FS 8810 (2,225.7–4,146'). Continuing east up the slope, you reach the crest and then begin a generally descending route north-northeast along the ridge down to a trailhead at FS 8810, reaching it 0.7 mile after crossing minor, east-heading FS 120. Walk east 50 yards to FS 8810's junction with

north-trending FS 23 and a trailhead for Mount Adams Wilderness (2,228.9–3,849').

RESUPPLY ACCESS

Hitch a ride for a 15-mile trip to Trout Lake, where hikers can

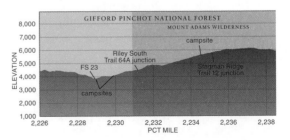

pick up mail, check and charge their electronics, and browse a thoughtfully complete selection of trail foods at the Trout Lake General Store. Some lodging is available but may not be located in the central townsite.

CAMPING From FS 23, the PCT heads 140 yards over to a creek, and 90 yards later you reach an old roadbed on which you could camp.

The trail then climbs north before traversing the slopes of a low summit and then briefly descending to a crossing of east-trending FS 521 (2,229.7–4,021').

CAMPING After hiking 0.25 mile north, you reach a few good campsites near a bridge over Swampy Creek.

Now you continue up an increasingly steep trail to the Mount Adams Wilderness boundary (2,230.1–4,181'), switchback northeast, head east, and finally drop gently southeast to a barely recognizable, often dry creek known as the White Salmon River.

WATER ACCESS

About 100 yards past it, you'll see a spring (2,232.5–4,820') gushing from thick vegetation 50 yards below the trail. This is your last reliable water until Sheep Lake, 6.5 miles later.

The trail then switchbacks, crosses the "river" in a shady bowl, switchbacks again, and then makes a long, snaking ascent to a junction with Stagman Ridge Trail 12 (2,235.1–5,812'), which starts a descent south. Pressing onward,

you climb east to a junction with Round the Mountain Trail 9 (2,235.5–5,901').

CAMPING SIDE TRIP This trail goes 0.25 mile east to Dry Lake Camp and then continues 5.5 miles to Timberline Camp, above the end of FS 8040. The easiest and most popular route to the summit of Mount Adams (12,276') starts there and climbs the south ridge. You should have no trouble attaining the summit in good weather, for this is the route that mule trains used in the 1930s. A climbing pass is required May–September.

GEOLOGY This massive andesitic stratovolcano, like the others you've seen, should still be considered active. Its last eruption may have been 1,000–2,000 years ago, but in May 1921 its near-surface magma generated enough heat to initiate a large snowslide that eradicated the forest on the slope below it.

On the high slopes east of the junction with Trail 9, you can see the White Salmon Glacier. Some PCT mountaineers prefer to climb Mount Adams via that icy route, which starts from this junction and crosses Horseshoe Meadow.

The PCT climbs northwest around a ridge that separates this glacier from the Pinnacle Glacier immediately north of it. This northward, round-the-mountain route is quite a contrast with that on Mount Hood; it stays at a relatively constant elevation, and where it climbs or descends, it usually does so on a gentle gradient. To the north and northwest, you can often see Goat Rocks and Mount Rainier.

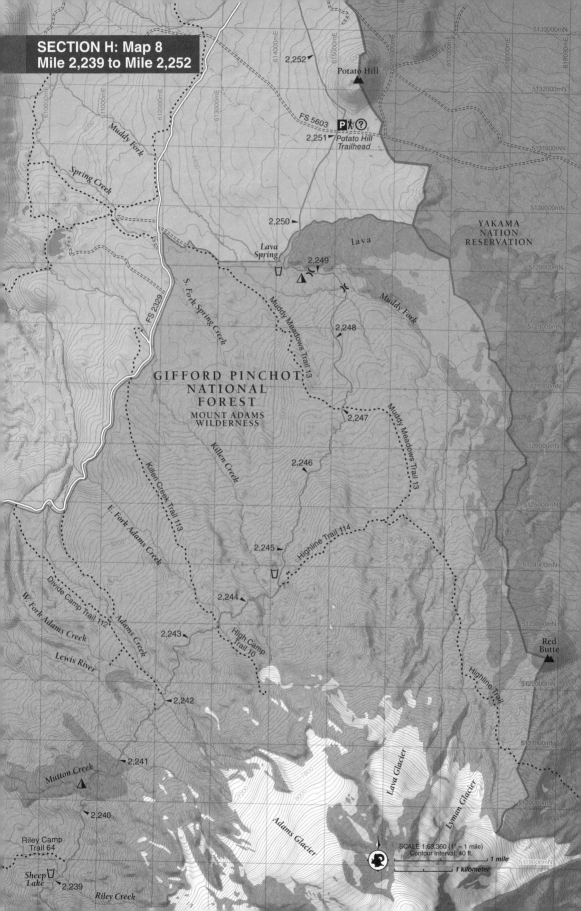

2,252

Potato Hill

FS 5603

2,251 ▸ Potato Hill
Trailhead

2,250 ▸

lava

YAKAMA
NATION
RESERVATION

Lava
Spring

2,249

lava

Muddy Fork

Muddy Fork

Spring Creek

Muddy Fork

4200

S. Fork Spring Creek

Muddy Meadows Trail 13

2,248

FS 2329

GIFFORD PINCHOT
NATIONAL
FOREST
MOUNT ADAMS
WILDERNESS

2,247

Muddy Meadows Trail 13

Killen Creek

2,246

5600

Killen Creek Trail 113

Highline Trail 114

2,245 ▸

E. Fork Adams Creek

2,244 ▸

High Camp Trail 10

Divide Camp Trail 112

Adams Creek

2,243 ▸

W. Fork Adams Creek

Lewis River

2,242

Red
Butte

Highline Trail

Lava Glacier

2,241 ▸

Mutton Creek

Adams Glacier

Lyman Glacier

2,240 ▸

Riley Camp
Trail 64

Sheep
Lake

2,239 ▸

Riley Creek

SCALE 1:63,360 (1" = 1 mile)
Contour Interval: 40 ft.

1 mile

1 kilometer

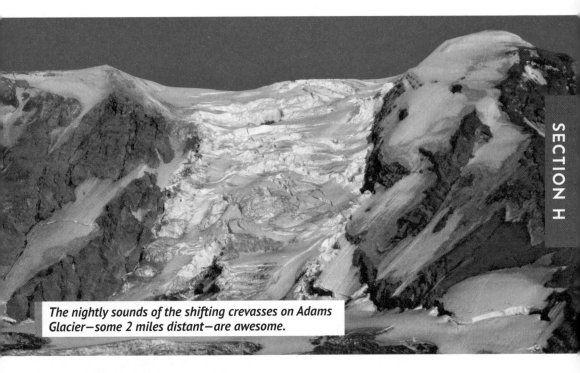

The nightly sounds of the shifting crevasses on Adams Glacier—some 2 miles distant—are awesome.

WATER ACCESS

After traversing to a saddle just east of Burnt Rock, the trail descends toward 70-yard-wide, 5-foot-deep Sheep Lake (2,239.0–5,783'), which is 40 yards northwest of the trail, and then reaches milky, jump-across Riley Creek (2,239.1–5,764').

Next on the menu, you approach Mutton Creek (2,240.4–5,893') and follow it up beside a geologically recent, rather barren lava flow over which you eventually head diagonally quite a distance up. The route then bounds from one wash to the next, crosses milky Lewis River (2,241.7–6,065'), and in 200 yards reaches a spur trail.

VIEWS This spur goes 110 yards north to a viewpoint from which you'll see distant, snowy Mount Rainier standing above a nearer, clear-cut–patched landscape.

The PCT quickly crosses some silty tributaries of West Fork Adams Creek before it curves north-northwest to a junction with Divide Camp Trail 112 (2,242.1–6,021'), which descends northwest toward FS 2329.

VIEWS Directly upslope from you is the overpowering, steeply descending Adams Glacier, which appears to be a gigantic, frozen waterfall. Along this journey

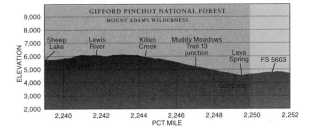

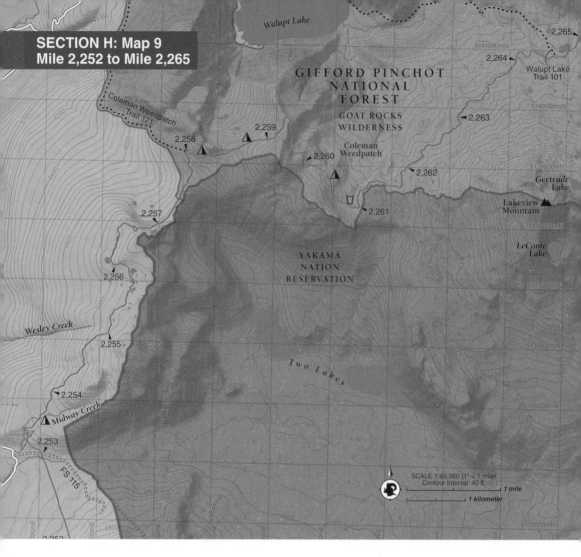

Walupt Lake

GIFFORD PINCHOT
NATIONAL
FOREST

GOAT ROCKS
WILDERNESS

Coleman
Weedpatch

Coleman Weedpatch
Trail 121

2,258

2,259

2,260

2,257

2,256

2,255

Wesley Creek

2,254

Midway Creek

2,253

FS 115

2,265

2,264

Walupt Lake
Trail 101

2,263

2,262

2,261

Gertrude
Lake

Lakeview
Mountain

LeConte
Lake

YAKAMA
NATION
RESERVATION

Two Lakes

SCALE 1:63,360 (1" = 1 mile)
Contour Interval: 40 ft.
1 mile
1 kilometer

north, glances back toward the massive peak will always single out this prominent feature.

The trail heads northeast across a 400-yard swath of bouldery glacier outwash sediments and then makes a tricky ford across silty Adams Creek. After climbing its bank, the route contours northeast past a 70-yard-wide pond and in minutes arrives at a junction with Killen Creek Trail 113 (2,243.4–6,115'), which starts beside a seasonal creek as it descends northwest toward FS 2329. Contour onward, descend to a large flat through which flows clear Killen Creek, and cross this creek's wooden bridge as it reaches a brink (2,244.3–5,924') and cascades merrily down 30 feet to a small meadow and a beautiful cluster of subalpine firs.

As you are about to head north away from Mount Adams, reflect upon another

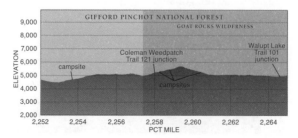

characteristic of this semicircular trail that distinguishes it from its counterpart on Mount Hood: the trail stays on the mountain's lower slopes, and you never feel like you've set foot on the mountain itself—the upper slopes don't begin until a "distant" 2,000 feet above you. In this respect, the trail resembles those around Mount Jefferson and the Three Sisters.

A short distance from this fragrant copse, the trail meets Highline Trail 114 (2,244.5–5,918'), which leads east toward the Yakama Nation Reservation.

WATER ACCESS

Just north of this junction, you spy a 70-yard pond 100 yards northwest. It is better to descend 80 feet down the slope to this pond than to continue onward to a second, readily accessible one that receives steady impact from packers.

The PCT passes the second pond (2,244.9–5,812') and becomes a rambling, evenly graded pathway that descends north-northeast into a subalpine fir/lodgepole-pine forest whose monotony is broken by an intersection with the Muddy Meadows Trail 13 (2,247.0–5,237') that starts east then south toward a junction 1.9 miles later with the Highline Trail.

WILDLIFE Meeting no traffic other than perhaps chickadees or juncos, you continue north and eventually reach a sturdy bridge across the 5-yard-wide Muddy Fork (2,248.6–4,745').

CAMPING Curving northwest, the path soon reaches and then parallels an alder-and-willow-lined, silty Muddy Fork west to its wooden bridge and a very good campsite (2,249.1–4,627') nestled between two of this creek's branches.

WATER ACCESS

A short distance farther, you round the nose of a recent lava flow and head north to the vibrant, crystal-clear waters gushing from trailside Lava Spring (2,249.5–4,522') at the foot of the flow. Because its water is among the best you'll find along the entire PCT, you might as well rest and enjoy it.

Leaving it, you follow the 40-foot-high edge of the flow a short way, leave Mount Adams Wilderness, and then climb gently through a predominantly lodgepole forest to a small trailhead parking lot a few yards north of paved FS 5603 (2,251.0–4,758'). From the lot, you walk northeast 50 yards along an old jeep road and then veer north-northeast along a trail that ascends gently toward Potato Hill (5,387'). Although motorized vehicles are specifically barred from the PCT, they or their tracks are likely to be encountered along this rather viewless stretch through second-growth forest. The trail quickly reaches the jeep road again, follows its northwest-curving path around Potato Hill, and then takes this dusty road north-northwest past huckleberries and mountain ash to a junction with FS 115 (2,253.0–4,502'). Walk 50 yards up a road, and then branch left for a grassy diagonal trek up a trail to a closed road that descends west-southwest 0.1 mile to FS 115. You'll walk across no more roads until US 12 near White Pass, almost 42 miles away.

CAMPING The trail starts west-northwest up toward Midway Creek (2,253.3–4,575'), which has an excellent, spacious campsite about 1,500 feet ahead, and then climbs through alternating forested and cleared land toward the crest.

As the gradient eases, you enter forest for good and follow a winding path that takes you past eight stagnant ponds. After leaving the last pond (2,256.1–5,081') on the left (west), you hike around the west slope of a knoll, descend gently to the west side of a broad saddle, and enter the Goat Rocks Wilderness (2,257.4–4,981'). Then climb moderately to a switchback (2,258.0–5,223'), from which Coleman Weedpatch Trail 121 descends 3.1 miles to Walupt Lake Horse Camp.

The trail climbs east to a saddle and passes two small ponds on the left. Then it climbs north to a prominent ridgecrest that stands directly south of Walupt Lake (3,926'). To the north you see the glistening summit of Old Snowy Mountain (7,900') in the heart of the Goat Rocks country, over whose slopes you must soon climb.

The route now winds southeast down auxiliary ridges and enters a forest of mountain hemlock, western white and lodgepole pine, and Alaska yellow cedar.

WATER ACCESS

You pass near two undesirable ponds before crossing a trickling creek (2,260.7–5,153') that you shouldn't overlook, for it contains the best water you'll taste for miles.

After descending gently east, you curve around boggy Coleman Weedpatch. You then arc east, north of an unseen lake, and follow the easy path northeast, through a dense

mountain-hemlock forest across the lower slopes of Lakeview Mountain (6,660'). As the trail veers east, the forest transforms into an open stand of lodgepoles, and the path finally curves southeast to a junction with Walupt Lake Trail 101 (2,264.6–4,964'), which goes 4 miles to its trailhead at Walupt Lake Campground.

Beyond the junction, the countryside is quite open, and the topography stretches out below as you hike the trail up the west slope of a long, north-trending ridge. Fireweed, yarrow, lupine, and pearly everlasting proliferate along the trailside before you reach the shady confines of a coniferous forest. Now you contour for several miles before reaching the diminutive headwaters of Walupt Creek (2,268.7–5,577'). Continue west up toward a saddle where you'll see shallow, clear, 130-yard-long Sheep Lake (5,710'). Just north of it, you meet a junction with Nannie Ridge Trail 98 (2,269.4–5,765').

Your route through the Goat Rocks country will take you on ridges high above glaciated canyons. Walupt Creek canyon was the first major one you've seen in this wilderness, and those north of it are even more spectacular. From this junction, you descend 0.3 mile before hiking diagonally up to a crest saddle. Now in Yakama Nation Reservation territory (2,270.9–6,079'), you head north across barren slopes that have snow patches through most of the summer. The trail steepens as it approaches often snowbound Cispus Pass (2,271.7–6,474'), where you leave the tribal lands.

PLANTS The timberline trail drops north and passes dwarfed specimens of mountain hemlock and subalpine fir as it descends toward the headwaters

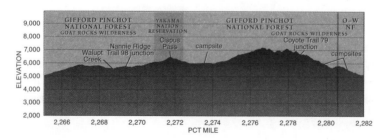

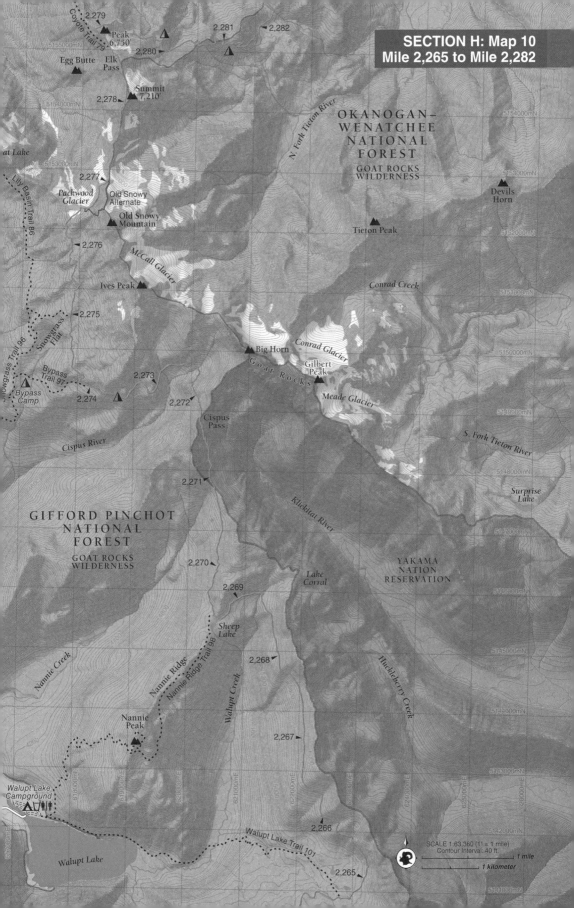

2,279

Coyote Trail 79

Peak
6,750'

2,281

2,282

2,280

Egg Butte

Elk
Pass

Summit
7,210'

2,278

OKANOGAN–
WENATCHEE
NATIONAL
FOREST

GOAT ROCKS
WILDERNESS

N. Fork Tieton River

at Lake

2,277

Packwood
Glacier

Old Snowy
Alternate

Old Snowy
Mountain

Devils
Horn

Lilly Basin Trail 86

2,276

McCall Glacier

Tieton Peak

Ives Peak

Conrad Creek

2,275

Snowgrass Trail 96

Snowgrass
Flat

Big Horn

Conrad Glacier

Gilbert
Peak

Goat Rocks

Bypass
Trail 97

2,273

2,272

Meade Glacier

Snowgrass Trail

Bypass
Camp

2,274

Cispus
Pass

S. Fork Tieton River

Cispus River

Surprise
Lake

2,271

Klickitat River

GIFFORD PINCHOT
NATIONAL
FOREST

GOAT ROCKS
WILDERNESS

2,270

Lake
Corral

YAKAMA
NATION
RESERVATION

2,269

Sheep
Lake

2,268

Nannie Creek

Nannie Ridge

Nannie Ridge Trail 98

Walupt Creek

Huckleberry Creek

Nannie
Peak

2,267

Walupt Lake
Campground

2,266

Walupt Lake Trail 101

2,265

SCALE 1:63,360 (1" = 1 mile)
Contour Interval: 40 ft.

1 mile

1 kilometer

Walupt Lake

SECTION H

of the Cispus River. The basin is much smaller than it first appears, and you quickly reach the easternmost tributary (2,272.4–6,146'). The scale of the canyon is put in true perspective when backpackers hike past miniature conifers that are now seen as only 30 feet high instead of 80, as you might suppose. After descending west, jump across the base of a splashing, 20-foot-high waterfall and then make a winding contour to a junction with Bypass Trail 97 (2,274.0–5,964').

CAMPING Bypass Trail 97 goes 0.6 mile west down to wind-shielded Bypass Camp, which lies on the east side of Snowgrass Creek.

SIDE TRIP Westward, Bypass Trail 97 continues 0.5 mile past Bypass Camp, for a total of 1.1 miles, to Snowgrass Trail 96, which offers the shortest route into the Goat Rocks area.

Northward, Trail 96 connects with the PCT north of your Bypass Trail 97 junction. Southwest, Trail 96 goes 3.6 miles to a fork from which the south branch goes over to a nearby hiker trailhead on spur road FS 405, and the north branch goes 0.5 mile to an equestrian trailhead near the end of FS 2150.

Leaving the Bypass Trail 97 junction, the PCT switchbacks up to a saddle, traverses slopes above Snowgrass Flat (no camping), and arrives at a junction with Snowgrass Trail 96 (2,275.0–6,404'). After a fairly steep climb north 0.2 mile, you see a 40-foot-high "Split Rock." This broke apart eons ago, and full-size conifers now grow in the gap between the two halves.

The route next climbs north-northeast past the rock and then switchbacks west over

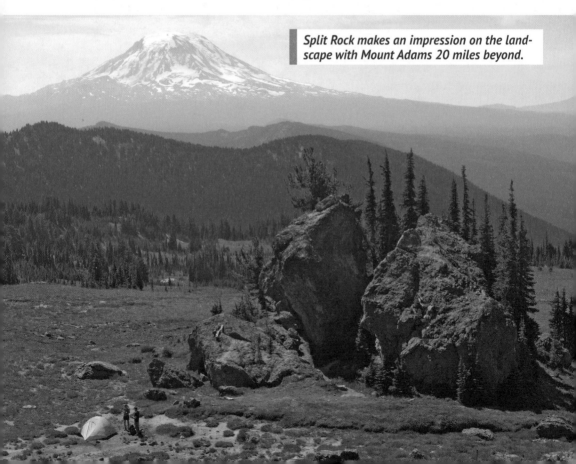

Split Rock makes an impression on the landscape with Mount Adams 20 miles beyond.

to a nearby ridge. From about this point north to Elk Pass and then east to the saddle above McCall Basin, you can expect to find quite a number of snowfields through most of the summer. About 0.75 mile past the Trail 96 junction, you tread across rocks with deep striations, convincing "fingerprints" of past glaciers. Climbing to the low west ridge of Old Snowy Mountain, you find the site of the former Dana May Yelverton Shelter (2,276.3–7,015'), which memorialized the hiker who died here in August 1962 of hypothermia. The shelter once provided protection from the area's frequent summer storms (no fires allowed). The 6-inch-high junipers here attest to the severity of this environment. Above lies the realm of rock and ice, the habitat of the alpine mountaineer.

As you climb briefly north from the shelter site, you may see one or two low windbreaks, neither giving you much protection if you are caught in a storm. Crossing a snowfield takes you to the brink of the severely glaciated, 3,000-foot-deep Upper Lake Creek canyon. This canyon will become even more impressive as this northbound trail provides even better views down and across it. To the northwest you see usually frozen Goat Lake (6,470') nestled in a classic glacial cirque at the southeast end of the Johnson Peak ridge.

At this brink, 0.25 mile beyond the shelter, the official PCT heads northeast along the gentle upper slopes of the Packwood Glacier. Typically this leg is mostly snowbound and potentially dangerous; the older PCT route, given as an alternate below, is sometimes passable for stock. When you start across these slopes, you leave the second-highest PCT point in Washington—7,095 feet.

ALTERNATE ROUTE From the trail up Old Snowy Mountain (2,276.6–7,095'), you have an almost full panorama of the Goat Rocks country.

From this brink, the old Cascade crest route makes short switchbacks east 0.4 mile to the north shoulder of Old Snowy Mountain. Up there, at 7,630 feet, you are almost as high as on the alternate hikers' route along Crater Lake's rim (Section C). From that point, you then have a steep descent 0.3 mile north to a saddle where you meet the PCT (2,277.0–7,095').

VIEWS Looking above the canyons to the northwest, you see the monarch of the Cascade Range, mighty Mount Rainier (14,410'), ruling above all the other stratovolcanoes. To the south is Mount Adams (12,276'), the crown prince and third-highest peak in the range (California's Mount Shasta, at 14,180 feet, rivals Mount Rainier in size). Off to Adams's west lies the youthful, onetime princess, Mount St. Helens (8,363'); before Mount St. Helens blew its top off in 1980, it was a symmetrical peak 9,677 feet in elevation.

The official PCT route cuts rather precariously across the upper part of Packwood Glacier before curving north down to a crest saddle (2,277.0–7,095'), where it rejoins the alternate route.

This Egg Butte section of the PCT, constructed with heroic efforts in 1953–54, now continues along the jagged ridge, contours around its "teeth," and provides alpine views across McCall Glacier toward Tieton Peak (7,768'), due east of Old Snowy. You reach a small saddle, from which the trail makes a precarious descent across a steep slope as it bypasses Summit 7,210. You can expect this narrow footpath to be snowbound and

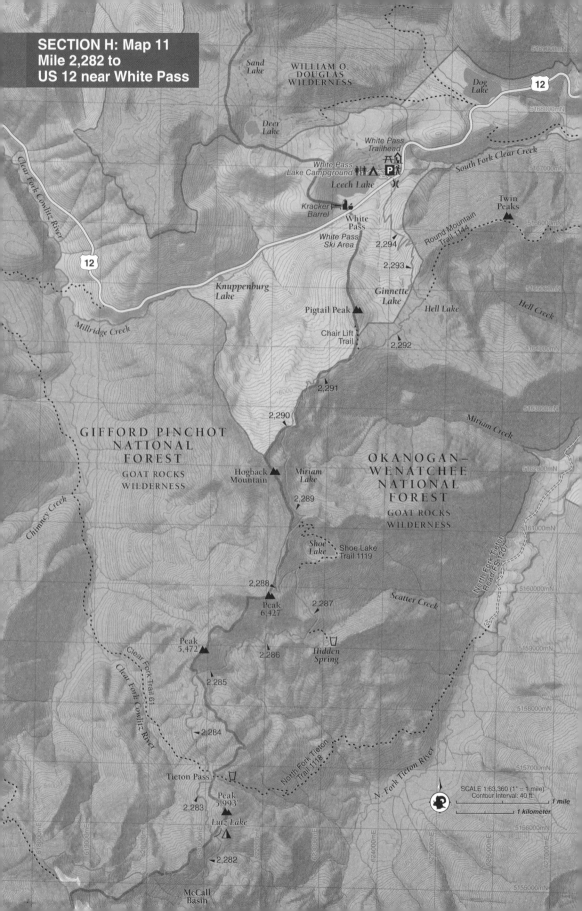

Sand
Lake

WILLIAM O.
DOUGLAS
WILDERNESS

Dog
Lake

12

Deer
Lake

White Pass
Trailhead

White Pass
Lake Campground

Leech Lake

South Fork Clear Creek

Twin
Peaks

Clear Fork Cowlitz River

Kracker
Barrel

White
Pass

White Pass
Ski Area

2,294

2,293

Round Mountain Trail 1144

12

Knuppenburg
Lake

Pigtail Peak

Ginnette
Lake

Hell Lake

Hell Creek

Millridge Creek

Chair Lift
Trail

2,292

2,291

2,290

GIFFORD PINCHOT
NATIONAL
FOREST

GOAT ROCKS
WILDERNESS

Chimney Creek

Hogback
Mountain

Miriam
Lake

2,289

Miriam Creek

OKANOGAN–
WENATCHEE
NATIONAL
FOREST

GOAT ROCKS
WILDERNESS

North Fork Tieton Road FS 1207

Shoe
Lake

Shoe Lake
Trail 1119

2,288

Peak
6,427'

2,287

Scatter Creek

Peak
5,472'

2,286

Hidden
Spring

Clear Fork Trail 61

2,285

Clear Fork Cowlitz River

2,284

North Fork Tieton Trail 1118

N. Fork Tieton River

Tieton Pass

2,283

Peak
5,993'

Lutz Lake

2,282

McCall
Basin

SCALE 1:63,360 (1" = 1 mile)
Contour Interval: 40 ft.

1 mile

1 kilometer

hazardous through most of July. Crampons may be required, particularly in early summer, and stock animals may be forced back. Reaching the ridge again, you follow it down to Elk Pass, where you meet the upper end of Coyote Trail 79 (2,278.6–6,690').

PLANTS Here the windswept whitebark pines stand chest-high at most, and the junipers creep just inches above the frost-wedged rocks.

Pushing toward supplies at White Pass, you first drop northwest, paralleling Coyote Trail 79 below you, and then in 0.3 mile angle east across the sometimes-snowy north slopes of Peak 6,750. You trade breathtaking views down Upper Lake Creek canyon to the northwest for views north down larger Clear Fork Cowlitz River canyon.

The trail descends east-southeast to the foot of the Elk Pass snowfield, down which hikers sometimes ski. Cross its runoff creek and several others, pass glacially striated bedrock, and then slip and slide down short, steep switchbacks etched on a narrow ridge. The grade abates and ends near a small pond at the foot of another snowfield. By late afternoon, the snowfields in this basin are melting at a good rate, as evidenced by the roar of the cascade to the west. From the pond, you switchback steeply but briefly up to a saddle.

CAMPING The PCT switchbacks east and almost touches a crest saddle (2,281.1–5,566'), on which you could set up an emergency bivy, and then it switchbacks down into forest cover. You hike over to a saddle that holds knee-deep Lutz Lake and several

small campsites (2,282.3–5,081'). Leave No Trace informs us that 200 feet is a good distance from water sources to camp.

Beyond this viewless spot, the trail descends north around the west slope of Peak 5,993 to Tieton Pass and a junction with the North Fork Tieton and Clear Fork Trails (2,283.4–4,778').

WATER ACCESS

From this junction, North Fork Tieton Trail 1118, which at 4.5 miles is the shortest trail approach to this pass, descends east before curving northeast down to North Fork Tieton Road 1207. You can usually find creek water by descending about 0.25 mile along this trail.

SIDE TRIP From this junction, Clear Fork Trail 61, starting a moderate descent west-northwest from Tieton Pass, takes a long way out (7.9 miles) toward US 12.

The PCT starts a gentle descent northwest, gradually makes a winding route north past two stagnant ponds, crosses east over the divide, and rounds Peak 5,472. Now you continue east on this viewless path until it climbs the southeast spur of Peak 6,427 and reaches a junction with Hidden Spring Trail 1117 (2,286.7–5,556').

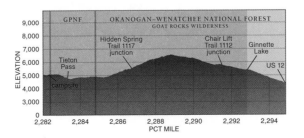

WATER ACCESS

Hidden Spring Trail 1117 heads east from the PCT. In 0.3 mile one or more short spur trails in this vicinity head east to Hidden Spring, which lies just above a beautiful meadow. Note that this is your last real opportunity for good water this side of US 12, 8.2 trail miles from the spring.

On the PCT, climb north then northwest, and where the Shoe Lake Trail 1119 bends northeast, branch west (2,287.6–6,104'). The PCT first curves southwest as it climbs toward Peak 6,427 and then curves north, leaving forest cover as it approaches a ridge. Cross this and then traverse steep slopes on the west side of Peak 6,547. These at first are bouldery and open, offering views west into steep Clear Fork Cowlitz River canyon, whose floor lies 0.5 mile below the trail. Boulders give way to firs and hemlocks and, through midsummer, some snow problems.

Soon you recross the ridge and have views southeast of Shoe Lake (no camping allowed) as you contour over to the other end of the Shoe Lake Trail, which was once the original route of the PCT. Overuse at the lake led to the creation of the newer route. In 90 yards you top a narrow ridge; from it you see Mount Rainier poking its head above Hogback Ridge, while Mount Adams just manages to lift its crown above Goat Rocks.

You make one switchback, descend a well-graded trail past a thumb above you and Miriam Lake below you, and then reach the stepped slope of Hogback Mountain (6,789'). Descending its northeast ridge, you have more views of Mount Rainier and cross the Goat Rocks Wilderness border twice within a mile. Then you enter forest once again, cross a vaguely defined saddle, and climb gently to a nearby junction with Chair Lift Trail (2,291.5–5,805').

From the junction, the PCT makes a viewless, winding descent northeast to a junction with little-used Round Mountain Trail 1144 (2,292.6–5,434'), which starts on a gentle descent east before curving north to the twin Peaks. Your route curves northwest; passes a small, stagnant pond; and reaches green, 100-yard-long Ginnette Lake (2,292.8–5,419'). You now leave Goat Rocks Wilderness, get a glimpse of the chairlift jeep road northwest of the trail, and then switchback down to a trailhead parking lot 50 yards south of US 12 (2,294.9–4,409'). (From the highway, the short road to the trailhead begins just 30 yards east of, and on the other side of the highway from, the Leech Lake spur road to White Pass Lake Campground.)

RESUPPLY ACCESS

About 200 yards up the Leech Lake spur road, where it bends from west to north, an old, closed road starts south and then quickly bends southwest for a rambling trek over to White Pass Village, reaching a north–south road that starts from the west side of the village. This usually soggy route is supposedly for campers, hikers, and equestrians, but hikers can safely walk southwest along the broad highway shoulder to reach the Kracker Barrel Store and White Pass Village.

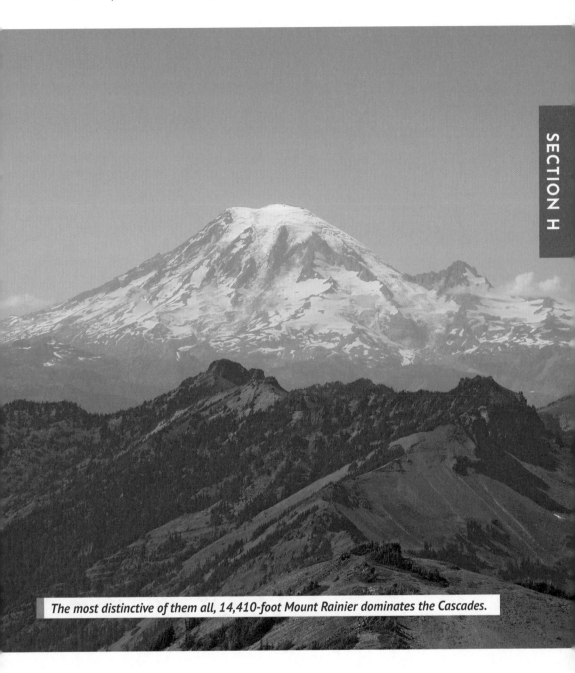

The most distinctive of them all, 14,410-foot Mount Rainier dominates the Cascades.

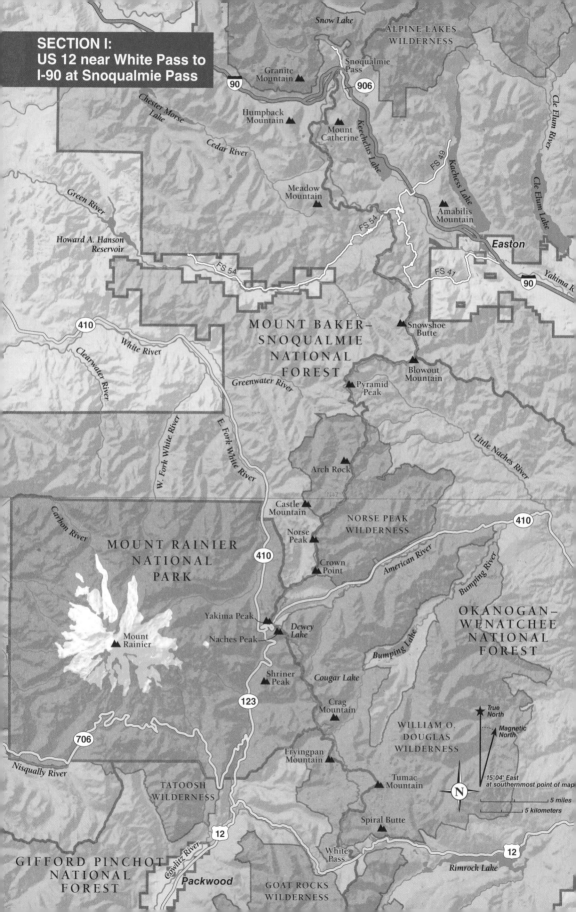

Snow Lake

ALPINE LAKES
WILDERNESS

90

Granite
Mountain ▲

Snoqualmie
Pass

906

Keechelus Lake

FS 49

Kachess Lake

Cle Elum River

Cle Elum Lake

Chester Morse
Lake

Humpback
Mountain ▲

Cedar River

Mount
Catherine ▲

Meadow
Mountain ▲

FS 54

Amabilis
Mountain ▲

Easton

Green River

FS 54

FS 41

90

Yakima R.

Howard A. Hanson
Reservoir

410

White River

Clearwater River

MOUNT BAKER–
SNOQUALMIE
NATIONAL
FOREST

Greenwater River

Snowshoe
Butte ▲

Blowout
Mountain ▲

Pyramid
Peak ▲

Little Naches River

W. Fork White River

E. Fork White River

Arch Rock ▲

N47

Castle
Mountain ▲

NORSE PEAK
WILDERNESS

410

Carbon River

MOUNT RAINIER
NATIONAL
PARK

410

Norse
Peak ▲

Crown
Point ▲

American River

Bumping River

OKANOGAN–
WENATCHEE
NATIONAL
FOREST

Yakima Peak ▲

Dewey
Lake

Naches Peak

Mount
Rainier ▲

123

Shriner
Peak ▲

Cougar Lake

Bumping Lake

Crag
Mountain ▲

WILLIAM O.
DOUGLAS
WILDERNESS

True
North

Magnetic
North

706

Fryingpan
Mountain ▲

Tumac
Mountain ▲

15°04' East
at southernmost point of map

Nisqually River

TATOOSH
WILDERNESS

N

5 miles

5 kilometers

Spiral Butte ▲

12

White
Pass

Rimrock Lake

12

GIFFORD PINCHOT
NATIONAL
FOREST

Cowlitz River

Packwood

GOAT ROCKS
WILDERNESS

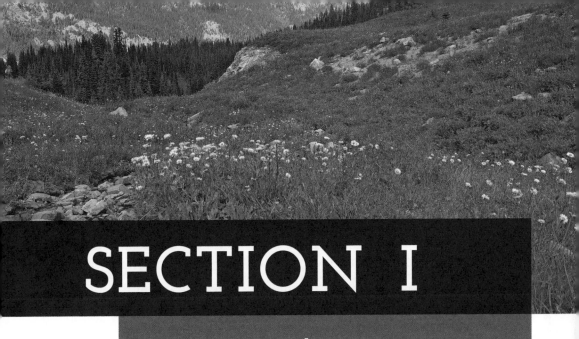

SECTION I

US 12 near White Pass to I-90 at Snoqualmie Pass

STARK CONTRASTS IN LAND USE separate this section of the Pacific Crest Trail (PCT) into two very different segments. The southern half is largely a subalpine parkland glistening with lakes cupped in forests and meadows. Most of this backcountry lies protected within the boundaries of two wilderness areas and Mount Rainier National Park. The northern half, on the other hand, being lower, is totally within the montane forest belt so favored by the lumber industry, and it blisters with a lot of barren earth, some of the most extensively clear-cut land in the West.

Moderate topography characterizes both halves of this section, and fit border-bound hikers can make good time. From White Pass, the trail sloshes through soggy muskeg country, crossing a plateau pocked with pools and lakes. As the Cascade divide rises into a knobby backbone, the trail follows it faithfully, swinging from saddle to subalpine saddle, passing within

Above: Asters, arnica, owl's clover, and lupine create a flash mob of color.

12 miles of massive Mount Rainier. Not quite one-third of the way through this section, at Chinook Pass, the broadest of these flower-rich saddles, WA 410 crosses the crest.

Halfway through this section, the craggy divide slopes below the subalpine zone, and though fir and hemlock forests dominate here, meadows and crest-top vistas keep the hiking varied and interesting. Still 40 miles from Snoqualmie Pass, the trail enters an area where much of the land was once owned by Plum Creek, the landholding subsidiary of Burlington Northern Railroad. The railroad received title to every other square mile during the railroad subsidies of the 1880s in return for laying tracks across Stampede Pass, so the forests have been mined, and nearly half of this last stretch goes through recovering clear-cuts laced with logging roads. Today, most of Plum Creek's holdings have been acquired by the U.S. Forest Service, King County, and the Nature Conservancy.

DECLINATION 15°04'E

USGS MAPS	
White Pass, WA	White River Park, WA (PCT barely enters map)
Raven Roost, WA	Stampede Pass, WA
Cougar Lake, WA	Norse Peak, WA
Lester, WA	Lost Lake, WA
Chinook Pass, WA	Noble Knob, WA
Blowout Mountain, WA	Snoqualmie Pass, WA

POINTS ON THE TRAIL, SOUTH TO NORTH

	Mile	Elevation in feet	Latitude/Longitude
US 12 near White Pass	2,294.9	4,409	N46° 38' 37.1687" W121° 22' 45.4575"
Beusch Lake	2,300.9	5,101	N46° 41' 44.0075" W121° 23' 49.7454"
Bumping River ford by Bumping Lake Trail junction	2,308.6	4,101	N46° 45' 49.6523" W121° 25' 32.7371"
WA 410 at Chinook Pass	2,323.5	5,434	N46° 52' 18.7611" W121° 30' 56.4455"
Bear Gap Trail junction	2,329.0	5,885	N46° 54' 59.8518" W121° 28' 20.4535"
Big Crow Basin Spring	2,334.1	6,237	N46° 57' 42.0828" W121° 27' 11.4931"
Arch Rock Spring spur trail junction	2,341.6	5,685	N47° 02' 08.3472" W121° 23' 48.8589"

POINTS ON THE TRAIL, SOUTH TO NORTH *(continued)*

	Mile	Elevation in feet	Latitude/Longitude
Little Bear Creek Trail junction on Blowout Mountain	2,356.9	5,329	N47° 08' 10.5089" W121° 18' 16.4342"
Sheets Pass	2,365.5	3,702	N47° 12' 55.4317" W121° 19' 29.3243"
Stampede Pass and FS 54	2,374.9	3,671	N47° 16' 59.7452" W121° 21' 04.5862"
I-90 at Snoqualmie Pass	2,393.1	3,000	N47° 25' 35.8773" W121° 24' 55.7528"

CAMPSITES AND BIVY SITES

Mile	Elevation in feet	Latitude/Longitude	Number of tents	Feature	Notes
2,295.1	4,500	N46° 38' 41.8740" W121° 23' 03.1380"	10	White Pass Lake Campground	Vault toilet
2,297.7	5,311	N46° 39' 35.5800" W121° 24' 49.4400"	3	Sand Lake Shelter	
2,301.8	5,194	N46° 42' 01.7682" W121° 23' 13.3363"	2	Pipe Lake	On southeast corner
2,307.3	4,639	N46° 44' 53.3389" W121° 25' 08.7842"	>4	Stream	On both sides of bridge
2,310.8	4,807	N46° 46' 14.5620" W121° 25' 41.8660"	2	Stream	
2,320.8	5,146	N46° 51' 25.7248" W121° 29' 17.2650"	>4	Dewey Lake	On right
2,325.7	5,766	N46° 53' 37.0021" W121° 30' 04.4275"	3	Sheep Lake	Surrounding lake
2,333.4	5,841	N46° 57' 15.3600" W121° 26' 18.9000"	4	Basin Lake	0.5 mile off-trail
2,347.0	4,770	N47° 05' 22.4823" W121° 23' 45.5015"	>10	Camp Ulrich	Outhouse, fire ring
2,367.7	4,652	N47° 13' 15.3409" W121° 21' 15.6378"	3		Flat spot near trail on right
2,379.8	3,553	N47° 17' 48.2400" W121° 25' 25.6200"	3	Stirrup Lake	0.5 mile off-trail
2,384.3	4,201	N47° 20' 39.7800" W121° 26' 12.0600"	5	Mirror Lake	
2,390.9.	3,178	N47° 24' 26.5800" W121° 25' 53.3400"	2	Lodge Lake	

WEATHER TO GO

In early season, snow clinging to north and east slopes between Bumping River and Blowout Mountain can make carrying an ice ax worthwhile.

SUPPLIES

For White Pass, see "Supplies" in the previous section. For Snoqualmie Pass, see "Supplies" in the next section.

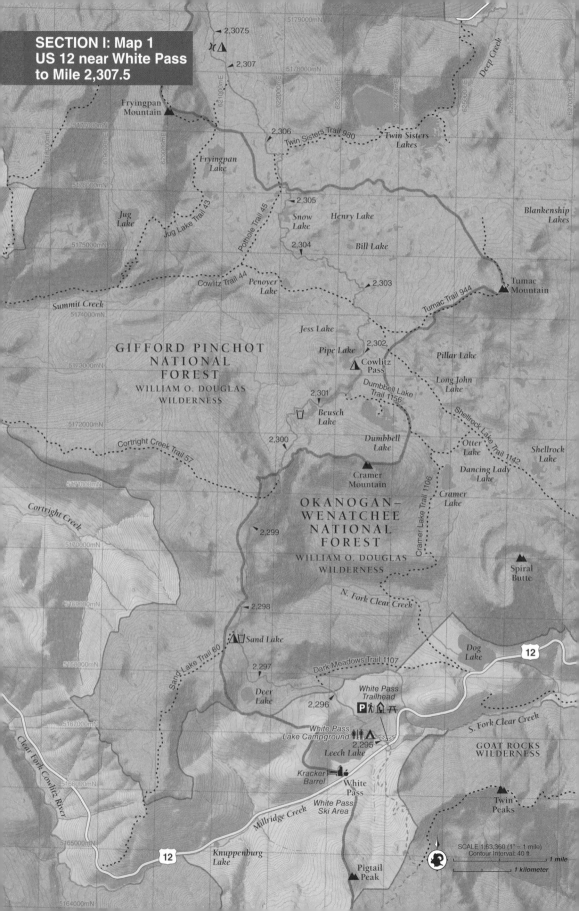

2,307.5

2,307

Fryingpan Mountain

Fryingpan Lake

2,306

Twin Sisters Trail 980

Twin Sisters Lakes

Blankenship Lakes

2,305

Jug Lake

Jug Lake Trail 43

Pothole Trail 45

Snow Lake

Henry Lake

2,304

Bill Lake

Cowlitz Trail 44

Penoyer Lake

2,303

Tumac Trail 944

Tumac Mountain

Summit Creek

Jess Lake

Pipe Lake

2,302

Cowlitz Pass

Pillar Lake

GIFFORD PINCHOT NATIONAL FOREST

WILLIAM O. DOUGLAS WILDERNESS

Dumbbell Lake Trail 1156

Long John Lake

2,301

Beusch Lake

Shellrock Lake Trail 1142

2,300

Dumbbell Lake

Otter Lake

Shellrock Lake

Cortright Creek Trail 57

Cramer Mountain

Dancing Lady Lake

Cortright Creek

2,299

OKANOGAN– WENATCHEE NATIONAL FOREST

Cramer Lake Trail 1106

Cramer Lake

WILLIAM O. DOUGLAS WILDERNESS

Spiral Butte

N. Fork Clear Creek

2,298

Sand Lake Trail 60

Sand Lake

Dog Lake

12

Dark Meadows Trail 1107

2,297

Deer Lake

White Pass Trailhead

S. Fork Clear Creek

2,296

P

White Pass Lake Campground

2,295

Leech Lake

GOAT ROCKS WILDERNESS

Kracker Barrel

White Pass

Clear Fork Cowlitz River

White Pass Ski Area

Twin Peaks

12

Millridge Creek

Knuppenburg Lake

Pigtail Peak

SCALE 1:63,360 (1" = 1 mile)
Contour Interval: 40 ft.

1 mile

1 kilometer

PERMITS

No wilderness permits are required along this section, unless you venture some distance west of the PCT into Mount Rainier National Park.

WATER

On the crest-top route between Government Meadow and Stampede Pass, water is scarce, partly because logging has obliterated some springs. By mid-July, few reliable and convenient water sources can be found, especially toward the end of this section.

SPECIAL CONCERNS

Mosquitoes can be especially bad in the marshy terrain north of White Pass.

In some of the logged areas, blowdowns and generally battered soil make following the trail less than easy, although few hikers get off route. The trail crosses many logging roads and follows a few for very short distances. Most of these crossings and followings are clearly posted with PCT emblems or diamonds, but a few might require a brief search.

US 12 NEAR WHITE PASS TO I-90 AT SNOQUALMIE PASS

>>> THE ROUTE

Hikers driving to White Pass will want to turn north off US 12 just 0.5 mile northeast of White Pass and park, after 0.2 mile, at the trailhead parking lot near Leech Lake. The PCT crosses US 12 (2,294.9–4,409') only 30 yards east of the Leech Lake PCT trailhead turnoff and passes an old shelter on its way to this parking lot.

Pulverized duff and horse apples evince this section's popularity with equestrians as you start from the lot in a gentle, switchbacking climb before entering William O. Douglas Wilderness at the next trail junction.

HISTORY A staunch conservationist, the late U.S. Supreme Court Justice William Douglas grew up near Yakima, and he hiked throughout the lands now named after him, loving the area enough to establish his home in Goose Prairie, on the Bumping River.

After leveling out in the fir-and-spruce forest, the PCT passes a junction with Dark Meadows Trail 1107 (2,296.1–4,816'), which descends east to Dog Lake. Resuming a gradual climb, you skirt a meadow, rise beside and then cross Deer Lake's outlet creek, and

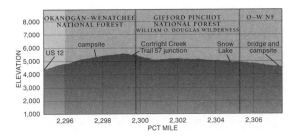

switchback up to a much larger meadow just before reaching Deer Lake (2,297.1–5,181').

WATER ACCESS

CAMPING Ahead, a barely ascending walk north through forest and lupine-rich glades brings you to Sand Lake (2,297.7–5,311'), where, from the base of the lake's peninsula, a spur leads south to a shelter that's barely large enough to sleep three.

Just beyond this spur, a sign points west to US 12, along obscure Sand Lake Trail 60. The PCT, however, continues north on an essentially level track, past the curious spikes of bear grass. The trail contours around a rocky knob to meet Cortright Creek Trail 57 (2,299.6–5,481') coming from the southwest. Under subalpine firs, the PCT starts winding down a few steep switchbacks.

WATER ACCESS

The brief descent ends at Beusch Lake (2,300.9–5,101'), the entry point onto the heart of the plateau that caps this part of the gentle divide between the Cowlitz and Yakima Rivers.

PLANTS For 6 miles now, the trail runs across hummocky flatlands riddled with ponds, puddles, mudholes, and muskeg. Patchily forested with droopy hemlocks and pointy subalpine firs, and carpeted with heather, huckleberry, and azalea, this area supports only acid-tolerant plants.

Turn east along the north shore of Beusch Lake and soon come to Dumbbell Lake Trail 1156 (2,301.4–5,136'), which forks south between two pools. From here, you curve north to pass within close view of Pipe Lake's bowl and then pass its long, slender stem, where there's a good picnic spot (2,302.0–5,197'). A few minutes north from here, the trail arcs northeast around a couple of grassy ponds and arrives at ill-defined Cowlitz Pass. In this open area, snags from an old fire stand over spirea and azalea and allow a view of Mount Rainier. A trail (2,302.5–5,168') heads east from here for Shellrock Lake.

The PCT soon turns northwest, reaches a junction with Cowlitz Trail 44 (2,302.7–5,128'), and starts a twisting, winding course, first northeast and then trending northwest. Although the topography map shows almost no contours through here, dozens of hillocks and gullies dimple this land, and the trail takes great pains to avoid every hint of meadow or soggy ground. On the way, you pass just north of one unnamed lake and wind into dark forest and then down to Snow Lake (2,304.8–4,940').

You cross Snow Lake's outlet and weave a north-trending course, barely descending. Peeking in and out of fir groves, you come to Twin Sisters Trail 980, tracking right (east), and then intersect Pothole Trail 45 (2,305.8–4,849'), which to the south meets Cowlitz Trail 44. Still avoiding meadows while trending northnorthwest, you hike just west of a creek that is gradually gathering water and momentum. The

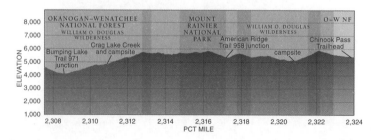

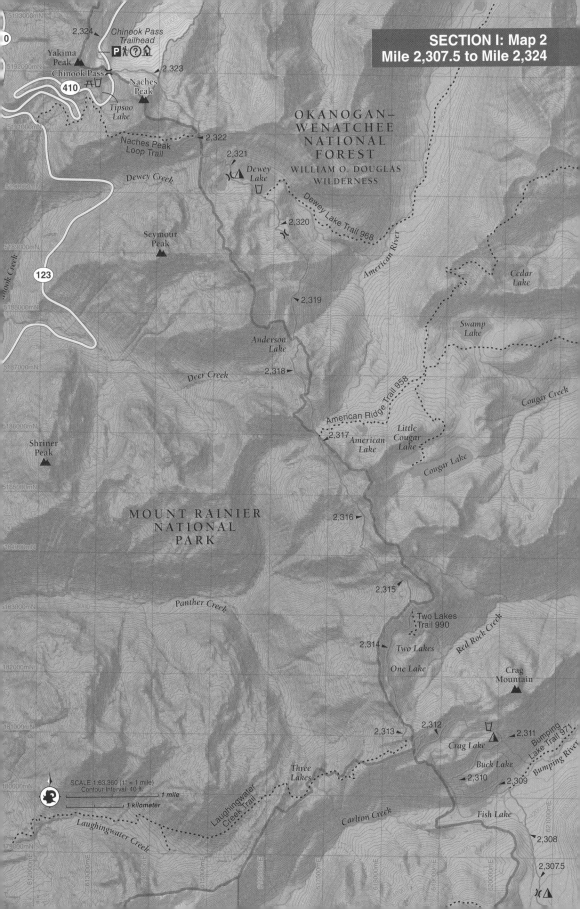

2,324

Chinook Pass
Trailhead

Yakima
Peak

2,323

Chinook Pass

410

Naches
Peak

Tipsoo
Lake

2,322

Naches Peak
Loop Trail

2,321

Dewey
Lake

OKANOGAN–
WENATCHEE
NATIONAL
FOREST

WILLIAM O. DOUGLAS
WILDERNESS

Dewey Creek

123

Seymour
Peak

2,320

Dewey Lake Trail 968

American River

Cedar
Lake

2,319

Anderson
Lake

Swamp
Lake

Deer Creek

2,318

American Ridge Trail 958

Cougar Creek

Shriner
Peak

2,317

American
Lake

Little
Cougar
Lake

Cougar Lake

MOUNT RAINIER
NATIONAL
PARK

2,316

2,315

Panther Creek

Two Lakes
Trail 990

Red Rock Creek

2,314

Two Lakes

One Lake

Crag
Mountain

2,313

2,312

2,311

Bumping Lake Trail 971

Crag Lake

Buck Lake

Bumping River

Three
Lakes

2,310

2,309

SCALE 1:63,360 (1" = 1 mile)
Contour Interval: 40 ft.

1 mile

1 kilometer

Laughingwater
Creek Trail

Carlton Creek

Fish Lake

Laughingwater Creek

2,308

2,307.5

track channels into a steady, gentle descent as you pass the forested slopes of Fryingpan Mountain and a junction with southbound Jug Lake Trail 43 (2,306.9–4,665').

CAMPING With more easy walking, you come to a wooden bridge over the Bumping River, where there are several campsites (2,307.3–4,604').

From this bridge, the PCT skirts east of a large meadow and decidedly drops off the Cowlitz–Yakima plateau. The steady descent ends at the outlet of Fish Lake (2,308.6–4,101'), headwaters of the Bumping River. Across this creek is a junction with Bumping Lake Trail 971, where the PCT cuts west to touch the north shore of long, shallow Fish Lake. The PCT promptly leaves the lakeside path and starts working up long switchbacks that take you above Buck Lake, across Crag Lake's outlet, and then back to a spur that drops to Crag Lake itself.

WATER ACCESS

As the PCT contours just beyond this spur, it passes a reliable, drinkable rill (2,311.3–5,042').

VIEWS A couple of more long, lazy switchbacks have you rising across meadowy slopes verdant with flowers such as aster, spirea, blueberry, and corn lily. Marveling at Mounts Rainier, Adams, and St. Helens, you then turn north around the Cascade divide and pass Laughingwater Creek Trail (2,312.9–5,712'), which drops southwest. Here, at the start of a long tour high along the Cascade backbone, you can, in good weather, look forward to miles of glorious, expansive views; in bad weather, you'll find yourself shrouded in clouds, exposed to the brunt of wet, westerly storms.

Contouring now, you soon recross the divide to traverse above One Lake and eventually meet Two Lakes Trail 990 (2,314.6–5,603'), which descends 0.3 mile to Two Lakes. Next the PCT makes a quick climb back to the west side, where you are now in Mount Rainier National Park, and the mountain's overwhelming presence hardly lets you notice the many wildflowers underfoot, of which partridge foot is the most common flower. You start another long trek, contouring through forest and meadow across a couple of spur ridges before dropping via abrupt switchbacks to a saddle and a junction with American Ridge Trail 958 (2,317.2–5,350'), which departs eastward. Here you look down the long, forested valley of the American River.

Now the PCT makes a brief climb north to cross a crest saddle, exiting and reentering the national park, and then contours through subalpine-fir groves before winding down to visit Anderson Lake (2,318.5–5,369'). Continuing north, the trail leaves the national park once again and barely climbs as it crosses a seasonal trickle, travels over scree, and rounds a spur ridge. It then arcs down toward Dewey Lake, first meeting Dewey Lake Trail 968 (2,320.4–5,158'), which branches east to the American River valley.

WATER ACCESS

CAMPING Just beyond the junction, Dewey Lake's expansive waters and numerous campsites along the shore-hugging PCT invite a pause (2,320.8–5,146'); be aware, however, that no campfires are allowed within 0.25 mile of the lake. Whenever possible, camp on durable surfaces such as flat granite or decomposing rock gravel. (Both are surprisingly comfortable and way cleaner than sand or grass.)

After rounding Dewey Lake's shore and bridging its inlet, the route climbs out of the soggy lake basin, working west through dark forest before emerging onto meadowland. After this, the trail switchbacks into the national park and immediately meets the Naches Peak Loop Trail (2,322.0–5,830'), a day hiker's path that reaches WA 410 only 0.3 mile south of Chinook Pass. The PCT now leaves the national park for good.

PLANTS Here is an introduction to amazingly colorful flora. Paintbrush, pasqueflower, lupine, avalanche lily, and a galaxy of other blossoms spill over the PCT.

The trail tops the rise and then descends, first abruptly and then in a long traverse past a tarn, exiting the William O. Douglas Wilderness (2,323.3–5,479') but remaining in the Okanogan-Wenatchee National Forest and heading on to WA 410's fairly steady traffic at Chinook Pass (2,323.5–5,434'). In this vicinity are junctions with a spur trail to the highway's rest area and a trail to Tipsoo Lake. From Chinook Pass, it's 68 miles east to Yakima, 41 miles northwest to Enumclaw, and 34 miles southwest to Paradise, the starting point for the challenging "standard" route to the top of Mount Rainier.

WATER ACCESS

The trail leaves the pass for a 0.3-mile descent to a picnic area beside Tipsoo Lake.

Beyond the footbridge over the highway, the PCT turns north onto an old roadbed, crosses a bench, and then, once more a trail, approaches traffic as it makes a rising traverse.

PLANTS This steep slope supports a scrubbier flora than that at Chinook Pass proper. Fireweed, huckleberry, manzanita, pearly everlasting, and bedraggled Alaska cedars, hardy plants all, testify to tougher conditions.

SECTION I

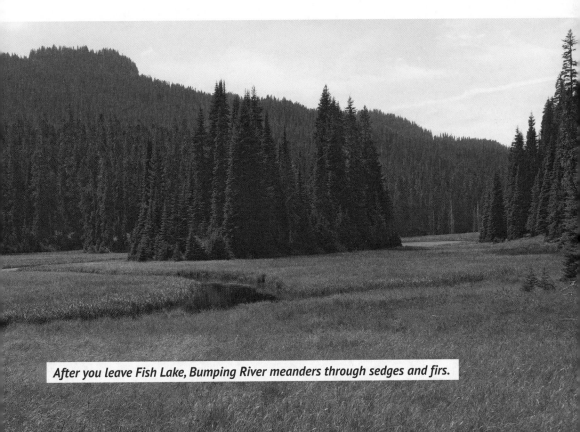

After you leave Fish Lake, Bumping River meanders through sedges and firs.

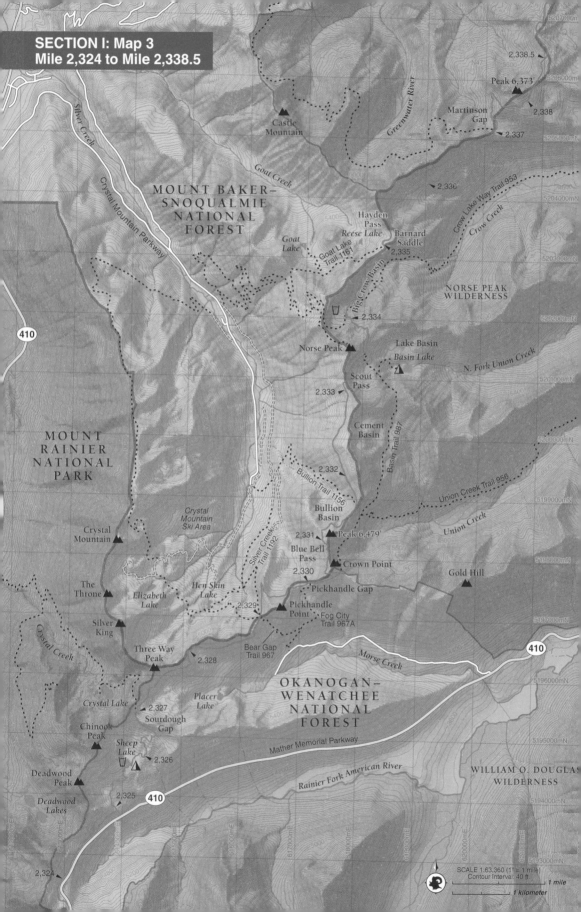

2,338.5

Peak 6,373'

Martinson Gap

2,338

2,337

Greenwater River

2,336

Crow Lake Way Trail 953

Crow Creek

Castle Mountain

Goat Creek

MOUNT BAKER–
SNOQUALMIE
NATIONAL
FOREST

Hayden Pass
Reese Lake

Barnard Saddle

2,335

Goat Lake

Goat Lake Trail 1161

Big Crow Basin

NORSE PEAK
WILDERNESS

Silver Creek

Crystal Mountain Parkway

2,334

Norse Peak

Lake Basin
Basin Lake

N. Fork Union Creek

Scout Pass

2,333

Cement Basin

Basin Trail 967

MOUNT
RAINIER
NATIONAL
PARK

2,332

Bullion Trail 1156

Union Creek Trail 956

Union Creek

Crystal
Mountain
Ski Area

Bullion Basin

2,331

Peak 6,479'

Blue Bell Pass

2,330

Crown Point

Gold Hill

Silver Creek Trail 1192

Crystal Mountain

Pickhandle Gap

The Throne

Hen Skin Lake

Elizabeth Lake

2,329

Pickhandle Point

Fog City Trail 967A

Silver King

Crystal Creek

Three Way Peak

2,328

Bear Gap Trail 967

Morse Creek

410

OKANOGAN–
WENATCHEE
NATIONAL
FOREST

Placer Lake

Crystal Lake

2,327

Sourdough Gap

Chinook Peak

Sheep Lake

2,326

Mather Memorial Parkway

Deadwood Peak

WILLIAM O. DOUGLAS
WILDERNESS

Deadwood Lakes

2,325

410

Rainier Fork American River

2,324

SCALE 1:63,360 (1" = 1 mile)
Contour Interval: 40 ft

1 mile

1 kilometer

410

WATER ACCESS

CAMPING The gradual ascent turns up a ravine and steepens into a couple of switchbacks before the trail reaches Sheep Lake (2,325.7–5,760'), a popular spot for day hikers and overnighters.

After following the lakeshore for a bit, the PCT starts upslope, weaving and switchbacking generally northeast across meadowy bowls and up into ptarmigan and pika country. It then travels under small crags to Sourdough Gap (2,326.9–6,385'). The names of this saddle and other features to the north recall the gold and silver prospectors who worked this region in the past.

Admiring Mounts Adams and St. Helens, you can savor here the start of another long stretch of high traverse, which is wonderfully scenic if the weather is good. Skidding down scree off the gap, you reach a switchback and, after another hairpin, settle into a long, gently descending trek near treeline. Placer Lake comes into view 600 feet below as you approach Bear Gap, where you find a major trail plexus (2,329.0–5,885'). From here, Silver Creek Trail 1192 drops northwest to civilization at Crystal Mountain Ski Area, Hen Skin Lake Trail 1193 starts southwest, and Bear Gap Trail 967 comes up from Morse Creek and WA 410 to the east. You, however, take the PCT in a slant across the gap. For the next mile and a half,

you cross between Okanogan-Wenatchee and Mount Baker–Snoqualmie National Forests. Your route now contours north, as you view ski lifts and condominiums well below, until the PCT turns southeast on its way around the steep flanks of Pickhandle Point.

Next the trail angles back across the crest at Pickhandle Gap and presently meets a trail (2,330.0–5,921') dropping east and bound for Fog City and Gold Hill. Then the PCT rises along the open south slopes of Crown Point and, at the breathtaking crest between Crown Point and Gold Hill, reaches the southern boundary of Norse Peak Wilderness, which your route borders for the next 4.5 miles. Here you also reach a junction with Basin Trail 987 (2,330.5–6,195'), dropping north off the crest 50 yards west of where you gain it. Follow the PCT on a steady climb west and then north around Crown Point, before long coming onto the narrow watershed divide at Blue Bell Pass.

FIRE From this saddle, the trail— damaged by the 2017 Norse Peak Fire from Pickhandle Gap to Louisiana Saddle—contours north and approaches the spur dividing Pickhandle and Bullion Basins.

Contour around Peak 6,479, which takes you to narrow Bullion Pass. Balancing astride this narrow saddle, you meet Bullion Basin Trail 1156 (2,331.7–6,125') descending to the west. As the crest rises to a summit again, you ascend along its west flank in a long, meadow traverse to Scout Pass.

VIEWS Here you have a view across Lake Basin's gentle parkland, bossed over by one of the area's larger crags.

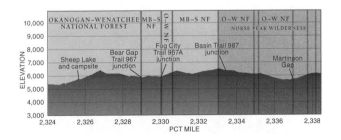

A gentle descent leads you across the head of Lake Basin, and you once again pass Basin Trail 987 (2,333.4–6,384').

CAMPING Basin Trail 987 descends to excellent camping at Basin Lake, 0.5 mile below. Camping off-trail at sites such as this helps to relieve some of the environmental pressures due to increased numbers of hikers.

Round the northeast spur of Norse Peak, and descend into Big Crow Basin.

WATER ACCESS

As you near the bottomland at the head of this basin, you pass 30 feet above a welcome and reliable spring (2,334.1–6,237').

Some 40 yards beyond this, you meet a junction with a westward-climbing trail and Crow Lake Way Trail 953, which passes an old shelter 0.5 mile away on its eastward descent. Next the PCT rounds Big Crow Basin, and then it rises along a bench and back to the crest at forested Barnard Saddle. After weaving through a couple of small, crest-line ravines, the PCT passes a junction with Goat Lake Trail 1161 (2,335.0–6,105'), which heads left (southwest). The PCT returns to the east side of the divide at Hayden Pass, and you get a view over Little Crow Basin. From the pass, the PCT stays within the Norse Peak Wilderness for several miles.

Your route makes a steep slant down into this basin and then gradually descends across its upper glades and fir forest. The PCT soon crosses an avalanche gully and continues slanting down and out of Little Crow Basin. Then it goes northeast for some time before making a brief climb to Martinson Gap and unmaintained Castle Mountain Trail 1188 (2,337.0–5,744'). Beyond this gap, the track turns northwest to angle up the slopes of Peak 6,373, passing an old burn. Next the trail pivots and arcs around the south and east slopes of Peak 6,373, recrosses the crest, and gradually settles onto the broadening Cascade divide, still presenting Mount Rainier's massive white dome through the scattered and stunted subalpine firs. Along this stretch, the PCT intersects Arch Rock Trail 1187 (2,339.6–5,941').

Beyond this junction, easy walking takes you to the Raven Roost Trail 951 (2,340.3–5,820'), which heads right (east) along a spur ridge toward Cougar Valley. The PCT contours east around a broad summit, passing through more blends of burned forest and meadow on the way to the spur trail (2,341.6–5,685') to Arch Rock Spring.

WATER ACCESS

At the end of this 200-yard-long spur, you find a perennial spring trickling from a pipe.

FIRE Beyond the junction, the PCT descends, and then it crosses a seasonal branch of the South Fork Little Naches River. This area is full of dead standing timber as a result of the 2017 Norse Peak Fire.

The route loses elevation along the broad crest to Louisiana Saddle (2,343.1–5,191'), from which obscure Louisiana Saddle Trail 945A

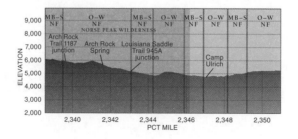

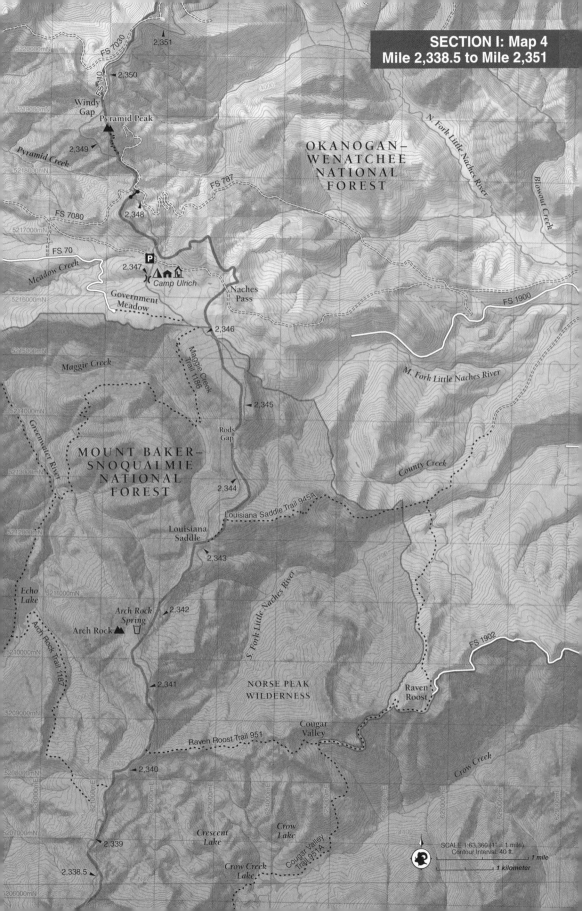

FS 7030

2,351

2,350

FS 110

Windy
Gap

Pyramid Peak

2,349

Pyramid Creek

FS 7080

FS 787

2,348

OKANOGAN–
WENATCHEE
NATIONAL
FOREST

N. Fork Little Naches River

Blowout Creek

FS 70

Meadow Creek

P

2,347

Camp Ulrich

Government
Meadow

Naches
Pass

FS 1900

2,346

Maggie Creek

Maggie Creek
Trail 1186

M. Fork Little Naches River

2,345

Rods
Gap

2,344

County Creek

MOUNT BAKER–
SNOQUALMIE
NATIONAL
FOREST

Greenwater River

Louisiana Saddle Trail 945A

Louisiana
Saddle

2,343

Echo
Lake

Arch Rock
Spring

2,342

S. Fork Little Naches River

Arch Rock Trail 1187

Arch Rock

FS 1902

2,341

NORSE PEAK
WILDERNESS

Raven
Roost

Cougar
Valley

Raven Roost Trail 951

Crow Creek

2,340

Crescent
Lake

Crow
Lake

Cougar Valley
Trail 951A

2,339

2,338.5

Crow Creek
Lake

SCALE 1:63,360 (1" = 1 mile)
Contour Interval: 40 ft.

1 mile

1 kilometer

heads east. The PCT continues descending to Rods Gap, from which it abruptly gains back 400 feet. After leveling out for a bit, your trail gently descends northwest and meets Maggie Creek Trail 1186 (2,346.2–4,856') heading west for a deep drop to the Greenwater River. Not much farther northwest, the PCT's descent takes you out of Norse Peak Wilderness; your descent ends at perennial Meadow Creek in Government Meadow.

CAMPING After bridging this creek, you go 100 yards to Camp Ulrich (2,347.0–4,770'), a large camping area with a conspicuous log cabin plus a fire ring and outhouse. This camp is named for Mike Ulrich, a trail worker in this area during the 1940s and '50s. On the shelter you may see a sign warning that the wrath of Mike's ghost will fall on anyone who harms the area's trees.

HISTORY From the back side of the shelter, you continue 200 yards north to a sign that recalls the first wagon trail to cross the Cascades east of Puget Sound. In 1853 the party, headed by David Longmire, rested here by Government Meadow before starting a rough descent into the Greenwater River canyon. By 1855 a military road was completed through this area, crossing gentle Naches Pass, 0.5 mile east.

From the sign, your path continues 40 yards to a parking area, and then you continue 80 yards on an east-southeast bearing to cross a jeep road (2,347.2–4,795') that provides access to a parking area.

Now you climb briefly to a minor gap and then make a winding traverse of 0.5 mile over toward Forest Service Road 787, which you keep on your right (east) as you trek 0.3 mile northwest to a junction (2,348.2–4,866'), from which a crest road starts northeast. Take this road just 20 yards to a resumption of trail tread, branching left; the winding crest road goes about 0.3 mile before giving rise to a short spur road. The PCT, more or less paralleling the crest road, also takes about 0.3 mile to reach the spur road. Just a few paces up this road, look for the resumption of trail tread, take it, and in 70 yards reach a junction with the Pyramid Peak Trail (2,348.6–5,012'). You could take this trail steeply up to the top, but the energy expended

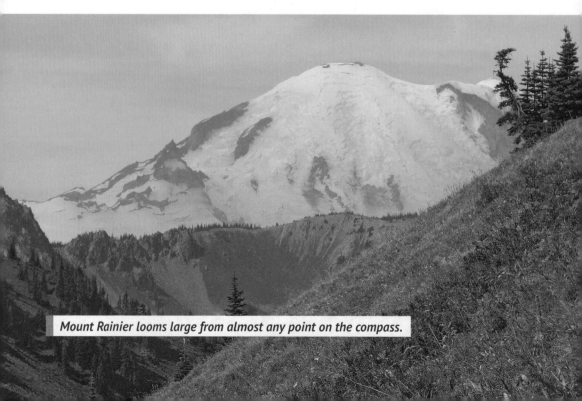

Mount Rainier looms large from almost any point on the compass.

isn't worth the effort. You'd see plenty of clear-cuts, and most folks will see more of them than they want to long before they reach Snoqualmie Pass. The PCT, traversing northwest through forest, offers glimpses of Mount Rainier, and then, after 0.5 mile, it goes northeast to offer a view or two of clear-cuts. On this tack, there is one short stretch that, when snowbound, could expose you to a fatal fall if you slip and go over the brink.

Leave the slopes of Pyramid Peak behind at Windy Gap and now begin a fairly long stretch across east- and south-facing slopes. You start with a 1-mile trek northeast and then go 0.5 mile east to a point where you cross a spur ridge.

From the spur ridge, hike about 0.25 mile northwest through untouched forest, but where the PCT curves north, you encounter a clear-cut and traverse partly through its upper section.

WATER ACCESS

Within forest again, you head northeast and soon hear a noisy spring (2,351.7–5,053') immediately below the tread.

In 240 yards, you go diagonally across an unpaved road (2,351.9–5,013'). Ahead, the PCT makes an east-northeast, usually viewless, descending traverse to another road (2,352.9–4,749'), which climbs 250 yards west to an old crest road. Onward, you contour 0.3 mile to a ravine and then gently ascend to a road-laced crest saddle (2,354.3–4,899'). Between two of these roads, the PCT starts a moderate-to-steep ascent southeast, levels off near the crest, follows it about 0.5 mile southeast, and then curves east-northeast to descend to a crossing of gravel FS 784 (2,355.4–4,967'). Down, FS 784 and then FS 1913 together descend an even 6 miles to FS 19, a paved, relatively heavily used road. Up, FS 784 goes 140 yards to often windswept Green Pass.

From the FS 784 crossing, the PCT climbs 150 yards northeast, and now you face the first significant climb in many miles: up the west ridge of Blowout Mountain. You follow a couple of switchbacks and then, viewing Goat Rocks and much of the broad Naches River drainage to the south, slant up to the ridgecrest, from which the obscure but signed Little Bear Creek Trail (2,356.9–5,329') drops off to the right (south). The PCT continues climbing, switchbacking once, and enters a small stand of subalpine firs, where you meet obscure Manastash Ridge Trail 1388 (2,357.6–5,557'), bound east for Mount Clifty and Quartz Mountain.

On the PCT, you climb a bit more to the crest of Blowout Mountain, where you get the most expansive views in some time, once again seeing Mount Rainier dominating the central Washington hinterlands. Now you follow the trail along a narrow summit ridge and look east down to view a marshy pond. The PCT then rounds the north summit of Blowout Mountain and switchbacks down through a dense fir forest to a junction with Blowout Mountain Trail 1318 (2,358.4–5,251').

North from this junction, a steep ridgeline descent ends your hiking through extensive, unmarred terrain as you emerge onto a vast, clear-cut landscape. For quite some time, the trail keeps on or near the ridge dividing the Yakima and Green Rivers. At first, it is barely east of deforested private land, but then it follows the flat but narrow ridge across a section line back into fully forested government land. The track eventually emerges from the woods just east of the crest, where you can see the PCT rising around barren Point 4,942, ahead, at the end of a logging road. The route barely touches this road and then contours before climbing 50 yards onto the adjacent crest. From this, it then switchbacks down, crossing two roads on its way to a major saddle (2,361.4–4,380').

From this saddle, the PCT reenters forest to make a long, lazily switchbacking descent to Tacoma Pass (2,364.1–3,455'). FS 52 crosses this

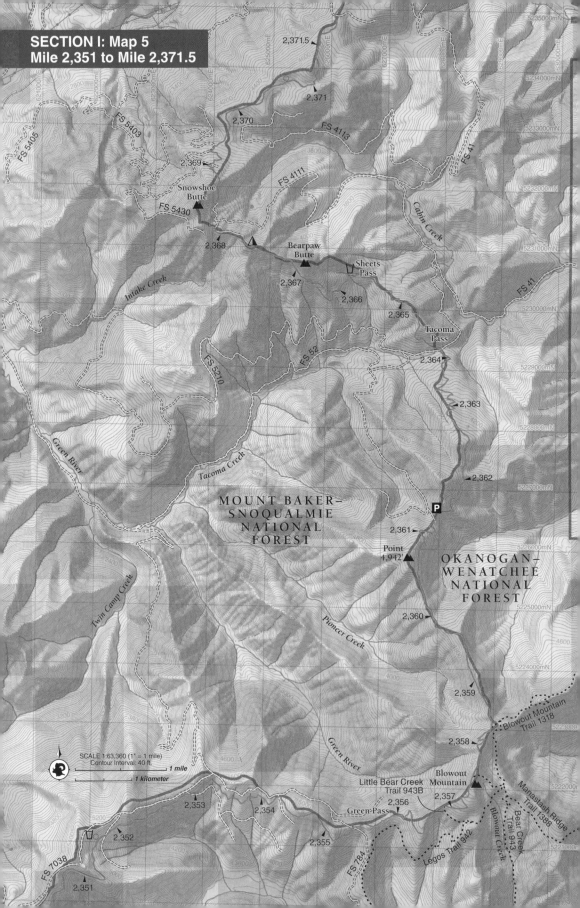

2,371.5

2,371

2,370

FS 4113

FS 41

FS 5403

FS 5405

2,369

FS 4111

Snowshoe
Butte

FS 5430

2,368

Bearpaw
Butte

Sheets
Pass

Cabin Creek

FS 41

Intake Creek

2,367

2,366

2,365

Tacoma
Pass

2,364

FS 52

2,363

FS 5210

2,362

Tacoma Creek

MOUNT BAKER–
SNOQUALMIE
NATIONAL
FOREST

P

2,361

Green River

Point
4,942'

OKANOGAN–
WENATCHEE
NATIONAL
FOREST

Twin Camp Creek

2,360

Pioneer Creek

2,359

Blowout Mountain
Trail 1318

2,358

Green River

2,353

2,354

Little Bear Creek
Trail 943B

Green Pass

2,356

2,357

Blowout
Mountain

Manastash Ridge
Trail 1388

Bear Creek
Trail 943

Blowout Creek

2,355

SCALE 1:63,360 (1" = 1 mile)
Contour Interval: 40 ft.

1 mile

1 kilometer

2,352

FS 784

Legos Trail 942

FS 7038

2,351

pass, and you jaywalk this logger's thoroughfare to ascend northwest into clear-cut land again. With Mount Rainier in full view, you now stride northwest along the divide as the PCT crosses one old logging road and then follows another one downhill 30 yards before crossing it.

WATER ACCESS

Now in forest, you cruise across Sheets Pass (2,365.5–3,702') and then climb and contour through pleasant woods to a seasonal creek (2,365.8–3,740'). This rill might carry water into mid-August of a wet year.

From here, the route turns south and climbs around the south ridge of Bearpaw Butte. Climbing in and out of the next clear-cut, you find the trail a bit grassy and overgrown, but you follow short hairpins trending northwest. As the PCT leaves the hairpins and goes northwest, you spot a stagnant pond about 300 feet below the trail.

The climb takes you to the crest, which the PCT follows northwest across an old log landing (where logs were gathered and sorted during a logging operation), across an old road, and then across another landing. Shortly the trail drops a few yards south to avoid a ridgetop road, and as it heads toward Snowshoe Butte, it makes the short climb back to cross the ridgetop road where the road curves. Next the trail turns north along the east slope of Snowshoe Butte and passes

through a corner of forested public land into more-razed earth on the butte's north ridge. A switchbacking descent takes you in and out of this clear-cut, across one road, and then lands you on a second road. Follow this second road 250 yards northeast downhill, leave it on the same side as that on which you entered it, and walk back into the forest onto a broad saddle (2,369.6–4,195').

As you then follow the low crest from here, the trail branches north-northeast; heads back into a clear-cut; and, at the crest of a small knob, turns east onto a track. Follow this 200 yards past an old slash pile and continue east, more or less directly up the adjacent ravine, passing a glade of corn lilies before reaching the edge of the clear-cut near the crest of a knob, where the trail turns north. The track goes just east of the knob's summit and then descends just east of the rounded divide to a pass where fast-growing grasses and shrubs, especially huckleberries, partly obscure the trail.

PLANTS Huckleberry and blueberry bushes favor cleared and burned land, so they cover a great deal of this country. By mid-August, most PCT hikers here develop a purple tongue from sampling the abundant fruit.

At the low point of the pass (2,371.9–4,329'), you cross a road. From here, make a short climb up the next knob north before starting a descent toward the Stampede Pass weather station, visible ahead. Steep switchbacks take you across a track and then across a more substantial road. The last switchback takes you into dense forest where an overgrown four-wheel-drive track might lead some hikers

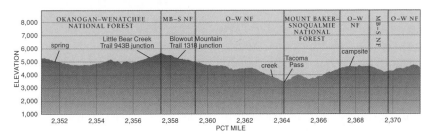

astray. Trail blazes help you head nearly straight down the divide to a notch, from which you ascend to hike along the east side of the next knob. You emerge from forest at a power-line cut and then soon reach another power-line cut with old log poles. A railroad tunnel runs deep beneath this latter cut.

A short distance farther, you cruise behind the weather station and cross its access road (2,373.9–3,924'). Now you follow the low Cascade divide as it turns west, crossing another road and then another power-line cut on your way through a regenerating forest of silver fir, Douglas-fir, lodgepole pine, white pine, and western hemlock. The trail makes a gradual descent to FS 54 (2,374.9–3,671') a couple hundred yards south of Stampede Pass.

The PCT next strikes steeply uphill, switchbacking through the second-growth forest. Soon after cresting the rise, the trail turns north, parallel to a logging road, and enters a former clear-cut. After a slight climb, the PCT cuts west across the divide and cruises through huckleberry prairies and across two logging roads. The trail barely descends into a ravine before contouring south out of it, and then it slants southwest down through thick fireweed and other pioneers of clear-cuts.

WATER ACCESS

The trail crosses a logging road and then empties onto and follows the same road to a hairpin (2,376.8–3,851'), where a rill might trickle through July.

Dropping from the road here, the PCT descends gradually, switchbacking across another logging road before reaching Dandy Pass. Here you enter forested land and circle halfway around a hill under the shade of a magnificent forest of giant, old-growth hemlocks. This mile-long arc is a now-rare glimpse at the quality of tree for which the Pacific Northwest is famous. Eventually you cross the section line and enter brushy country again, just shy of a saddle. You turn north here and skirt the saddle to cross and then parallel a logging road.

WATER ACCESS

In a few minutes, you come to a creek (2,379.0–3,512') that probably cascades year-round. A rough, rocky traverse north from here, paralleling and then dropping across a road, brings you to an even more certain stream, Stirrup Creek (2,379.8–3,447').

CAMPING Along the south bank of this stream, Stirrup Lake Trail 1338 runs 0.5 mile through an old clear-cut up to the lake, where you can find a pleasant campsite barely in the trees.

Climbing gradually from here among tall cedars, the trail crosses a well-graded logging road and rounds a ridge before striking northwest on a level traverse through a 1989 clear-cut. Note what kind and how much growth has occurred since then.

WATER ACCESS

Eventually, the trail reenters forest and heads to the dribbling headwaters of Meadow Creek (2,382.0–3,670').

From here, work up a couple of hairpins, gaining 350 feet to a ridgeline that overlooks the mostly clear-cut headwaters of North Fork Cedar River, a major feeder into Seattle's water

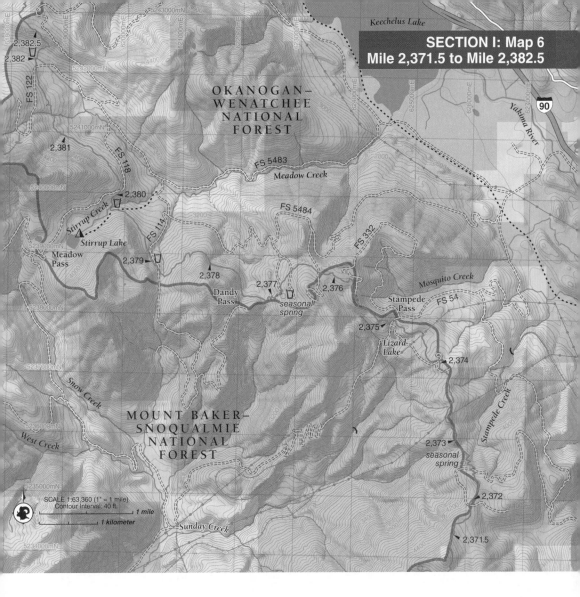

supply. At the valley's head, you see Yakima Pass cupping Twilight Lake, which, at the bottom of an overly logged amphitheater, looks like a forlorn island of natural beauty trying to hide behind a relict forest curtain.

From the pass—part of an old American Indian route—the PCT strikes northwest directly uphill, crosses an unmaintained route, and then cuts northeast to ford the creek that issues from Mirror Lake.

WATER ACCESS

The trail then slants down to the pass, crossing a logging road en route, and skirts Twilight Lake along its west shore (2,383.4–3,582').

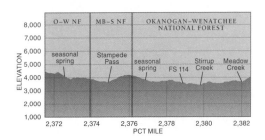

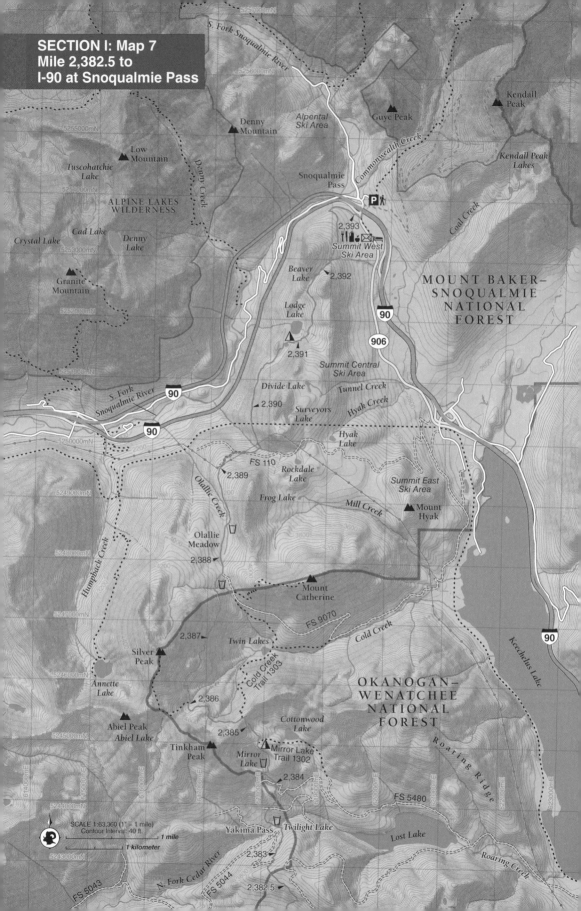

S. Fork Snoqualmie River

Kendall Peak

Denny Mountain

Alpental Ski Area

Guye Peak

Kendall Peak Lakes

Low Mountain

Tuscohatchie Lake

Denny Creek

Snoqualmie Pass

Commonwealth Creek

Coal Creek

ALPINE LAKES WILDERNESS

Crystal Lake

Cad Lake

Denny Lake

2,393

Summit West Ski Area

MOUNT BAKER–SNOQUALMIE NATIONAL FOREST

Granite Mountain

Beaver Lake

2,392

Lodge Lake

90

2,391

906

Summit Central Ski Area

S. Fork Snoqualmie River

90

Divide Lake

2.390

Surveyors Lake

Tunnel Creek

Hyak Creek

90

Hyak Lake

FS 110

2,389

Rockdale Lake

Frog Lake

Summit East Ski Area

Olallie Creek

Humpback Creek

Olallie Meadow

2,388

Mill Creek

Mount Hyak

Mount Catherine

FS 9070

Cold Creek

2,387

Twin Lakes

Keechelus Lake

Silver Peak

Cold Creek Trail 1303

OKANOGAN–WENATCHEE NATIONAL FOREST

90

Annette Lake

2,386

Cottonwood Lake

Abiel Peak
Abiel Lake

2,385

Roaring Ridge

Tinkham Peak

Mirror Lake

Mirror Lake Trail 1302

2,384

FS 5480

SCALE 1:63,360 (1" = 1 mile)
Contour Interval: 40 ft.

1 mile

1 kilometer

Yakima Pass

Twilight Lake

Lost Lake

2,383

Roaring Creek

FS 5043

FS 5044

2,382.5

WATER ACCESS

Just beyond this first ford, the PCT turns across the end of a logging road and then climbs steeply to cross and recross the outlet creek on the way to Mirror Lake (2,384.3–4,201'). Suddenly, you've entered a refuge of undisturbed mountain landscape: craggy Tinkham Peak overlooks the sapphire waters that periodically ripple with feeding trout, and the rimming fir forest invites secluded access to a scenic swim—in warm weather, anyway.

CAMPING After passing some campsites on the way around the east shore of this lake, you exit the lake basin and meet Mirror Lake Trail 1302 (2,384.6–4,231') coming up from the Lost Lake trailhead only 1.2 miles to the southeast.

Here the PCT merges with Cold Creek Trail 1303, continues north for a bit, and then climbs some steep hairpins to a spur of Tinkham Peak. At a junction (2,385.1–4,524'), Cold Creek Trail 1303 drops away north from the PCT, which turns west on a hillside below andesite bluffs. Soon you cross a small creek on the way down to a soggy bowl with a couple of tiny ponds and a rug of marsh marigolds. Next the PCT turns north and passes an unmaintained trail that climbs west to Silver Peak. The route then

begins a very steep, rocky climb of its own as it traverses the slopes of Silver Peak.

WATER ACCESS

This climb takes you to a tiny side valley behind a knob, from which you make a steep and then a moderate descent among silver firs to a perennial creek (2,387.7–3,896').

After crossing this creek, the PCT continues north, soon entering a clear-cut that allows a view of Chair Peak and its satellites across the gash of the Snoqualmie River valley. Then the trail descends to and follows Olallie Creek.

WATER ACCESS

You cross a road and then a feeder of Olallie Creek and finally cross to the east bank of Olallie Creek itself (2,388.3–3,634').

Along the creek, you pass through a patch of forest and then break back into logged land, where you hear the roar of I-90 some 1,400 feet below. Soon you follow a logging road a few yards north before descending from it, traversing under power lines, and dropping onto the power-line access road (2,389.1–3,364'). The PCT follows this road west and downhill 0.4 mile, past a spur road climbing east, and then drops beside Rockdale Creek, which tumbles under a canopy of maples and firs. Cross the creek, turn north under power lines, proceed across talus slopes dotted with vine maple, and then enter deep fir-and-cedar forest for a long, flat traverse.

Eventually, the steep slope you cross levels into a bench, and the path skirts a small pond where an unsigned track branches northwest. Quickly the PCT then comes to a sign

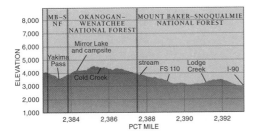

pointing out a 100-yard spur to Lodge Lake (2,390.9–3,168').

CAMPING Down this spur, you'll find the lake's campsites. Some are close to the PCT, although a number of them, popular with overnighters, are set around the shallow, muskeg-rich lake. Locate tent sites as far away from the PCT in order to not detract from other hiker's vistas.

The PCT rises as it rounds Lodge Lake's bowl and then traverses slopes up past a creek ford to cross a forested saddle and enter a swale holding Beaver Lake. Here the trail passes under ski lifts of the Snoqualmie Pass ski area before starting a long, descending arc down the groomed ski slopes. The trail slowly curves far to the west, presenting views of I-90 and the complex of cute buildings at Snoqualmie Pass below the craggy peaks across the valley. The latter promise a more ruggedly scenic and pristine section of PCT to the north. A final switchback quickly takes you down to a trailhead (2,392.8–3,019') at the end of a broad road with ample room for parking.

The next set of directions may seem confusing as you read them, but the route is plain when you're actually there. On this road, you make a curving descent 250 yards east to a very broad snow-parking area that branches southeast, then continue 150 yards straight ahead to a point where you branch northeast for a 40-yard descent down a road to a longer road. This goes 140 yards southeast to the main road, which curves north 130 yards to pass under I-90 (2,393.1–3,000'). Here Section I ends by the freeway's West Summit exit.

RESUPPLY ACCESS

If you're a long-distance hiker, you may first want to head southeast along the main freeway frontage road, which is WA 906. Along it you'll find a choice of eating establishments, groceries, and lodgings. About 0.4 mile along this road, on the left, is the Snoqualmie Pass Post Office, housed within a gas station.

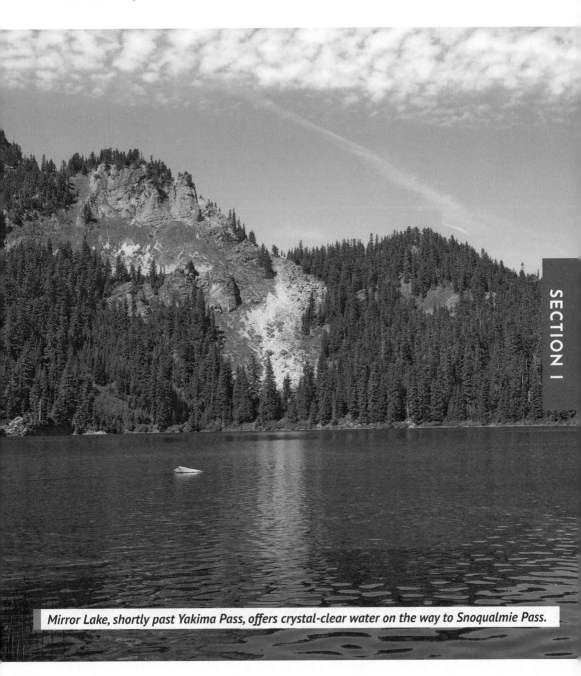

Mirror Lake, shortly past Yakima Pass, offers crystal-clear water on the way to Snoqualmie Pass.

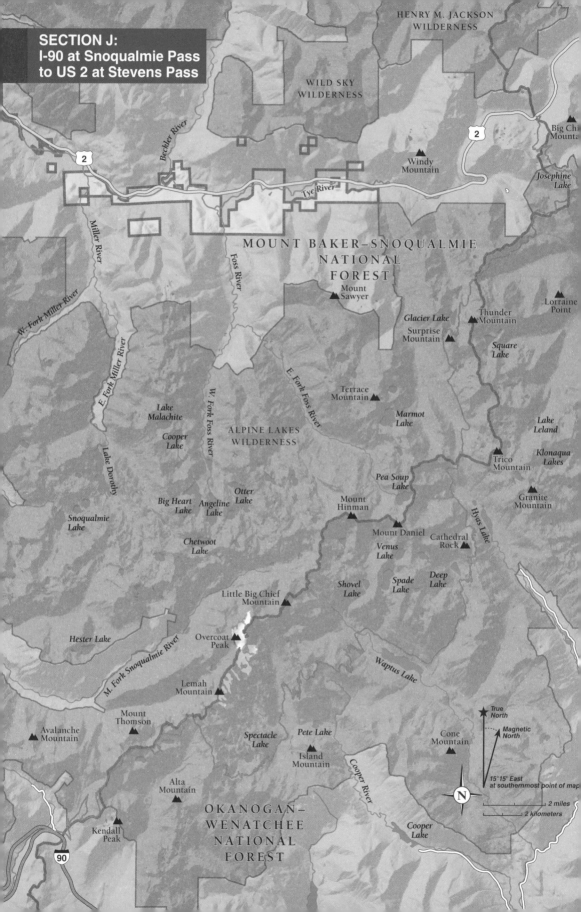

HENRY M. JACKSON
WILDERNESS

WILD SKY
WILDERNESS

Beckler River

2

Big Chi
Mounta

Windy
Mountain

Josephine
Lake

Tye River

Miller River

MOUNT BAKER–SNOQUALMIE
NATIONAL
FOREST

Foss River

W. Fork Miller River

Mount
Sawyer

Lorraine
Point

Glacier Lake

Thunder
Mountain

E. Fork Miller River

Surprise
Mountain

Square
Lake

Terrace
Mountain

E. Fork Foss River

Lake
Malachite

W. Fork Foss River

ALPINE LAKES
WILDERNESS

Marmot
Lake

Lake
Leland

Cooper
Lake

Klonaqua
Lakes

Lake Dorothy

Trico
Mountain

Pea Soup
Lake

Otter
Lake

Granite
Mountain

Big Heart
Lake

Angeline
Lake

Mount
Hinman

Snoqualmie
Lake

Hyas Lake

Chetwoot
Lake

Mount Daniel

Cathedral
Rock

Venus
Lake

Shovel
Lake

Spade
Lake

Deep
Lake

Little Big Chief
Mountain

Hester Lake

Overcoat
Peak

M. Fork Snoqualmie River

Waptus Lake

Lemah
Mountain

True
North

Mount
Thomson

Magnetic
North

Avalanche
Mountain

Spectacle
Lake

Pete Lake

Cone
Mountain

Island
Mountain

Cooper River

15°15' East
at southernmost point of map

Alta
Mountain

N

2 miles

OKANOGAN–
WENATCHEE
NATIONAL
FOREST

2 kilometers

Kendall
Peak

Cooper
Lake

90

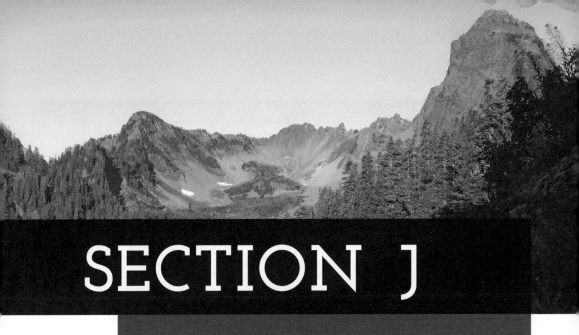

SECTION J

I-90 at Snoqualmie Pass to US 2 at Stevens Pass

FROM HIGH TRAVERSES ALONG CRAGGY CRESTS to meadowland tours past swimmable lakes and forest walks near churning rivers, this section bisects a spectacular variety of Cascades backcountry, making for a classic, weeklong backpack in the land of Alpine Lakes Wilderness.

From Snoqualmie Pass, the Pacific Crest Trail (PCT) climbs directly to the crest-top crags and boldly traverses among them. Confronted by Chikamin Peak and brutal Lemah Mountain, it relinquishes the divide, swerving east to where summer storms generally dissipate into clear skies. On this stretch, the route dips into and climbs out of two major watersheds, Lemah Creek and the Waptus River. It then works its way back to and weaves along the descending divide, visiting a number of memorably scenic lake basins on its way to Stevens Pass. In all, this section will challenge your legs, lift your spirits, and confirm your reasons for backpacking.

Above: Glacial cirques and volcanic plugs are common in the Cascades.

DECLINATION 15°15'E

USGS MAPS

Snoqualmie Pass, WA	Polallie Ridge, WA
Chikamin Peak, WA	Stevens Pass, WA
Scenic, WA	Mount Daniel, WA

POINTS ON THE TRAIL, SOUTH TO NORTH

	Mile	Elevation in feet	Latitude/Longitude
I-90 at Snoqualmie Pass	2,393.1	3,018	N47° 25' 35.8773" W121° 24' 55.7528"
Ridge Lake and Gravel Lake	2,400.3	5,280	N47° 27' 44.3507" W121° 22' 02.5084"
Lemah Creek	2,413.8	3,198	N47° 28' 35.7114" W121° 15' 42.4458"
Waptus Burn Trail junction	2,422.9	5,171	N47° 29' 55.4541" W121° 12' 46.8216"
Waptus River	2,427.8	3,027	N47° 31' 01.2866" W121° 12' 30.7189"
Deep Lake	2,434.8	4,379	N47° 32' 24.2777" W121° 08' 16.4508"
Start of Cathedral Pass Trail alternate route	2,437.8	5,527	N47° 33' 01.7483" W121° 07' 46.0313"
Deception Pass	2,442.8	4,478	N47° 35' 36.8474" W121° 08' 25.7101"
Deception Lakes outlet creek	2,446.2	5,006	N47° 37' 49.4500" W121° 08' 44.6793"
Mig Lake	2,456.7	4,662	N47° 42' 10.1600" W121° 05' 10.4400"
Lake Susan Jane	2,459.8	4,577	N47° 43' 19.8241" W121° 03' 57.9363"
US 2 at Stevens Pass	2,464.1	4,053	N47° 44' 46.4028" W121° 05' 18.6332"

CAMPSITES AND BIVY SITES

Mile	Elevation in feet	Latitude/Longitude	Number of tents	Feature	Notes
2,397.5	4,841	N47° 26' 02.9863" W121° 23' 20.1230"	2		
2,400.3	5,280	N47° 27' 43.1568" W121° 21' 58.2941"	>4	Gravel Lake	
2,402.4	5,070	N47° 28' 06.7017" W121° 20' 43.3723"	2	Joe Lake	Flat spot near trail on right
2,407.8	4,922	N47° 27' 10.5393" W121° 17' 44.8910"	2	Near Mineral Creek Trail	
2,414.5	3,240	N47° 29' 08.7057" W121° 15' 32.8984"	4	Near stream and Lemah Meadow	West of trail
2,422.5	5,255	N47° 30' 05.4766" W121° 13' 02.2088"	2	Nearby creek	1 on left, 1 on right
2,427.7	3,045	N47° 31' 01.4480" W121° 12' 28.6094"	2	Waptus River	Flat spot near trail on right
2,430.0	3,234	N47° 30' 23.6644" W121° 10' 12.4950"	2	Waptus Lake	Below trail on right
2,433.3	4,222	N47° 31' 25.7721" W121° 08' 10.3442"	2	Spinola Creek	Bivy on right
2,434.8	4,379	N47° 32' 24.2800" W121° 08' 16.3700"	>4	Deep Lake	

CAMPSITES AND BIVY SITES *(continued)*

Mile	Elevation in feet	Latitude/ Longitude	Number of tents	Feature	Notes
2,437.8	5,540	N47° 33' 04.1498" W121° 07' 50.3402"	3	Near junction with Cathedral Pass Trail	East of PCT
2,439.8	4,589	N47° 33' 50.2771" W121° 08' 02.1075"	3	Stream nearby	Flat spot near trail on right
2,444.7	4,467	N47° 36' 44.4143" W121° 08' 13.3502"	>4	Stream nearby	
2,449.8	5,036	N47° 39' 13.1838" W121° 08' 26.4689"	2	Glacier Lake	Bivy on left and right
2,453.3	5,263	N47° 41' 00.1602" W121° 06' 55.8290"	2	Seasonal creek nearby	
2,456.7	4,662	N47° 42' 10.1600" W121° 05' 10.4400"	2	Mig Lake	Vault toilet
2,459.8	4,577	N47° 43' 19.6397" W121° 04' 00.3998"	2	Lake Susan Jane	On north shore, vault toilet

SUPPLIES

A host of services is available at the settlement of Snoqualmie Pass. From the West Summit exit off I-90, a frontage road heads southeast through the settlement, and you'll first encounter The Summit Deli and a gas station, which, besides dispensing fuel, is the local Greyhound bus stop. In front of it is The Aardvark Express, which serves cold, hopped beverages and interesting homemade victuals. Adjacent to it is another restaurant, Summit Pancake House, followed by the Summit Inn. You'll find more services, but the most important may be Lee's Summit Grocery, just next door, which has the Snoqualmie Pass Post Office (98068) inside and Bob's Espresso in the parking lot.

At this section's end, the Stevens Pass Ski Resort accepts and holds hikers' packages; for details visit stevenspass.com. The closest town to this pass is Skykomish (post office 98288), about 14 miles west, with lodging and restaurants.

PERMITS

None are required along this section, but the U.S. Forest Service asks that all hikers self-register at the post just beyond the Snoqualmie Pass trailhead.

SPECIAL CONCERNS

Snow typically lingers through mid-August on some of the steep traverses during the first 15 miles, making for some treacherous ravine crossings.

I-90 AT SNOQUALMIE PASS TO US 2 AT STEVENS PASS

>>>THE ROUTE

To reach the trailhead, eastbound drivers take the West Summit exit off I-90 and turn left to immediately cross under I-90. Westbound drivers take the East Summit exit, follow the frontage road (WA 906) briefly through the settlement of Snoqualmie Pass, and then, by the West Summit exit off-ramp, cross under I-90. On the road north of I-90, you'll quickly reach a spur road that branches right, climbing to the nearby main trailhead parking lot and its adjacent equestrian parking lot.

This section begins PCT mileage from I-90 (2,393.1–3,018'). On the road north of it, you walk just a few yards to a footpath starting up the road's cut. If you're on foot, take this path, which winds up to the far end of the trailhead parking lot (2,393.3–3,016'). Here, you are joined by those on horseback or starting from the lot. With fir and hemlock above you and bunchberry, spring beauty, huckleberry, and devil's club at your feet, cross an abandoned road, and before long start climbing three long, well-graded switchbacks. They lift you around a ridge, away from the freeway noise and into the Alpine Lakes Wilderness (2,395.1–3,853'), high above Commonwealth Creek. As the trail traverses above this valley's floor, the route crosses a tributary right below a spraying waterfall and then comes to a junction with Commonwealth Basin Trail 1033 (2,395.6–3,786').

SIDE TRIP Heading up Commonwealth Creek, Commonwealth Basin Trail 1033 takes you to Red Pass in about 2.6 miles.

From the junction, the PCT resumes climbing on newer tread, heading for high country that was seldom visited before the completion of this PCT segment in 1978.

To the west and north, Chair Peak, Snoqualmie Mountain, Red Mountain, and other summits already hint at the alpine terrain awaiting as the trail next switchbacks south. Returning into deeper forest, you continue climbing steadily on another switchback leg, up to the divide between the Snoqualmie and Yakima Rivers. Along here, you glimpse Kachess Lake to the southeast and then immediately angle back onto the west flank of the steepening divide to continue the ascent.

| VIEWS | Before long, the route emerges onto talus, and the high country opens up all around you. Besides the craggy, multicolored peaks to the west, Mount Rainier rises like a huge apparition to the south. Even if bad weather obscures this view, you will still find your spirits lifted by brilliant pockets of paintbrush, columbine, spirea, valerian, tiger lily, and other flowers. The PCT continues rising gradually, with dwarfed mountain hemlocks clinging to trailside craglets and more peaks coming into view to the north, including Mount Thomson and distant Mount Stuart. Cross to the east side of the crest, from which level hiking shows you Chikamin Ridge at the head of Gold Creek Valley, and Alta Mountain and the amazing cliffs of Rampart Ridge draw your eye across the valley.

WATER ACCESS

Water might seep from late snow patches on this trail, but otherwise, this airy section, often just a ledge blasted from the rocky crest, is fairly dry. But soon the trail rounds a narrow spur ridge well above glistening Alaska Lake, and then it cuts down to the crest saddle (2,400.3–5,280') between Ridge and Gravel Lakes.

CAMPING You'll find campsites on the west shore of Gravel Lake, the northwestern of the two lakes. Camping is also allowed at Ridge Lake, but be sure to camp at designated sites only at both lakes. Camp on dirt and let the plants grow in this sensitive subalpine environment. The more-secluded bivy sites at Gravel Lake give hikers the opportunity to employ the Leave No Trace principle of camping out of sight of others.

From the north side of Ridge Lake, the PCT takes off on a talus traverse around the rim of the cirque holding Alaska Lake and then climbs some as it rounds the sharp east ridge of Alaska Mountain. Next, steep switchbacks that hold snow into August take you down the north slope of this peak, and then a traverse leads you to a narrow, forested saddle (2,402.5–4,500') between Joe and Edds Lakes. These lakes lie, respectively, 400 feet below to the east and 800 feet below to the west.

WILDLIFE The trail slants off the saddle into a meadowy ravine and then rises across the open, rocky south flank of Huckleberry Mountain. As you turn left (north) around the east side of this peak, which is a summer pasture for wary mountain goats, you enter a beautiful hanging vale.

Here, with a full view of Mount Rainier, the trail meets a stream that cascades among

continued on page 284

SECTION J

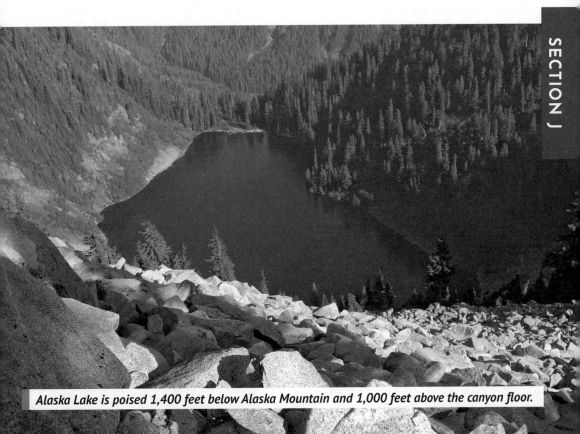

Alaska Lake is poised 1,400 feet below Alaska Mountain and 1,000 feet above the canyon floor.

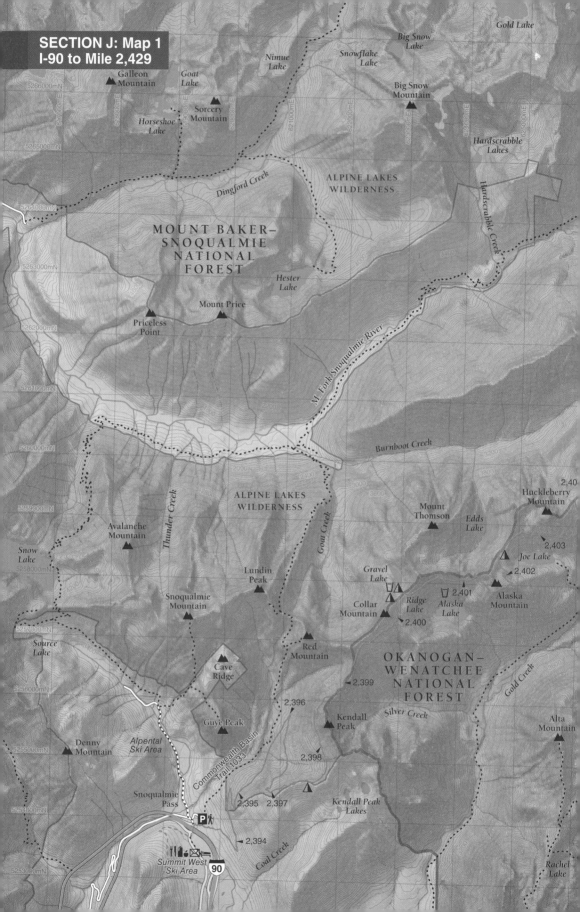

Gold Lake

Big Snow Lake

Snowflake Lake

Nimue Lake

Goat Lake

Galleon Mountain ▲

Sorcery Mountain ▲

Horseshoe Lake

Big Snow Mountain ▲

Hardscrabble Lakes

Hardscrabble Creek

Dingford Creek

ALPINE LAKES WILDERNESS

MOUNT BAKER–SNOQUALMIE NATIONAL FOREST

Hester Lake

Mount Price ▲

Priceless Point ▲

M. Fork Snoqualmie River

Burnboot Creek

Huckleberry Mountain ▲ 2,40

ALPINE LAKES WILDERNESS

Mount Thomson ▲

Edds Lake

Thunder Creek

Avalanche Mountain ▲

Snow Lake

Goat Creek

Lundin Peak ▲

Gravel Lake

2,403 ◄

△ Joe Lake

2,402

Snoqualmie Mountain ▲

Collar Mountain ▲

Ridge Lake

□ 2,401

Alaska Lake

Alaska Mountain ▲

2,400 ◄

Source Lake

Red Mountain ▲

OKANOGAN–WENATCHEE NATIONAL FOREST

Cave Ridge ▲

2,399 ◄

Gold Creek

2,396 ◄

Kendall Peak ▲

Silver Creek

Alta Mountain ▲

Guye Peak ▲

Denny Mountain ▲

Alpental Ski Area

Commonwealth Basin Trail 1033

2,398 ◄

△

Snoqualmie Pass

2,395 ► ◄ 2,397

Kendall Peak Lakes

🅿 🥾

2,394 ◄

🍴🏨📷🏠

Summit West Ski Area

Coal Creek

90

Rachel Lake

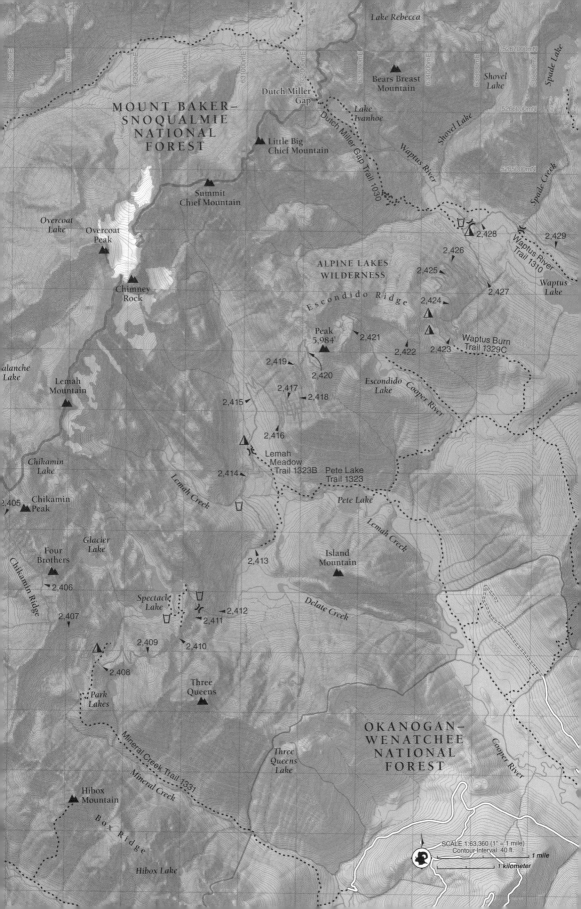

Lake Rebecca

Shovel Lake

Spade Lake

Bears Breast Mountain

Lake Ivanhoe

Dutch Miller Gap

MOUNT BAKER–
SNOQUALMIE
NATIONAL
FOREST

Little Big Chief Mountain

Summit Chief Mountain

Overcoat Lake

Overcoat Peak

Chimney Rock

Shovel Lake

Waptus River

Spade Creek

2,428

2,429

Waptus River Trail 1310

2,426

2,425

2,427

Waptus Lake

ALPINE LAKES
WILDERNESS

Escondido Ridge

2,424

2,421

2,422 2,423

Waptus Burn Trail 1329C

Peak 5,984'

2,419

2,420

Escondido Lake

Cooper River

Avalanche Lake

Lemah Mountain

2,415

2,417

2,418

2,416

Chikamin Lake

Lemah Meadow Trail 1323B

2,414

Lemah Creek

Pete Lake Trail 1323

Pete Lake

Lemah Creek

2,405

Chikamin Peak

Glacier Lake

Four Brothers

2,406

2,413

Island Mountain

Delate Creek

Chikamin Ridge

2,407

Spectacle Lake

2,412

2,411

2,409

2,410

2,408

Park Lakes

Three Queens

OKANOGAN–
WENATCHEE
NATIONAL
FOREST

Mineral Creek Trail 1331

Mineral Creek

Three Queens Lake

Cooper River

Hibox Mountain

Box Ridge

SCALE 1:63,360 (1" = 1 mile)
Contour Interval: 40 ft.

1 mile

1 kilometer

Hibox Lake

continued from page 281

rock slabs and heather gardens. At the head of this ravine, you pass a couple of small pools before coming to the crest at Huckleberry Saddle (2,403.9–5,560'), which is a broad pass with a fragile carpet of bilberries. This scenic gap has remained nearly pristine largely because the **U.S. Forest Service prohibits camping here.**

| VIEWS | Short switchbacks among dwarfed hemlocks take you above the saddle, allowing views of Mount Index and the Olympic Mountains in the distant northwest. This climb then leads to a traverse below the tip of a crag to Needle Sight Gap (2,404.4–5,930'). After a glimpse through this notch beyond Burnboot Creek to distant Glacier Peak, the PCT turns southeast for a long alpine traverse along the meadow and rocky southwest face of Chikamin Ridge.

| WILDLIFE | Whole platoons of marmots may whistle loudly and then scurry from approaching hikers as the latter make their way across this headwall of Gold Creek, from which they can admire the placid sheen of Joe Lake, the twin thumbs of Huckleberry Mountain and Mount Thomson, and the miragelike dome of Mount Rainier. On the way, the trail crosses a few steep chutes that usually shelter slippery snow well into midseason.

After climbing gently on the last third of this traverse, the PCT reaches Chikamin Pass (2,406.9–5,651'), where you can look across Park Lakes' basin to Three Queens; Box Ridge; and, in the distant northeast, the granite pyramid of Mount Stuart. Now descend a couple of switchbacks into the lake basin, where mosquitoes swarm in the subalpine meadows much more thickly than at the breezy crests you just left.

| CAMPING | Once on gentler ground, the route passes campsites, then a junction with southbound Mineral Creek Trail 1331 (2,407.9–4,911'), where there is an access spur that leads to some campsites.

Weaving through this hummocky plateau, which actually straddles the divide between Mineral Creek and Delate Creek, you follow the PCT generally east and then northeast around the bowl of the northernmost Park Lake. With the lake behind you, climb a pair of switchbacks to pass some ponds and gain a northwest spur of Three Queens (2,408.7–5,350'). Here you can look north over turquoise Spectacle Lake to the spiny, metamorphic fangs, hanging glaciers, and alpine waterfalls of Lemah Mountain. The rolling Wenatchee Mountains rise in the more distant east.

Now start a bone-jarring, 2,000-foot descent, twisting and pounding down literally scores of

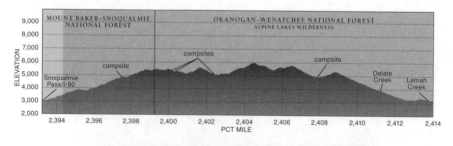

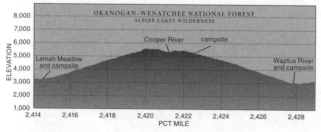

tight switchbacks—hairpins that continue from a chute on the east side of a knob down to the runout of Three Queens' avalanche slopes. (The official estimate is 42; only because 42 is, well, you know, the answer to everything.)

WATER ACCESS

As the trail drops into thicker forest, you pass Spectacle Lake Trail 1306 (2,410.3–4,430'), which forks north to the lake, and below this junction, you walk on a sturdy bridge across roaring Delate Creek (2,411.2–3,941').

The last series of switchbacks finally drops you onto a bottomland forest with fern glades, and later you cruise past eastbound Pete Lake Trail 1323 (2,413.1–3,245').

WATER ACCESS

Northbound, the PCT rounds a small knob and then gently descends northwest to the trunk stream of Lemah Creek (2,413.8–3,198').

From here, the trail continues north, rising over a small moraine and then dropping to cross a bridge over North Fork Lemah Creek. Immediately after climbing out of this stream's ravine, the PCT meets Lemah Meadow Trail 1323B (2,414.4–3,228'), which climbs northwest from Pete Lake.

CAMPING The PCT continues north past a campsite (2,414.5–3,240'), gradually leaving behind Lemah Creek, and then passes through forest and meadow and across a freshet. The trail then comes to a spot (2,415.2–3,370') from which it embarks on a 2,200-foot climb to the top of Escondido Ridge,

a climb best started early in the morning if it's to be a warm day.

Not far into this climb, you cross a couple of seasonal streams, but beyond those you must count on vistas through the cedar, hemlock, and vine-maple forest to inspire you on. Brief though these are, the impressive alpine views of Lemah Mountain, Chikamin Ridge, and Three Queens broaden with every switchback.

Eventually the montane forest wanes, and smaller mountain hemlocks and subalpine firs spread around you as the trail turns up a ravine into a secluded cirque with a chilly tarn (2,419.9–5,520') where **camping is prohibited.** Switchback once more, and contour southeast through subalpine parkland. Continue around Peak 5,984 to reach another cirque, **where camping is also prohibited,** and cross the inlet (2,421.2–5,300') of the lowest of a chain of crystalline tarns before starting a gradually rising traverse across the next ridge.

CAMPING From the top of this ridge, the PCT arcs around a sheltered vale, jumping its creek and passing a campsite a few hundred yards farther southeast (2422.5–5,255'). Next you exit this meadowy glen and emerge onto the edge of Escondido Ridge, where you have a view over Waptus Lake and beyond to ever-closer Mount Stuart.

Along the ridge, you find Waptus Burn Trail 1329C (2,422.9–5,171'), which continues down the ridge while the PCT switchbacks down and begins a 2,200-foot descent to the Waptus River.

VIEWS A grand alpine panorama oversees these well-graded switchbacks. Across the valley, long waterfalls drain the lofty Mount Daniel–Mount Hinman massif, and at the valley's head, the impressive sedimentary slabs of Bears Breast Mountain thrust skyward. As you stomp down the first switchbacks, pointy subalpine firs give way to open brush (a scar from the 1929 Waptus Burn fire); then you traverse north to the main bank of switchbacks, the last three touching a cascading stream.

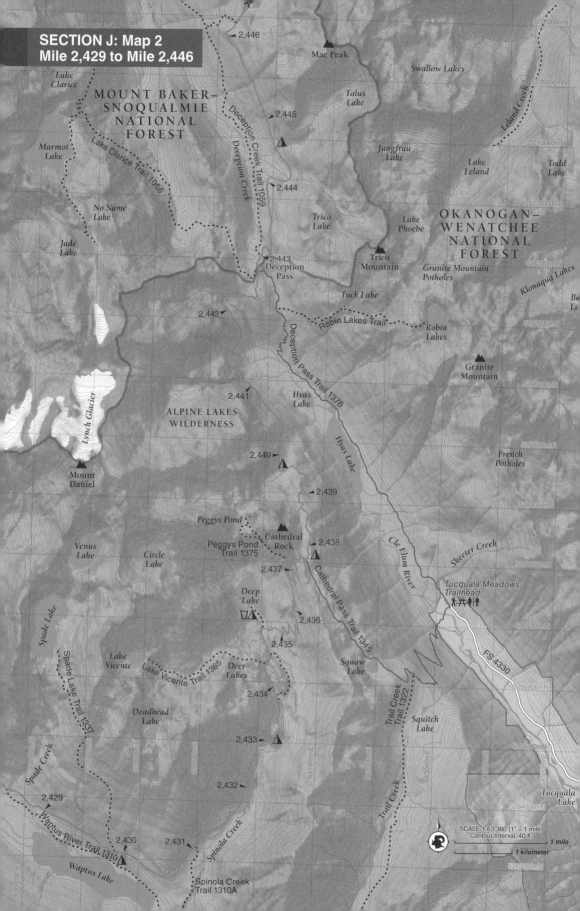

MOUNT BAKER–
SNOQUALMIE
NATIONAL
FOREST

OKANOGAN–
WENATCHEE
NATIONAL
FOREST

ALPINE LAKES
WILDERNESS

Mac Peak

Swallow Lakes

Lake Clarice

Talus Lake

Leland Creek

Marmot Lake

Lake Clarice Trail 1066

Deception Creek Trail 1059

Jungfrau Lake

Lake Leland

Todd Lake

No Name Lake

Deception Creek

2,446

2,445

2,444

Trico Lake

Lake Phoebe

Jade Lake

2,443
Deception Pass

Trico Mountain

Granite Mountain Potholes

Klonaqua Lakes

2,442

Tuck Lake

Robin Lakes Trail

Robin Lakes

Granite Mountain

Lynch Glacier

2,441

Deception Pass Trail 1376

Hyas Lake

French Potholes

Mount Daniel

2,440

2,439

Hyas Lake

Peggys Pond

Peggys Pond Trail 1375

Cathedral Rock

2,438

2,437

Skeeter Creek

Cle Elum River

Tucquala Meadows Trailhead

Venus Lake

Circle Lake

Deep Lake

2,436

Cathedral Pass Trail 1345

Spade Lake

Spade Lake Trail 1337

Lake Vicente

Lake Vicente Trail 1365

Deer Lakes

2,435

2,434

Squaw Lake

FS 4330

Deadhead Lake

2,433

Squitch Lake

Trail Creek Trail 1322

Spade Creek

2,432

Trail Creek

Tucquala Lake

2,429

Waptus River Trail 1310

2,430

2,431

Spinola Creek

Waptus Lake

Spinola Creek Trail 1310A

SCALE 1:63,360 (1" = 1 mile)
Contour Interval: 40 ft.

1 mile

1 kilometer

CAMPING Western red cedar droops over the trail as it empties onto the broad valley floor and comes to a campsite at northwest-bound Dutch Miller Gap Trail 1030 (2427.7–3,045').

WATER ACCESS

You won't find water until 0.1 mile later, at the Waptus River (2,427.8–3,027').

A girder bridge gets you across this cold torrent, and you turn downstream. The PCT then winds northeast past a connection to Dutch Miller Gap Trail 1030 and continues under Douglas-firs that rise above a carpet of ferns and vanilla leaf. As you start rising off the valley floor, you cross Spade Creek and meet Waptus River Trail 1310 (2,428.6–3,111').

SIDE TRIP Waptus River Trail 1310 comes up from campsites 0.75 mile away at Waptus Lake and ultimately from the Cle Elum River, about 12 miles away.

CAMPING The PCT proceeds on a gently rising traverse above the valley, well shaded under spruce, fir, and cedar boughs, but you get the occasional blue glints of large Waptus Lake below. On the way, the path crosses a couple of fairly reliable streams. Between them, Spade Lake Trail 1337 climbs north, and north of Waptus Lake at the second stream, there are campsites (2,430.0–3,234').

Eventually, your trail turns left (north) into the Spinola Creek valley and meets Spinola Creek Trail 1310A (2,431.0–3,348'), which climbs about 1 mile from the outlet of Waptus Lake. Through alternating patches of forest, meadow, and talus, the trail steepens somewhat and even switchbacks in several places as it works up this valley, keeping some distance above the creek. A second series of switchbacks gets you around a knob and onto a bench from which Cathedral Rock marks your direction.

Now in a meadowy subalpine realm, you continue north and, not long after crossing a feeder creek, meet Lake Vicente Trail 1365 (2,434.3–4,441'), which ascends west. The PCT immediately turns through a small gap and then follows the bank of now-quiet Spinola Creek, soon crossing another tributary.

WATER ACCESS

CAMPING A bit farther north, the PCT approaches Deep Lake's indigo surface and its access trail (2,434.8–4,379'), which leads to several nearby campsites.

The PCT forks right (east), wades Deep Lake's ankle-deep outlet, and heads for the east side of Deep Lake's basin to begin a 1,200-foot climb to Cathedral Pass. Well-graded switchbacks take you far above the lake to the scraggly outliers of the subalpine-fir forest, where you get a new perspective of the alpine bluffs of Mount Daniel. From the last hairpin, Peggys Pond Trail 1375 (2,437.5–5,526') forks northwest

SECTION J

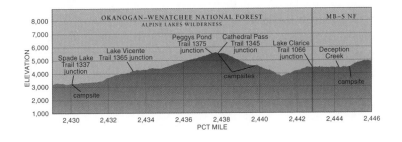

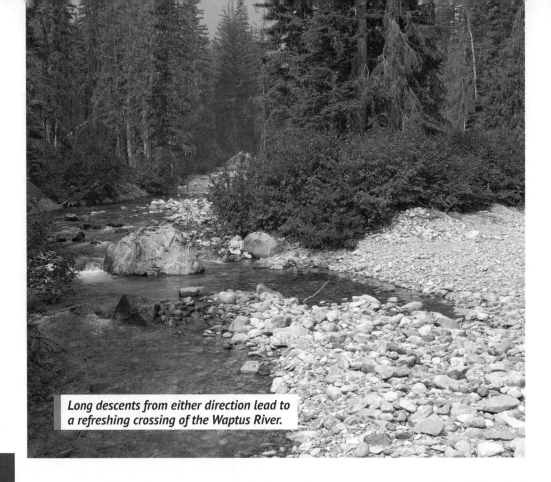

Long descents from either direction lead to a refreshing crossing of the Waptus River.

to Peggys Pond. Under towering Cathedral Rock, the trail tops a crest at Cathedral Pass for a view across the upper Cle Elum River valley to the gray, alpine uplands of Granite Mountain. From the pass, the Rainier View spur trail heads south down the ridge, while the PCT descends briefly east onto a parkland bench with a few campsites and a few small tarns (2,437.8–5,540'). To lessen your visual impact to other hikers, whenever possible, set up camp about 200 feet from the trail.

CAMPING

From here, Cathedral Pass Trail 1345, the old PCT, drops south 2,000 feet to the Cle Elum River. You can take the PCT, where there is a potentially treacherous stream crossing, or the Cathedral Pass and Deception Pass Trails as a long alternate route. In our opinion, the stream crossing in question is rarely dangerous enough for the average backpacker to warrant the 9.2-mile detour on the old PCT route. Still,

it's drawn on map J2 (page 286) and described below for those who may want to take it.

ALTERNATE ROUTE From the junction (2,437.8–5,527'), take Cathedral Pass Trail 1345 right (southeast) 2.1 miles to its junction with Trail Creek Trail 1322. Continue on Cathedral Pass Trail and switchback 2.2 miles northeast to meet Deception Pass Trail 1376 at Tucquala Meadows Trailhead. From there climb 4.9 miles northwest on Deception Pass Trail to rejoin the PCT at Deception Pass. This route is 4.2 miles longer than the PCT.

Wandering around hillocks as it continues north, the PCT proceeds in the shadow of Cathedral Rock along the edge of the scenic bench. It then starts twisting down a ridgeline, steepening as it goes, until it traverses into montane forest, where it makes a couple of longer switchbacks.

| CAMPING | These end at a bench that has shady campsites at a junction of two streams (2,439.8–4,589'). Avoid camping nearer than 200 feet to the stream whenever possible.

North of this bench, the trail continues descending steadily across slopes forested in complex patches of mountain hemlock and subalpine fir, then red cedar, Douglas-fir, and alder. The route crosses one creek and then comes to a second, which is potentially treacherous (2,441.1–3,806'). This stream, which drains Mount Daniel's northeast slopes, is swift and cold, and you'll want to wear shoes or boots to cross its stony bed. As at all stream crossings, you should assess the stream depth and current speed along with any other safety issues prior to crossing. Before the sun gets high, or on a cloudy day, the ford—quite variable—has twice been a bit downstream from the point where you encounter the stream and may not be more than a shin-deep cool-off for a few short strides.

From this ford, the trail ascends steadily across avalanche swaths and two or three more streams. The last, where the trail turns east at the head of the Cle Elum drainage, will likely require another, less vigorous footbath (2,442.2–4,236'). The gradual climb turns north again in a forest of unusually large subalpine firs and tops out at Deception Pass (2,442.8–4,478') to meet the end of the alternate route described previously.

Here at Deception Pass, a number of trail options confront the hiker. The old PCT (now Deception Pass Trail 1376) comes up from the Cle Elum River and Hyas Lake to rejoin the PCT. Marmot Lake Trail 1066 branches west, and Deception Creek Trail 1059 forks north for Deception Creek, meeting US 2 about 6 miles east of Skykomish. Beyond these junctions, the PCT heads north-northeast.

Now the PCT contours around a knob to drop to nearby Deception Creek, a small stream

in a deep and eroding drainage. Continue out of the gully on a level track, getting a glimpse back to the glimmering heights of Mount Daniel and its massive Lynch Glacier.

| CAMPING | Next you round a ridge; jump one stream; and then, near a large campsite (2,444.7–4,467'), jump another stream as you continue through cedar-and-fir forest. The PCT starts a long, gradual, northward rise above the valley of Deception Creek, eventually rounding a ridge to meet Deception Creek Trail 1059, which drops west.

WATER ACCESS

About 0.1 mile east of this junction, you cross the outlet (2,446.2–5,006') of Deception Lakes and then follow the west shoreline of the narrow lower lake. Although these lakes offer fine swimming and a pleasant rest, their accessibility means that much of their shorelines have been beaten to dust by visitors.

Just as it nears the upper lake, the PCT climbs northwest and enters a draw, at the end of which an unsigned and unmaintained trail drops off to the east. You, on the other hand, angle northwest uphill and around a ridge to resume the ascent high above Deception Creek. Now, however, you can see northwest beyond a checkerboard of clear-cuts to the jagged teeth of Mount Index, Mount Baring, and Three Fingers, as well as across the valley, where Lake Clarice nestles against Terrace Mountain. Turn up a steep slope and, with a few switchbacks, surmount it at Pieper Pass (2,448.2–5,933'). From here, the abandoned Cascade Crest Trail follows the ridgecrest north, but the PCT turns east toward inviting Glacier Lake and then drops off the pass for a braking descent.

SECTION J

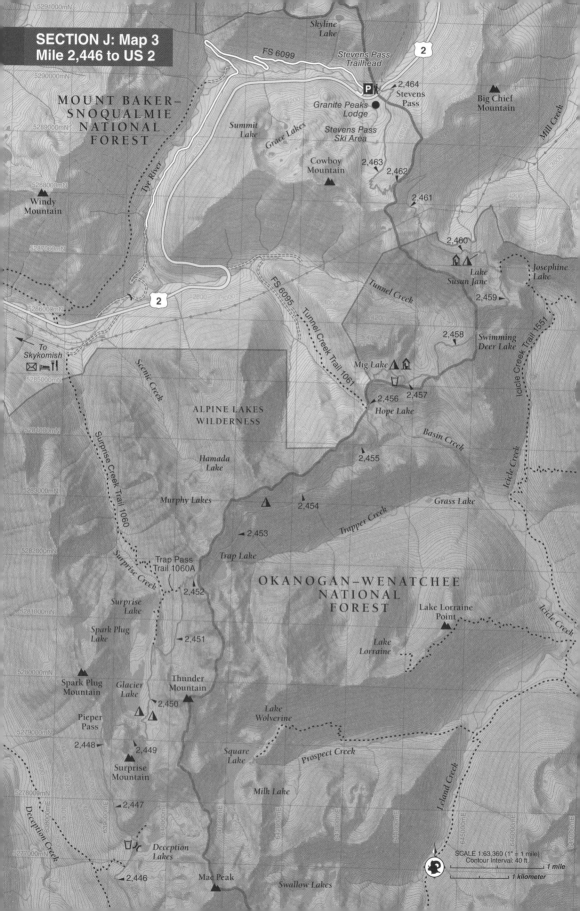

Skyline Lake

FS 6099

Stevens Pass Trailhead

2

2,464 Stevens Pass

Big Chief Mountain

Mill Creek

MOUNT BAKER–
SNOQUALMIE
NATIONAL
FOREST

Granite Peaks Lodge

Summit Lake

Grace Lakes

Stevens Pass Ski Area

Tye River

Cowboy Mountain

2,463

2,462

2,461

Windy Mountain

2,460

Lake Susan Jane

Josephine Lake

2

Tunnel Creek

2,459

To Skykomish

FS 6095

2,458

Swimming Deer Lake

Icicle Creek Trail 1551

Tunnel Creek Trail 1061

Scenic Creek

ALPINE LAKES
WILDERNESS

Mig Lake

2,457

2,456

Hope Lake

Basin Creek

Icicle Creek

2,455

Hamada Lake

Murphy Lakes

2,454

Grass Lake

Surprise Creek Trail 1060

2,453

Trapper Creek

Trap Pass Trail 1060A

Trap Lake

OKANOGAN–WENATCHEE
NATIONAL
FOREST

Lake Lorraine Point

2,452

Surprise Creek

Surprise Lake

2,451

Lake Lorraine

Icicle Creek

Spark Plug Lake

Spark Plug Mountain

Glacier Lake

Thunder Mountain

2,450

Lake Wolverine

Pieper Pass

2,448

2,449

Square Lake

Prospect Creek

Leland Creek

Surprise Mountain

2,447

Milk Lake

Deception Creek

Deception Lakes

2,446

Mac Peak

Swallow Lakes

SCALE 1:63,360 (1" = 1 mile)
Contour Interval: 40 ft.

1 mile

1 kilometer

Steep switchbacks take you down to a small bench with a tarn and a view of distant Glacier Peak, and then you wind among the granite boulders of a lower bench before descending a talus slope to the cirque floor.

CAMPING From here, you descend into the forest past campsites (2,449.8–5,036') that are above the southeast shore of Glacier Lake. Beyond this, you cross a creek and hike around the bottom of a talus slope as you parallel Glacier Lake's glistening east shore 50–100 feet above it. Then continue away from the lake past a narrow pond and shortly meet Surprise Creek Trail 1060 (2,450.6–4,863'), which heads north about 4 miles to meet US 2 about 8 miles east of Skykomish. At the junction, the PCT pivots right (southeast) to arc around the head of a ravine and start a rising traverse north.

This traverse takes you through forests and rocky fields, ever higher above Surprise Lake and ever closer to gnarly crags atop the crest. It ends where the PCT joins Trap Pass Trail 1060A (2,451.6–5,080') in the middle of a bank of steep switchbacks and then grinds up the rest of the switchbacks to the Cascade divide at Trap Pass. With Trap Lake seemingly a straight drop south, you switchback and traverse down and across its steep cirque wall to a sharply descending access trail (2,452.7–5,350') to the lake.

CAMPING After leaving the lake's bowl, the PCT keeps to flowery avalanche slopes and shady forested slopes high above Trapper Creek. At a small bench, it passes a few small campsites beside a seasonal creek (2,453.3–5,263') and then climbs briefly to a notch. From here, you slant and switchback

down through steep forest and across another bench, dropping before long to gentle terrain at overused Hope Lake (2,455.9–4,385').

SIDE TRIP From here, at a curiously low spot in the Cascade crest, Tunnel Creek Trail 1061 drops 1.4 miles northwest to Forest Service Road 6095, which descends 1.2 miles to US 2.

WATER ACCESS

CAMPING North from the turbid waters of Hope Lake, you climb through fir-and-hemlock forest onto a somewhat-swampy parkland plateau on which you turn east to the north end of Mig Lake (2,456.7–4,662'). By midsummer, this shallow lake warms to a pleasant swimming temperature. You'll also find camping and a vault toilet here.

East of Mig Lake, the PCT drops to a crest saddle, rounds a knob, and curves around a swampy pond.

Onward, climb around a forested ridge and confront steeper climbing beneath cliff bands, topping out at an unnamed crest saddle. Here a slice of Swimming Deer Lake tempts you to drop 300 feet through very steep forest, but more-accessible water is just down the trail,

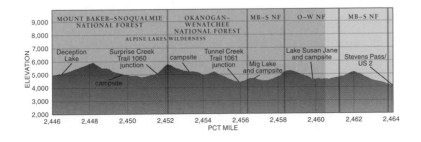

which contours east to a spur ridge and then drops along a rill in a grassy swale to the rim of Josephine Lake's cirque (2,459.3–4,940'). From here, Icicle Creek Trail 1551 descends around the cirque to the turquoise lake's outlet.

CAMPING From the Icicle Trail junction, the PCT proceeds northwest down a ravine and then down a talus slope to several campsites and a vault toilet on the north shore of Lake Susan Jane (2,459.8–4,577'). With power lines and the crest of Stevens Pass Ski Area in sight at this pretty and accessible lake, a wilderness-accustomed PCT hiker strongly senses reentry into civilization.

Next the trail traverses west under steep but well-flowered bluffs where snow lingers across the track until August. Soon after crossing a tumbling stream, the trail passes near the edge of the swath cut for the immense power lines overhead. These buzzing cables carry renewable hydroelectricity from the rural Columbia basin east of the Cascades to the cities of the coast. A couple of rough roads run through the logged swath, and you depend on trail signs to follow the climbing, switchbacking path across the former roadbeds.

North of the power lines, the trail continues climbing, taking long, meadowy switchbacks up to the Cascade crest at a saddle (2,462.0–5,160') near the top of a chairlift. Steeper, tighter switchbacks then take you down beneath this and other chairlifts to lower-angled slopes, from which you make a long, descending traverse north, crossing a creek on your way to four-lane US 2.

The trail ends at a parking area, and you head southwest through it as it quickly narrows to a road and is joined by another short road coming in from the left. On this road, you momentarily reach US 2 (2,464.1–4,053').

RESUPPLY ACCESS

This spot is only 100 yards north-northeast of signed Stevens Pass (4,056') and its obvious ski area. If you are picking up a resupply package at the resort, return to the trail by exiting Granite Peaks Lodge and using the pedestrian bridge leading to the parking lot on the north side of US 2 and the PCT trailhead, just past the green-roofed building.

SECTION J

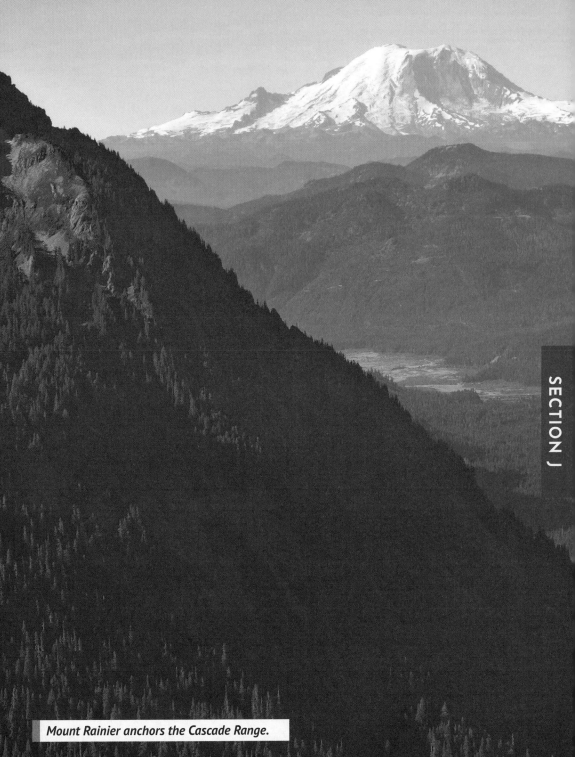

Mount Rainier anchors the Cascade Range.

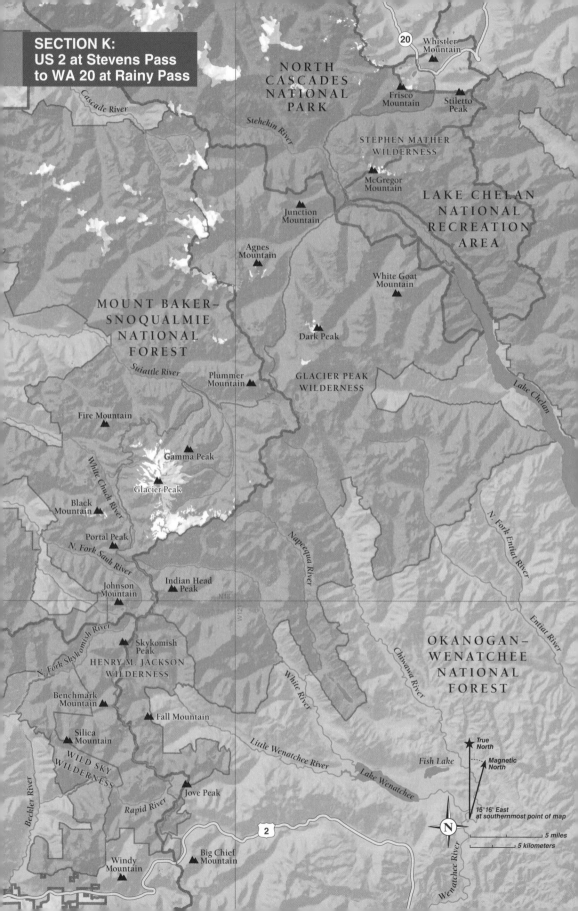

20 Whistler Mountain

NORTH CASCADES NATIONAL PARK

Frisco Mountain

Stiletto Peak

Cascade River

Stehekin River

STEPHEN MATHER WILDERNESS

McGregor Mountain

LAKE CHELAN NATIONAL RECREATION AREA

Junction Mountain

Agnes Mountain

White Goat Mountain

MOUNT BAKER– SNOQUALMIE NATIONAL FOREST

Suiattle River

Plummer Mountain

Dark Peak

GLACIER PEAK WILDERNESS

Lake Chelan

Fire Mountain

Gamma Peak

White Chuck River

Glacier Peak

Napeequa River

N. Fork Entiat River

Black Mountain

Portal Peak

N. Fork Sauk River

Indian Head Peak

N13

Entiat River

W12

N. Fork Skykomish River

Johnson Mountain

Skykomish Peak

HENRY M. JACKSON WILDERNESS

OKANOGAN– WENATCHEE NATIONAL FOREST

Chiwawa River

White River

Benchmark Mountain

Fall Mountain

Silica Mountain

WILD SKY WILDERNESS

Little Wenatchee River

Fish Lake

★ True North

Magnetic North

Beckler River

Rapid River

Jove Peak

Lake Wenatchee

15° 16' East
at southernmost point of map

2

Windy Mountain

Big Chief Mountain

N

5 miles

5 kilometers

Wenatchee River

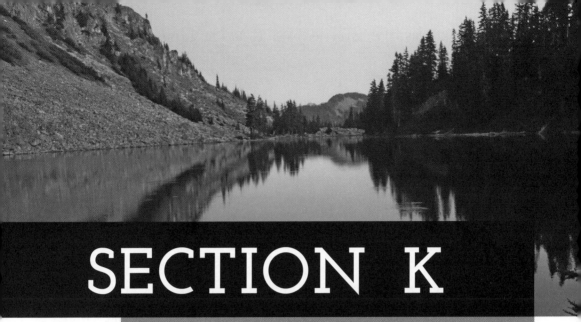

SECTION K

US 2 at Stevens Pass to WA 20 at Rainy Pass

IN THIS SECTION, you will travel across a very rugged section of the North Cascades. This stretch ranks second only to *Pacific Crest Trail: Southern California*'s John Muir Trail section in difficulty and provides a definite challenge. Traversing around Glacier Peak, you will descend to and then labor up a number of deep-floored canyons that radiate from that peak. Unfortunately, a nice contouring trail, such as the one around Mount Adams, is impossible to route around Glacier Peak proper, for such a trail would be too snowbound and too avalanche-prone.

Not only does this section have rugged topography, but it also sometimes has dangerous fords; cold, threatening weather; and persistent insects. Why, then, do thousands of backpackers flock to Glacier Peak Wilderness? Well, perhaps it's because it is a real wilderness and not, like so many others, a wilderness in name only. This area's intimidating, snowy terrain, contrasted with lovely, fragile wildflower gardens, will draw you back time and again.

Above: Dusk falls on Lake Valhalla.

DECLINATION 15°16'E

USGS MAPS

Stevens Pass, WA	Poe Mountain, WA
Gamma Peak, WA	McGregor Mountain, WA
Labyrinth Mountain, WA	Glacier Peak East, WA
Suiattle Pass, WA	McAlester Mountain, WA
Captain Point, WA	Glacier Peak West, WA
Agnes Mountain, WA	Washington Pass, WA
Bench Mark Mountain, WA	Lime Mountain, WA
Mount Lyall, WA	

POINTS ON THE TRAIL, SOUTH TO NORTH

	Mile	Elevation in feet	Latitude/Longitude
US 2 at Stevens Pass	2,464.1	4,053	N47° 44' 46.4028" W121° 05' 18.6332"
Lake Janus	2,473.9	4,146	N47° 49' 30.4074" W121° 05' 56.6944"
Wenatchee Pass	2,481.2	4,245	N47° 52' 23.3699" W121° 09' 20.3770"
Junction with Meadow Creek Trail to Pear Lake	2,482.5	4,860	N47° 52' 44.6697" W121° 09' 57.9003"
Lake Sally Ann	2,493.5	5,476	N47° 57' 37.0132" W121° 09' 11.7733"
Indian Pass	2,498.2	4,973	N47° 59' 46.7973" W121° 07' 17.3514"
Reflection Pond	2,500.2	5,588	N48° 01' 04.0701" W121° 07' 42.7899"
White Pass	2,502.0	5,904	N48° 01' 59.7995" W121° 08' 55.2384"
Red Pass	2,503.8	6,488	N48° 02' 45.9799" W121° 10' 39.9528"
Kennedy Creek	2,512.3	3,942	N48° 07' 20.2269" W121° 10' 39.3992"
Fire Creek Pass	2,520.2	5,820	N48° 09' 39.0414" W121° 09' 33.5780"
Suiattle River bridge	2,540.6	2,318	N48° 12' 26.6999" W121° 04' 44.8681"
Cloudy Pass Trail junction to alternate route and Holden	2,551.8	5,906	N48° 12' 10.8571" W120° 56' 23.4781"
Hemlock Camp	2,559.5	3,552	N48° 15' 27.0122" W120° 55' 38.1994"
Agnes Creek trailhead on Stehekin Valley Road	2,571.8	1,662	N48° 22' 47.0243" W120° 50' 22.4874"
Bridge Creek trailhead on Stehekin Valley Road	2,577.1	2,180	N48° 25' 56.6245" W120° 52' 18.2232"
WA 20 at Rainy Pass	2,591.1	4,855	N48° 30' 53.2653" W120° 44' 01.9904"

CAMPSITES AND BIVY SITES

Mile	Elevation in feet	Latitude/ Longitude	Number of tents	Feature	Notes
2,478.6	5,580	N47° 50' 44.9599" W121° 09' 16.2166"	3	Grizzly Peak	
2,481.2	4,245	N47° 52' 24.6897" W121° 09' 23.8929"	3	Wenatchee Pass	Bivy on both sides of trail
2,482.5	4,860	N47° 52' 45.9701" W121° 09' 56.3004"	>4	Pear Lake	Water access

CAMPSITES AND BIVY SITES (continued)

Mile	Elevation in feet	Latitude/ Longitude	Number of tents	Feature	Notes
2,486.7	4,777	N47° 54' 44.4401" W121° 10' 44.5998"	2	Creeks nearby	
2,489.2	4,165	N47° 55' 42.3046" W121° 10' 38.3711"	3	Pass Creek	Mice may create holes in gear; vault toilet
2,493.5	5,476	N47° 57' 39.3602" W121° 09' 08.0600"	3	Lake Sally Ann	Toilet, water access
2,505.5	5,453	N48° 03' 10.9076" W121° 09' 23.9955"	2	Creek nearby	Bivy on each side
2,506.8	4,741	N48° 03' 52.4577" W121° 09' 27.5372"	2	Creek nearby	
2,508.8	3,961	N48° 05' 10.6278" W121° 09' 52.4460"	2	Baekos Creek	Fire ring
2,520.8	5,455	N48° 09' 58.9044" W121° 09' 27.9767"	>4	Mica Lake	Above lake; sheltered sites; water access
2,521.3	5,161	N48° 10' 03.6842" W121° 09' 17.0078"	4		Several good spots here; backcountry toilet nearby
2,531.5	5,724	N48° 09' 40.3425" W121° 06' 02.9300"	>8	Near Dolly Creek	On left in shade
2,535.2	3,619	N48° 10' 06.8524" W121° 04' 32.2749"	3	Vista Creek	On right with fire ring
2,540.5	2,324	N48° 12' 26.6238" W121° 04' 46.1308"	4	Suiattle River	Water access
2,540.6	2,333	N48° 12' 28.3645" W121° 04' 43.6913"	3	Suiattle River	Water access
2,543.2	2,812	N48° 11' 47.2072" W121° 02' 41.4472"	>4		On both sides
2,549.1	4,492	N48° 11' 18.0566" W120° 58' 03.3479"	>4	Near Miners Creek	
2,552.4	5,806	N48° 12' 11.6690" W120° 56' 34.4447"	3		Signed site on left; fire ring
2,553.9	5,046	N48° 12' 55.4144" W120° 57' 00.8019"	2	Deep canyon	Signed site on right
2,555.5	5,377	N48° 13' 51.4882" W120° 56' 42.9511"	2		Signed site on right
2,557.1	4,724	N48° 14' 33.0599" W120° 57' 20.0788"	2		Signed site on left; fire ring
2,562.3	2,876	N48° 17' 34.0450" W120° 55' 48.7840"	>10	Cedar Camp	South Fork Agnes Creek
2,563.8	2,749	N48° 18' 34.0755" W120° 55' 13.4840"	>4	Swamp Creek Camp	Water access
2,566.8	2,206	N48° 20' 39.3806" W120° 54' 13.8699"	>4	Pass Creek	Vault toilet nearby
2,571.9	1,611	N48° 22' 46.9632" W120° 50' 22.4514"	2	High Bridge Campground	Other side of bridge; vault toilet, picnic table, fire pit, corral, bear-proof box
2,576.8	2,101	N48° 25' 47.8613" W120° 52' 06.7625"	>6	Bridge Creek Camp	Vault toilet, picnic tables, bear-proof box; creek nearby
2,579.7	2,580	N48° 27' 24.1760" W120° 50' 37.4149"	2	North Fork Camp	Vault toilet; bear wire
2,585.3	3,512	N48° 27' 56.1801" W120° 44' 28.3998"	>2	Hideaway Camp	Vault toilet, fire ring
2,586.2	3,632	N48° 28' 05.6467" W120° 43' 11.0456"	>2	Fireweed Camp	Just off trail; vault toilet, bear wire

SECTION K

SUPPLIES

See "Supplies" in the previous section for the facilities at Stevens Pass, this section's starting point. There are no other on-route supply points. However, upon reaching the Stehekin River near the end of the section, you can take a shuttle bus, $8 each way in 2020, over to Stehekin, which has a resort, a post office (98852), a hiker-oriented store, and an information center. If you need boots, clothes, or other special items, you can take a ferry from Stehekin to Chelan and then return.

Mazama, while off the trail about 22 miles east on WA 20, is definitely worth a splurge. Rooms for two at the Mazama Country Inn (800-843-7951, mazamacountryinn.com) are comfortable, and the gourmet foods from The Mazama Store (509-996-2855, themazamastore.com) are worth the calories. Call ahead for reservations. Meals can be prepared at the store 7 a.m.–6 p.m., and hiker-specific foods may be available in small quantities. The Mazama Store also accepts hiker packages.

PERMITS

A wilderness permit is required for all backcountry stays in North Cascades National Park. The Pacific Crest Trail (PCT) enters the park about 0.3 mile south of the High Bridge Ranger Station and leaves the park about 3.2 miles south of WA 20's Rainy Pass. If you're heading north on the PCT and don't already have a wilderness permit, you can get one in Stehekin at the Golden West Visitor Center or the Stehekin ranger station (in early or late season, when the visitor center is closed). If you're heading south on the PCT from Rainy Pass, then get a permit from the Wilderness Information Center at the Marblemount ranger station (if coming from the west) or from the Methow Valley Visitor Center in Winthrop (if coming from the east). While in the park, you are required to camp in designated trailside camps only. If you don't have a permit, you may find that you also won't have a campsite! Hikers with PCTA-issued long-distance hiking permits may camp at the Bridge Creek campsite without acquiring a separate North Cascades National Park permit.

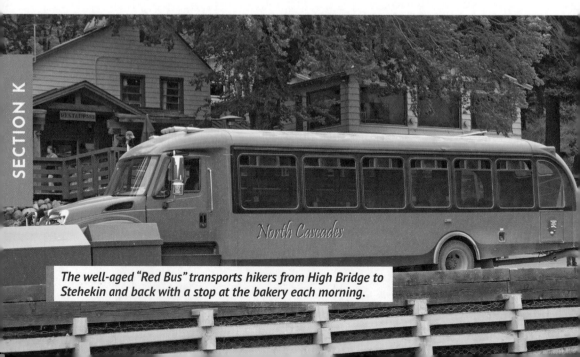

The well-aged "Red Bus" transports hikers from High Bridge to Stehekin and back with a stop at the bakery each morning.

SPECIAL CONCERNS

In this section of heavy rain and avalanches, bridges are periodically washed away. Generally, they are replaced within a year or two, but this is no consolation to you if you encounter a bridgeless stream. In particular, if either the bridge across White Chuck River or the one across Suiattle River is gone, the ford may be dangerous.

Additionally, this section is located in the central part of Washington's North Cascades (a part of the greater Cascade Range), extending roughly from Snoqualmie Pass north to the Canadian border, and is composed largely of granitic and metamorphic rocks. These rocks aren't the problem, but the snowfall they collect is: the North Cascades accumulate more snow than anywhere else in the United States. In the 2016–17 snow season, the Mount Baker Ski Area, lying west of the PCT, recorded 866 inches—more than 72 feet—of snow. What this means for you, the trekker, is that even in a normal year, you may encounter a lot of snow-covered trail, which slows you down and sometimes causes you to get off route. Don't try hiking across snow in a whiteout; you may get lost.

A final problem is bears, which are quite common from Stehekin north up the Stehekin River and up Bridge Creek. The National Park Service recommends using a bear-proof canister to protect your food, and proper food storage is required within North Cascades National Park. Bears are important members of the North Cascades wildlife community, and the park has labored to ensure that visitors don't have an adverse impact on bears by inadvertently feeding them backpacker food. The park has provided bear-proof food-storage boxes and food-hanging devices along the PCT from High Bridge to Twisp Pass Trail. Please use these for your food storage whenever you camp in order to protect the bear population. For tips on how to avoid negative encounters with bears, see pages 29–31.

US 2 AT STEVENS PASS TO WA 20 AT RAINY PASS

>>> THE ROUTE

Look for the trailhead about 250 yards north-northeast of Stevens Pass (4,056') on US 2 (2,464.1–4,053'), by the east side of a power substation. The PCT begins on a maintenance road that contours north across granitic terrain.

| PLANTS | On this open, bushy stretch, you pass an assortment of aster, bleeding heart, bluebells, columbine, fireweed, lupine, monkeyflower, paintbrush, parsnip, and Sitka valerian before curving west into a forested environment. You reach a 3-yard-wide tributary (2,466.6–3,881') of Nason Creek, which you continue up, entering the Henry M. Jackson Wilderness (2,467.5–4,169') before reaching a meadow through which Nason Creek flows. Here grow cinquefoil, shooting stars, red heather, and grass, all of which will die after three to four nights of tent coverage. Vegetated meadows should not be considered a site for camping, but their sandy or rocky margin may be satisfactory. Mosquitoes and several species of biting flies, common in northern Washington through midsummer, will not bother you if the day is cold or misty.

Now within Henry M. Jackson Wilderness, the trail climbs past a second small meadow and then switchbacks up to a saddle (2,469.6–5,030'), from which you can look down at beautiful Lake Valhalla and across it at the challenging west face of dark-gray Lichtenberg Mountain (5,844'). Descending north from the saddle, you reach another meadow and a spur trail (2,469.9–4,900') that descends southeast past a signed toilet site 200 yards to the northwest shore of deep, cool, sparkling Lake Valhalla (4,830').

The PCT now climbs east to a saddle, snowbound through late July, and then steadily descends northeast to Union Gap and a junction with Smithbrook Trail 1590 (2,471.7–4,688'), which descends east 0.7 mile to Forest Service Road 6700. From the gap, the PCT descends northwest along a lower slope of Union Peak (5,696') before turning north and ascending to a delightful, singing cascade (2,473.5–4,200').

WATER ACCESS

Tree frogs and evening grosbeaks may join in a twilight chorus as you approach shallow Lake Janus (2,473.9–4,146'), which is somewhat disappointing after Lake Valhalla. The warmer temperatures of this semiclear lake, however, do allow you a comfortable dip. Just northwest is the clear outlet creek.

Beyond this creek, the PCT switchbacks west up to a ravine on your left. In 0.25 mile, the trail reaches the crest; traverses a short, northeast slope with a view due north of distant, regal Glacier Peak (10,541'); and then reaches a saddle. A moderate descent northwest leads to a meadow (2,476.3–5,070'), from which a faint trail leads 40 yards northeast and then descends a moderately steep ravine toward Glasses Lake (4,626'). Your

path then follows a winding crest route up past outcrops of mica schist before it reaches the upper west shoulder (2,478.6–5,580') of Grizzly Peak (5,597').

From it you hike north along the ridge, round another summit, and then cross a saddle. Leaving it behind, the trail descends moderately across a west slope, passes well above shallow Grizzly Lake (4,920'), crosses the crest, and reaches a shadeless, grassy flat.

CAMPING Descending north on a sometimes soggy, moderate-to-steep trail, you reach the crest again and then switchback down it to broad, forested Wenatchee Pass (2,481.2–4,245'), where there are a couple of small campsites. Climbing north to a flat, you reach a junction with Top Lake Trail 1506 (2,481.9–4,581'), which curves east 0.5 mile to that lake (4,590').

WATER ACCESS

The PCT heads west to a ravine whose west side is composed of large boulders. Gushing from them is the outlet of Pear Lake, which is dammed behind them. Climb several short switchbacks, pass through a saddle with a view of Glacier Peak, and then climb a few more hairpins to a ridgeline, the edge of Pear Lake's cirque (2,482.5–4,860') at its junction with Meadow Creek Trail 1057.

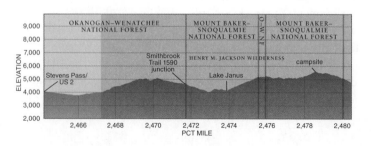

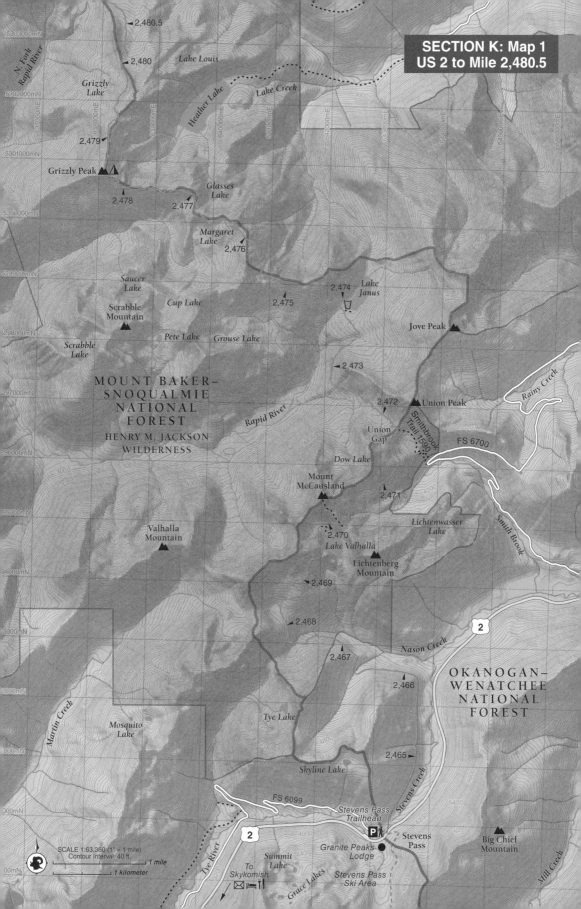

2,480.5

Lake Louis

2,480

N. Fork Rapid River

Grizzly Lake

Lake Creek

Heather Lake

2,479

Grizzly Peak ▲▲ ⚠

2,478

2,477

Glasses Lake

Margaret Lake

2,476

Saucer Lake

Cup Lake

Scrabble Mountain ▲

2,475

2,474

Lake Janus

Scrabble Lake

Pete Lake

Grouse Lake

Jove Peak ▲

MOUNT BAKER– SNOQUALMIE NATIONAL FOREST

HENRY M. JACKSON WILDERNESS

2,473

Rapid River

2,472

Union Peak ▲

Rainy Creek

Union Gap

Smithbrook Trail 1590

FS 6700

Dow Lake

Mount McCausland ▲

2,471

Lichtenwasser Lake

Smith Brook

Valhalla Mountain ▲

2,470

Lake Valhalla

Lichtenberg Mountain ▲

2,469

2,468

2,467

2,466

Nason Creek

② (2)

OKANOGAN– WENATCHEE NATIONAL FOREST

Martin Creek

Mosquito Lake

Tye Lake

2,465

Skyline Lake

Stevens Creek

FS 6099

Stevens Pass Trailhead

🅿

Stevens Pass

Big Chief Mountain ▲

Tye River

② (2)

Summit Lake

To Skykomish

Granite Peaks Lodge ●

Stevens Pass Ski Area

Grace Lakes

Mill Creek

SCALE 1:63,360 (1" = 1 mile)
Contour Interval 40 ft.

1 mile

1 kilometer

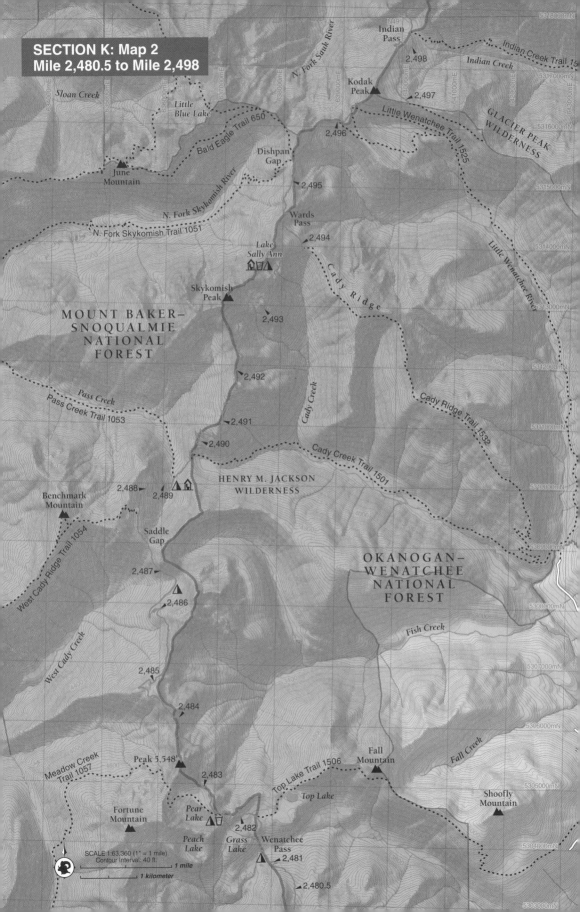

Sloan Creek

Little
Blue Lake

N. Fork Sauk River

Indian
Pass

2,498

Indian Creek Trail 15

Indian Creek

Kodak
Peak

2,497

2,496

Bald Eagle Trail 650

Dishpan
Gap

Little Wenatchee Trail 1525

GLACIER PEAK
WILDERNESS

June
Mountain

2,495

N. Fork Skykomish River

N. Fork Skykomish Trail 1051

Wards
Pass

2,494

Cady Ridge

Little Wenatchee River

Lake
Sally Ann

Skykomish
Peak

2,493

MOUNT BAKER–
SNOQUALMIE
NATIONAL
FOREST

2,492

Cady Creek

Pass Creek

Pass Creek Trail 1053

2,491

2,490

Cady Ridge Trail 1532

2,488

2,489

HENRY M. JACKSON
WILDERNESS

Cady Creek Trail 1501

Benchmark
Mountain

OKANOGAN–
WENATCHEE
NATIONAL
FOREST

West Cady Ridge Trail 1054

Saddle
Gap

2,487

2,486

Fish Creek

West Cady Creek

2,485

2,484

Fall
Mountain

Fall Creek

Meadow Creek
Trail 1057

Peak 5,548'

2,483

Top Lake Trail 1506

Top Lake

Shoofly
Mountain

Fortune
Mountain

Pear
Lake

2,482

Peach
Lake

Grass
Lake

Wenatchee
Pass

2,481

2,480.5

CAMPING From here, Meadow Creek Trail (formerly the PCT) heads west down to excellent campsites at the nearby, cliff-backed lake.

The PCT climbs northwest just below the crest of the ridge—a moraine—allowing glimpses down to the aquamarine lake, and then it weaves between mossy boulders atop the moraine. Next a switchback drops you to a notch where you leave the cirque and start a traverse around Peak 5,548. Scattered hemlocks stand over the trail until it rounds the peak and becomes a path blasted through huge granitic talus blocks. With pikas sounding off at your passage, continue traversing to a tier of tight, steep hairpins that work past a cliff and up to the crest (2,484.1–5,350').

On the west side of the crest, climb a bit more, and then settle into a contouring ramble. As you round the meadowy bench of a point (5,440'), you can see the country ahead through Saddle Gap to Skykomish Peak and Glacier Peak and west to the Monte Cristo peaks. For a stretch, the trail passes right below the scattered trees and glades of the crest line, and then it angles downslope into denser forest, passing one more talus slope before weaving down some switchbacks.

CAMPING From these, it resumes a contouring course and reaches a pair of adjacent, fairly reliable creeks and a large campsite (2,486.7–4,777').

Now the PCT climbs northwest gradually across steep slopes to a sign that claims water is available not far downslope. Just up the trail from here, you reach Saddle Gap (2,487.4–5,002').

Beyond the gap, you curve north down to a junction with West Cady Ridge Trail 1054 (2,487.7–4,930'), which climbs west on its way to North Fork of the Skykomish River.

CAMPING After descending north toward a prominent knob of metamorphic rock, the trail makes two long switchbacks down to 3-yard-wide Pass Creek. Immediately after crossing it on stepping-stones, you meet Pass Creek Trail 1053 (2,489.1–4,165'), which descends north alongside the creek. In 0.1 mile you come across another campsite with a toilet. These save the trail's water quality and should be used when possible.

The PCT climbs northeast and shortly arrives at Cady Pass, from which Cady Creek Trail 1501 (2,489.6–4,303') departs east before dropping to that creek. Camping is not recommended at this forested pass.

A long ascent—a taste of what's to come—now begins as the PCT switchbacks north up to a metamorphic ridge and reaches its crest. This strenuous ascent rewards you near its top with scenic views south and east. After descending slightly to a granitic saddle, the trail rounds the east slope of a knob (5,642') and then reaches another saddle. Beyond it, trailside snow patches can last into August.

WATER ACCESS

CAMPING Next you contour across the east slope of rugged Skykomish Peak (6,368'), where this

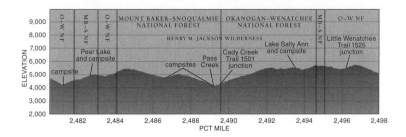

twisting course takes you around granitic knobs and into ravines—a couple with creeks—and eventually brings you to Lake Sally Ann (2,493.5–5,476'). This beautiful lake has attracted many over the years, and the U.S. Forest Service has lined off much of the beaten-down spots, built a privy, and laid revegetation netting. Camping here is a privilege that, if abused, could be revoked by the USFS. Follow Leave No Trace ethics, and check your impact on other hikers.

Beyond the lake, the PCT curves down past creeklets to a junction with Cady Ridge Trail 1532 (2,493.9–5,385').

Beyond this junction, the sometimes-snowbound trail climbs northwest across a slope of greenish mica schist, glistening white-vein quartz, and speckled adamellite before switchbacking up to Wards Pass (2,494.6–5,700'). Turning north, you then hike along a crest route that takes you down the soggy, volcanic soils of Dishpan Gap, where North Fork Skykomish Trail 1051 descends west and, just beyond, Bald Eagle Trail 650 (2,495.2–5,600') veers north-northwest.

WILDLIFE The PCT veers right (northeast) and crosses the southeast slope of Peak 5,892 to a ridgecrest with an open slope of grass, cinquefoil, and fawn lilies. Don't be surprised to see deer here.

Following the crest east across this glaciated country, you quickly arrive at a saddle, from which a spur trail contours south to Little Wenatchee Trail 1525. You head diagonally up the northwest slope of a triangular summit and then reach a junction with Little Wenatchee Trail 1525 (2496.2–5,496'), which contours southeast.

VIEWS The PCT heads north toward Kodak Peak (6,121') and then climbs east across its flowery, picturesque south slope of metamorphic rocks, where the distant view includes Mount Rainier, Chimney Peak, Mount Daniel, and the Stuart Range.

Upon your arrival at Kodak Peak's east ridge (2,496.9–5,660'), Glacier Peak comes into view to the north and an unmaintained trail strikes east-southeast along this ridge, the southern boundary of Glacier Peak Wilderness and the northern boundary of Henry M. Jackson Wilderness.

The trail turns northwest and descends across open slopes, July snowfields, and a couple of rivulets before curving north and switchbacking past stalwart hemlocks down to Indian Pass (2,498.2–4,973').

Ascending to the PCT from the southeast is faint Indian Creek Trail 1502. From its junction, you arc northwest up to a southwest spur of Indian Head Peak (7,442') and then climb north to a ridge and a junction with an older trail that traverses the north slopes of Indian Head Peak. Staying on the PCT, you descend to Lower White Pass (2,499.8–5,411'), from which the old Cascade Crest Trail once descended northeast; today the trail is called White River Trail 1507.

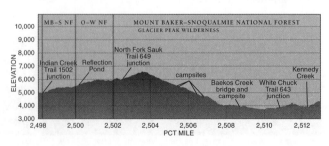

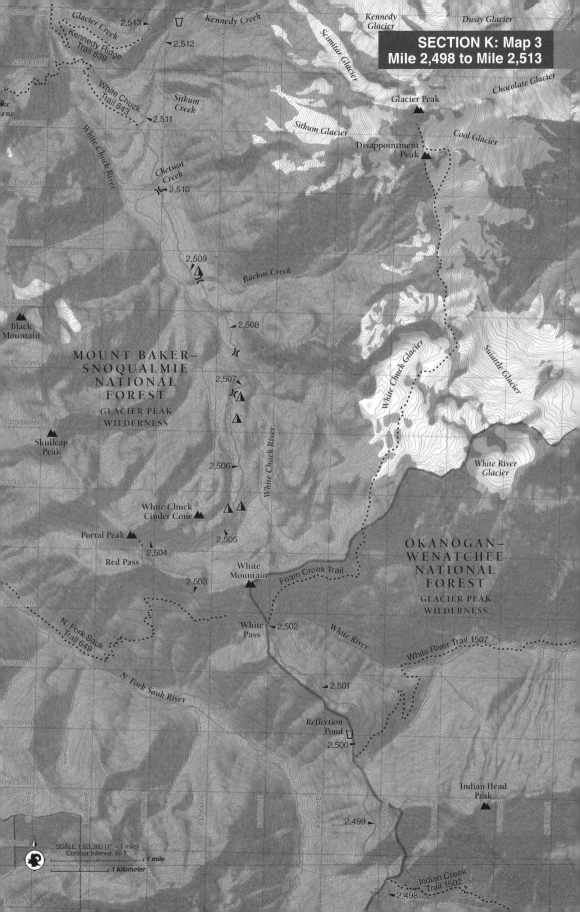

Glacier Creek

Kennedy Creek

Kennedy Glacier

Dusty Glacier

2,513

2,512

Kennedy Ridge Trail 639

Scimitar Glacier

Glacier Peak

Chocolate Glacier

White Chuck Trail 643

Sitkum Creek

2,511

Sitkum Glacier

Disappointment Peak

Cool Glacier

White Chuck River

Chetwot Creek

2,510

2,509

Backos Creek

2,508

White Chuck Glacier

Suiattle Glacier

Black Mountain

MOUNT BAKER–
SNOQUALMIE
NATIONAL
FOREST

GLACIER PEAK
WILDERNESS

2,507

2,506

White Chuck River

White River Glacier

Skulleap Peak

White Chuck
Cinder Cone

2,505

Portal Peak

2,504

Red Pass

White Mountain

OKANOGAN–
WENATCHEE
NATIONAL
FOREST

GLACIER PEAK
WILDERNESS

2,503

Foam Creek Trail

N. Fork Sauk
Trail 649

White
Pass

2,502

White River

White River Trail 1507

N. Fork Sauk River

2,501

Reflection
Pond

2,500

Indian Head
Peak

2,499

Indian Creek
Trail 1502

2,498

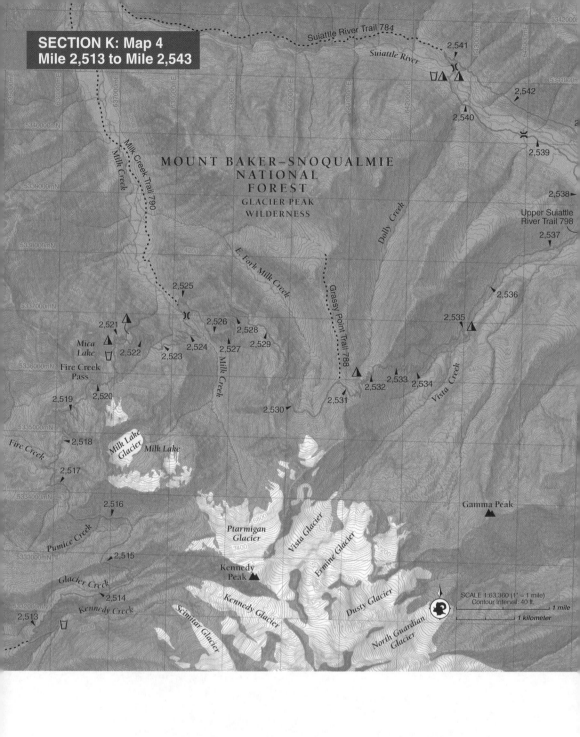

Suiattle River Trail 784

Suiattle River

2,541

2,542

2,540

2,539

MOUNT BAKER–SNOQUALMIE
NATIONAL
FOREST
GLACIER PEAK
WILDERNESS

2,538 ►

Dolly Creek

Upper Suiattle
River Trail 798

2,537

Milk Creek Trail 790

Milk Creek

E. Fork Milk Creek

2,525

Grassy Point Trail 788

2,536

2,535

2,521

2,526

2,528

Mica
Lake

2,522

2,524

2,527

2,529

2,523

2,531

2,532 2,533 2,534

Vista Creek

Fire Creek
Pass

2,519

2,520

Milk Creek

2,530

2,518

Fire Creek

Milk Lake
Glacier

Milk Lake

2,517

Gamma Peak

2,516

Ptarmigan
Glacier

Vista Glacier

Ermine Glacier

Pumice Creek

2,515

Glacier Creek

Kennedy
Peak

Dusty Glacier

2,514

SCALE 1:63,360 (1" = 1 mile)
Contour Interval: 40 ft.

1 mile

Kennedy Creek

2,513

Scimitar Glacier

Kennedy Glacier

North Guardian
Glacier

1 kilometer

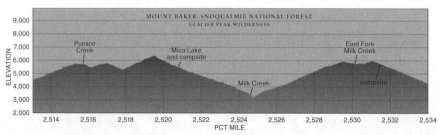

MOUNT BAKER–SNOQUALMIE NATIONAL FOREST
GLACIER PEAK WILDERNESS

ELEVATION

9,000
8,000
7,000
6,000
5,000
4,000
3,000
2,000

Pumice
Creek

Mica Lake
and campsite

Milk Creek

East Fork
Milk Creek

campsite

2,514 2,516 2,518 2,520 2,522 2,524 2,526 2,528 2,530 2,532 2,534

PCT MILE

WATER ACCESS

The PCT climbs a ridge north to the shores of semiclear Reflection Pond (2,500.2–5,588'), where you can gather water for purifying, and then traverses the snowbound northeast slopes up to a junction at White Pass (2,502.0–5,904'). No camping is allowed along the crest at White Pass.

Here, Foam Creek Trail begins a curving traverse northeast to Foam Basin, while another spur trail leads west down to the ridgecrest, where snowmelt is reliable.

WILDLIFE Continuing along the PCT, you follow its contouring path west-northwest to a fork, from which North Fork Sauk Trail 649 (2,502.5–6,011') descends steeply west. The meadow here has such an abundance of flowers and insects, it's no wonder that birds fly north to feast on them. Flycatchers hover and snatch insects from midair as you start a steady climb west-northwest on the PCT.

The trail becomes dusty as it approaches a small summit (6,650') affording an excellent panorama of the Monte Cristo massif and of prominent Sloan Peak. The path then turns north and shortly reaches the gray, garnet-biotite gneiss rocks of marmot-inhabited Red Pass (2,503.8–6,488').

VIEWS The view from here is nothing short of spectacular.

Above you and 5 miles northeast is a towering volcano, Glacier Peak (10,541'), which last erupted about 12,500 years ago. Below is the perennially snow-clad upper canyon of the White Chuck River. To the distant south is lofty, glistening Mount Rainier (14,410'), which is cloaked in snow, giving it the appearance of a giant stationary cloud that reigns eternally over the distant forest. If you're heading south, you'll definitely remember your climb to this pass.

CAMPING The PCT first switchbacks and then descends along the base of the east ridge of Portal Peak. When this section of trail is snowbound, most hikers slide directly down the steep but safe upper snowfield and then head downcanyon (east) until they reach the visible trail. Keeping north of the headwaters, the PCT descends toward a lone, 3-foot-high cairn on a low knoll, turns north, and then descends to a saddle between a 20-foot-high hill to the east and a high slope to the west. Some campsites are on the hill (2,505.5–5,453'). Just 250 yards north, you pass another campsite; farther down, you can see others along the banks of the rumbling White Chuck River below and to the east.

CAMPING You may spot a blue grouse and its chicks as you descend alongside a swelling creek that the PCT crosses three times via bridges. Leaving the last crossing and its campsites (2,506.8–4,741'), the trail switchbacks down toward the White Chuck River, parallels it above its west bank, and then crosses it (2,507.7–4,076') to the east via a wide, planked horse bridge. Leave the river's side, follow an undulating route north, and then descend to a log crossing of cold, roaring Baekos Creek (2,508.7–3,944'), whose north bank contains much green mica schist. Follow the base of its high north bank downstream 0.1 mile to several small tent sites and, in a short bit, switchback over the creek, and then descend to level ground and a number of log crossings over small creeks.

MOUNT BAKER–SNOQUALMIE NATIONAL FOREST
GLACIER PEAK WILDERNESS

Vista Creek and campsite — Upper Suiattle River Trail 798 junction — Dolly Creek — Suiattle River Trail 784 junction — campsites

ELEVATION: 8,000 / 7,000 / 6,000 / 5,000 / 4,000 / 3,000 / 2,000 / 1,000

PCT MILE: 2,534   2,536   2,538   2,540   2,542

SECTION K

While gathering water at Chetwot Creek (2,510.0–3,741'), you'll notice that the vegetation opens enough to afford views southwest to broad Black Mountain glacier, which spreads across the upper rim of a side canyon. Continuing north, you reach Sitkum Creek and make a log crossing of it (2,511.4–4,150'). From Sitkum Creek, a long climb lies ahead.

GEOLOGY As you enjoy a brief descent northeast, you pass small outcrops above that are rich in quartz and biotite, Miocene-age granitic intrusions.

WATER ACCESS

You reach chilly, glacier-fed Kennedy Creek (2,512.3–3,942'), a 10-yard-wide torrent that sometimes has to be forded because bridges built across it have a tendency to be wiped out by avalanches. Without a bridge, the ford would be treacherous. The current cubist bridge handles all but the highest water for now.

After crossing the creek, climb southwest along a path cut through unstable morainal material that in turn is being undercut by the creek. Soon you reach a junction with Kennedy Ridge Trail 639 (2,512.7–4,168'). Now the real climb begins as you ascend six short, steep switchbacks past huge andesite blocks to the lower crest of Kennedy Ridge. You struggle upward, stopping several times to catch your breath and admire the scenery. In spots, this crest is no wider than the trail. The gradient eases off, and you eventually reach Glacier Creek (2,514.5–5,300'), which occasionally has an avalanche roar down its canyon, destroying all the trees in its path.

SIDE TRIP For mountaineers, the shortest climb to Glacier Peak's summit (10,541') begins here. Should you try, bring rope, crampons, and an ice ax.

GEOLOGY Leaving the creek, you switchback north and then climb northwest past adamellite boulders. After a short, steep descent northeast, the trail contours in that direction to cross Pumice Creek

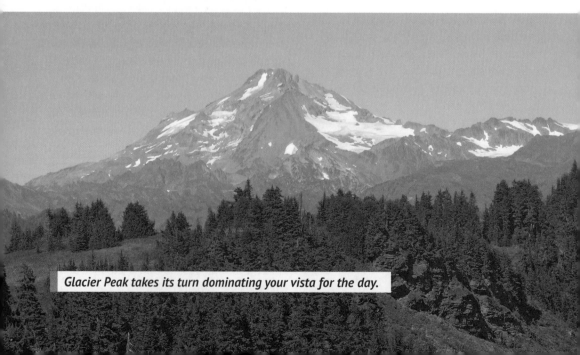

Glacier Peak takes its turn dominating your vista for the day.

(2,515.7–5,684'), whose bed contains metamorphic, granitic, and volcanic rocks. You might try to identify all three types and decipher their stories. The trail descends west and then contours over to a ridge. North of it, the PCT descends even more and then crosses a branch of Fire Creek (2,517.8–5,279') just below its fork upstream.

VIEWS Now you make one final effort, and voilà: a magnificent panorama of the North Cascades unfolds around you as you gain access to Fire Creek Pass (2,520.2–5,820').

GEOLOGY The North Cascades of Washington contain hundreds of glaciers, which account for about half of all the glacier area existing within the contiguous United States. The range's great number of fairly high summits, coupled with its year-round barrage from storms, accounts for its vast accumulation of ice and snow. Chances are that you'll encounter at least one storm, lasting only a few days if you're lucky, before you reach the Canadian border.

WATER ACCESS

CAMPING The usually snowbound route switchbacks down a ridge north-northeast to a ford of the outlet of usually frozen Mica Lake, where you'll find some small bivy sites (2,520.8–5,455').

From Mica Lake's shore, you can see dozens of unappealing switchbacks you'll have to climb to surmount the next ridge.

CAMPING As you descend farther, you must boulder-hop wide, shallow Mica Creek, just east of which is a good but open campsite (2,521.3–5,161') on a small bench. Continue to switchback east and reach another creek (2,522.8–4,400').

From it, the unrelenting descent takes you down to deep, 5-yard-wide Milk Creek. In 1974 a bridge replaced a log crossing, but that bridge was wiped out by an early-summer avalanche in 1975. Another bridge was built, but it became the next spring sacrifice when it was destroyed in 2003. The current bridge, sited upstream from its predecessors, lasted through the huge snowmelt in 2017, so it has a good chance of a long service life.

Immediately beyond this crossing, the PCT meets unmaintained Milk Creek Trail 790 (2,524.8–3,289'), descending north. When you leave the creek, take your time switchbacking up the east wall of this canyon. If the day is drizzly, the "fog drip" on the flowers of this heavily vegetated slope will saturate you from the thighs down. Ahead grow miles of this vegetation that you must hike through. However, as consolation, there are no flies or mosquitoes around to bother you in this weather. When you finally finish this creekless ascent and reach the ridgecrest (2,529.3–5,950'), a marmot may greet you; if not, you can at least rest here.

After a short, negligible climb, the trail contours the east slope of this ridge and leaves behind its outcrops of densely clustered, light-colored Miocene dikes, sills, and irregular masses. As you enter the East Fork Milk Creek basin, these outcrops give way to ancient metamorphic rocks. Along the south wall of this basin, the PCT passes just below a small knoll.

Beyond this point, the trail shortly crosses a 100-yard-wide boulder field that is laced with creeklets. The route now climbs gently northeast to another ridge (2,530.9–6,100'), from which Grassy Point Trail 788 descends for about a mile through meadows and affords views of the north face of Grassy Point.

CAMPING The PCT switchbacks slightly up the ridge, contours southeast across it, and then starts the first of 59 switchbacks down to Vista Creek. After a few of these, you reach the Dolly Vista campsite (2,531.5–5,724') beneath a few protective

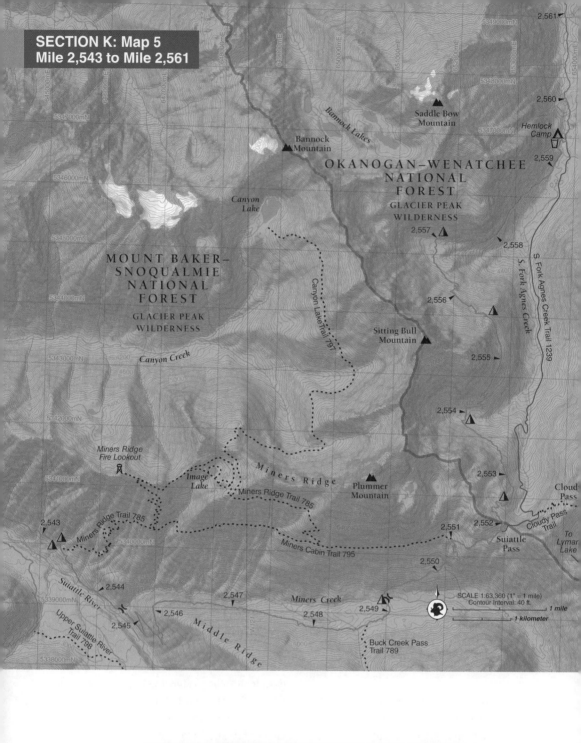

Bannock Lakes

Saddle Bow
Mountain

2,561 ►

2,560 ►

Hemlock
Camp

2,559 ►

Bannock
Mountain

**OKANOGAN–WENATCHEE
NATIONAL
FOREST**

**GLACIER PEAK
WILDERNESS**

Canyon
Lake

2,557 ►

2,558

S. Fork Agnes Creek Trail 1239

S. Fork Agnes Creek

**MOUNT BAKER–
SNOQUALMIE
NATIONAL
FOREST**

**GLACIER PEAK
WILDERNESS**

2,556 ►

Sitting Bull
Mountain

2,555 ►

Canyon Creek

Canyon Lake Trail 797

2,554 ►

Miners Ridge
Fire Lookout

Image
Lake

Miners Ridge

Plummer
Mountain

2,553 ►

Cloud
Pass

2,543 ►

Miners Ridge Trail 785

Miners Ridge Trail 785

2,552 ►

Cloudy Pass
Trail

Miners Cabin Trail 795

2,551 ►

Suiattle
Pass

To
Lymar
Lake

2,550 ►

Suiattle River

2,544 ►

2,547 ►

Miners Creek

2,549 ►

Upper Suiattle River
Trail 798

2,546 ►

2,548 ►

2,545 ►

Middle Ridge

SCALE 1:63,360 (1" = 1 mile)
Contour Interval: 40 ft.

1 mile

1 kilometer

Buck Creek Pass
Trail 789

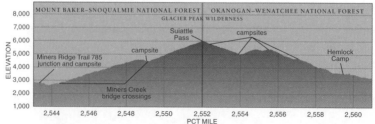

mountain hemlocks. A vault toilet is immediately north on a side trail downhill.

CAMPING From the campsite, the PCT switchbacks northeast down through open forest to a saddle on Vista Ridge. Starting down into deep Vista Creek canyon, you're grateful to be descending rather than ascending the last 38 switchbacks. By the last switchback, 50 yards from the creek, the trail has left behind most of the "rainforest," and it continues 100 yards northeast to a large campsite (2,535.2–3,619') near Vista Creek. From it, the PCT descends into a Douglas-fir forest with an understory of huckleberry shrubs, ferns, and Oregon grapes.

The trail curves east and the gradient eases as you approach a crossing of wide, silty Vista Creek (2,537.5–2,884'). The PCT eschews the crossing of Vista Creek, instead turning away from it, heading north for a mile, and then turning downstream and coming abreast of the cream-colored Suiattle River on its northwest track downstream. Continue through this fir-dominated forest, crossing a narrow stream on a footbridge and 0.75 mile later fording wide Dolly Creek (2,540.0– 2,409'). If you are stopping at the river for the night, consider gathering water at one of these streams, as the Suiattle's water is full of silt and can be difficult to filter.

PLANTS As you make your way north to the new bridge spanning the Suiattle, your path slips past the trunks of massive old-growth trees in this large forest of towering Pacific yews, Douglas-firs, and western hemlocks. The opportunity to regard these spectacular old-growth trees is rare, so take this time to enjoy a brief change of pace among them. Many of these awesome giants have a diameter of up to 12 feet and an assortment of large and colorful fungi on their trunks. This fragile ecosystem will benefit from your observance of Leave No Trace principles: take only memories, and leave only footprints.

WATER ACCESS

CAMPING Generous space for camping lies at either end of the brilliantly engineered bridge over the Suiattle River (2,540.6–2,318').

CAMPING Reach the east end and turn directly north, then northwest, to the junction with Suiattle River Trail 784 (2,540.9–2,508'), where a 180-degree redirect at a switchback sends you southeast, comfortably gaining elevation. You continue through a small old-growth stand, dominated by Douglas-fir but joined by some Pacific yew and western hemlock, that is no less spectacular in size than those in its larger counterpart to the south. After crossing a freshwater-laden ravine seemingly every 500 feet, you continue southeast, crossing some more evenly spaced wet ravines. You'll see some bivy sites 175 feet before the Miners Ridge Trail 785 junction (2,543.3–2,819').

The trail persists southeast. Descend nearly to the riverbed's elevation, and slog along in deep sand and over clustered tree roots between runoff streams as you hike opposite Gamma Creek. In another 0.5 mile, a stout log with comforting handrails is your bridge across Miners Creek (2,544.4–2,752').

The next trail segment, straight ahead, makes long, easy switchbacks up to the lower edge of Middle Ridge and then climbs east up its north slope to a junction with Buck Creek Pass Trail 789 (2,548.6–4,628'), which climbs 5 miles south to the pass.

CAMPING The PCT continues 0.25 mile east to a creek and then 0.25 mile north to the second crossing of Miners Creek (2,549.2–4,483'). You can camp nearby, just south of the creek.

From the creek's horse bridge, the PCT makes an initial jog downstream and then passes

SECTION K

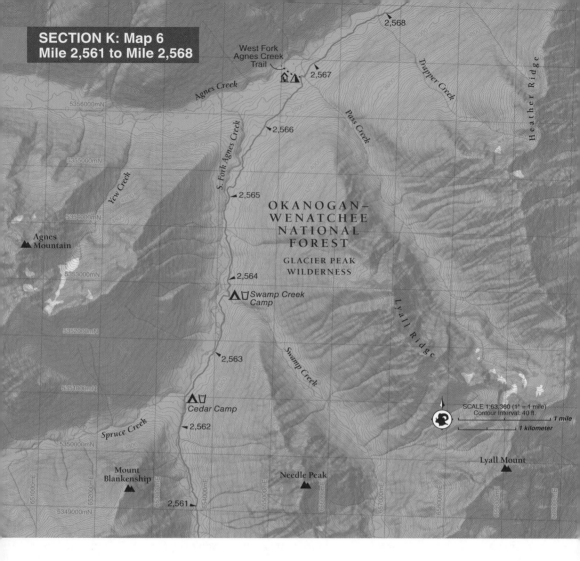

West Fork
Agnes Creek
Trail

2,567

Agnes Creek

Trapper Creek

Heather Ridge

2,568

Pass Creek

2,566

S. Fork Agnes Creek

2,565

OKANOGAN–
WENATCHEE
NATIONAL
FOREST

GLACIER PEAK
WILDERNESS

Yew Creek

Agnes
Mountain

2,564

Swamp Creek
Camp

Lyall Ridge

2,563

Swamp Creek

Cedar Camp

SCALE 1:63,360 (1" = 1 mile)
Contour Interval: 40 ft.

1 mile

1 kilometer

2,562

Spruce Creek

Lyall Mount

Mount
Blankenship

Needle Peak

2,561

more than half a dozen creeks and creeklets as it climbs east. Switchbacks ultimately take you 950 feet higher to a junction with the old PCT route, Miners Cabin Trail 795 (2,551.0–5,486'). You continue to climb east, soon getting southwest views of majestic Glacier Peak and southern views of Fortress Mountain and the deep canyon below it.

The route turns north and soon reaches a junction with the Cloudy Pass Trail (2,551.8–5,906'). If you've been having snow problems, you may want to start down this trail rather than stay on the PCT.

ALTERNATE ROUTE Follow the Cloudy Pass Trail about 0.5 mile to its

junction with the South Fork Agnes Creek Trail 1239 (the older PCT route), where you turn north and travel about 5 miles down South Fork Agnes Creek to rejoin the newer 7.7-mile-long PCT segment at Hemlock Camp.

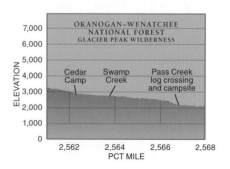

OKANOGAN–WENATCHEE
NATIONAL FOREST
GLACIER PEAK WILDERNESS

ELEVATION

Cedar
Camp

Swamp
Creek

Pass Creek
log crossing
and campsite

PCT MILE

SIDE TRIP From its junction with South Fork Agnes Creek Trail, the Cloudy Pass Trail continues east about 1 mile to Cloudy Pass, then southeast another mile to Lyman Lake. There, you can connect to the Hart and Lyman Lake Trail, which travels east about 8 miles to Holden.

CAMPING The PCT continues onward over Suiattle Pass, to the crest (2,552.0–5,990'). Switchbacks, often accompanied by snow patches, descend to a creeklet, from which a spur trail climbs north-northwest to a meadow campsite (2,552.4–5,806'). The PCT now takes you on a fairly scenic, rollercoaster route in and out of two deep side canyons. The trip is downhill all the way to the first of these (2,553.9–5,056'), with a campsite. Leaving this cirque and its giant rockfall boulders, which have buried the creek, you switchback about 400 feet up on the Agnes Creek canyon wall. After a traverse north, the trail bends into the second side canyon, where you encounter a signed campsite (2,555.5–5,377').

You pass up to a dozen more creeklets as you descend to a bridged creek on the floor of the second side canyon. About 300 yards past it, you meet another spur trail (2,557.1–4,724'), this one climbing steeply to a sheltered site for four small tents that has a view and spring-fed creeklet. You then drop east, briefly switchback west, and turn east again.

WATER ACCESS

Now the PCT makes a generally moderate descent to Agnes Creek, the forested route punctuated with bushy wildflower patches that allow views and an unfair amount of deadfall that provides colorful

conversation. At last you ford Agnes Creek and in about 150 yards reach Hemlock Camp (2,559.5–3,552'), where the older PCT route, given as an alternate on the previous page, rejoins the newer PCT. This camp has falling tree hazards and is unsafe for camping.

CAMPING Continuing north, the PCT stays near the creek through a forest of western hemlock, Engelmann spruce, western red cedar, Douglas-fir, and western white pine. You descend past Mount Blankenship (5,926') to the west and Needle Peak (7,885') to the east before reaching Cedar Camp near Spruce Creek (2,562.3–2,876'). At this site, you'll find only log stumps around a fire pit, but it's still a nice camp.

The canyon grows ever deeper as you trek north, catch a glimpse of the blue-green waters of South Fork Agnes Creek, and then contour over to signed and well-equipped Swamp Creek Camp (2,563.8–2,749').

SIDE TRIP Here, beside the 7-yard-wide torrent, Swamp Creek Trail 712 begins a 3-mile climb along the creek toward Dark Glacier, which is tucked in a deep amphitheater.

CAMPING Leaving Swamp Creek Camp, you cross the creek on a log with a hand rail, progress north to the rim of

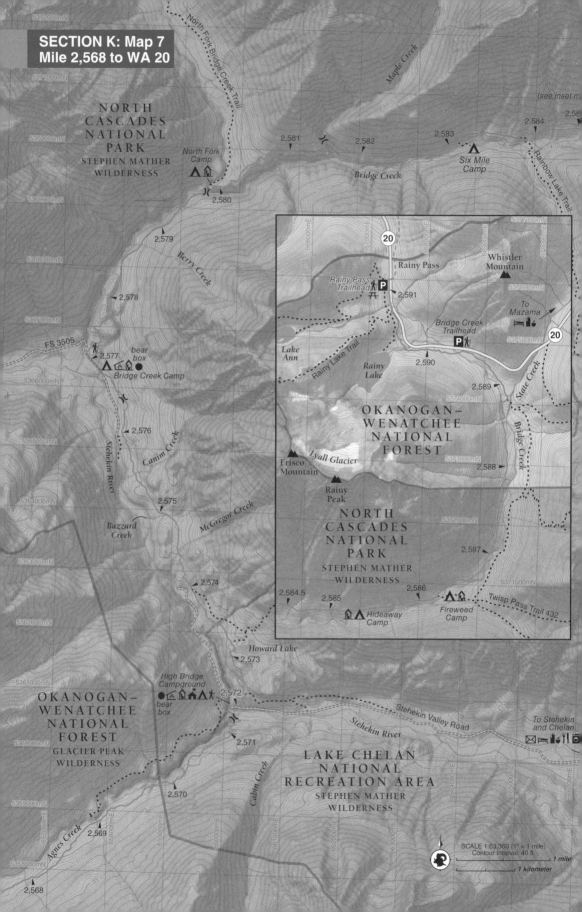

NORTH FORK BRIDGE CREEK TRAIL

North Fork Bridge Creek Trail

Maple Creek

(see inset)

NORTH
CASCADES
NATIONAL
PARK
STEPHEN MATHER
WILDERNESS

North Fork Camp

2,581

2,582

Bridge Creek

2,583

2,584

2,58

Six Mile
Camp

Rainbow Lake Trail

2,580

2,579

Berry Creek

20

Rainy Pass

Whistler
Mountain

Rainy Pass
Trailhead

2,591

2,578

Lake
Ann

Rainy Lake Trail

Bridge Creek
Trailhead

To
Mazama

20

FS 3505

2,577   bear
box

Bridge Creek Camp

Rainy
Lake

2,590

State Creek

2,589

Stehekin River

2,576

Canim Creek

OKANOGAN–
WENATCHEE
NATIONAL
FOREST

2,588

Bridge Creek

Lyall Glacier

Frisco
Mountain

Rainy
Peak

2,575

McGregor Creek

Buzzard
Creek

NORTH
CASCADES
NATIONAL
PARK
STEPHEN MATHER
WILDERNESS

2,587

2,574

2,584.5

2,585

2,586

Hideaway
Camp

Fireweed
Camp

Twisp Pass Trail 432

Howard Lake

2,573

High Bridge
Campground

bear
box

2,572

OKANOGAN–
WENATCHEE
NATIONAL
FOREST
GLACIER PEAK
WILDERNESS

2,571

Stehekin Valley Road

Stehekin River

To Stehekin
and Chelan

2,570

Cabin Creek

LAKE CHELAN
NATIONAL
RECREATION AREA
STEPHEN MATHER
WILDERNESS

Agnes Creek

2,569

SCALE 1:63,360 (1" = 1 mile)
Contour Interval: 40 ft.

1 mile

1 kilometer

2,568

the inner gorge of South Fork Agnes Creek, and then gradually curve down to a junction with West Fork Agnes Creek Trail 1272 (2,566.8–2,206'), which descends west-northwest to that creek. Several fair campsites and a toilet are just west of this junction above the west bank of Pass Creek. These are the last campsites you'll see within Glacier Peak Wilderness.

GEOLOGY You'll soon leave the granitic rocks of the Cloudy Pass batholith behind and walk upon schist and gneiss that date back to Jurassic times or earlier. The overpowering canyon through which you are hiking bears a strong resemblance to deep Kings Canyon in the Sierra Nevada of California, except that this one supports a much denser growth of flowers, shrubs, and trees.

Hiking northeast, you pass seasonal Trapper Creek (2,567.9–2,120') and then approach Agnes Creek, which, like its South Fork, possesses an inner gorge. The undulating trail goes right out to the gorge's brink at several spots and then descends to switchback down to the boundary of North Cascades National Park, where a massive bridge stands 40 feet above roaring Agnes Creek (2,571.6–1,560'), which at this point is larger than most rivers you've seen along the PCT. Now within the Lake Chelan National Recreation Area–Stephen Mather Wilderness, you cross the 27-yard-long bridge, climb a low ridge, and then contour northwest to the Agnes Creek trailhead at a bend in Stehekin Valley Road (2,571.8–1,662').

CAMPING Just 35 yards up the road is High Bridge Campground, with a shelter and outside tables. Water can be obtained by walking back down the road to the high bridge and then descending steep, short switchbacks north to the west bank of the Stehekin River.

RESUPPLY ACCESS

You can descend Stehekin Valley Road 200 yards to the High Bridge Ranger Station, which is immediately northeast of a bend in the Stehekin River. During the summer, shuttle buses from the Stehekin resort area, 10.6 miles downstream, depart about four times daily. The schedule changes from year to year—and even during the season—so check at the High Bridge Ranger Station (or on a posted sign nearby) for the current schedule. The shuttle buses take about an hour to reach the High Bridge stop, and the one-way fee between Stehekin and High Bridge was $8 in 2020. Bus service continues from here to Cottonwood Camp, 11.4 miles upriver, so it's possible to ride a total distance of 22 miles.

If you're like most hikers, you'll be weary by the time the PCT reaches the Agnes Creek trailhead, and you'll welcome the opportunity to relax overnight in Stehekin. The North Cascades Lodge

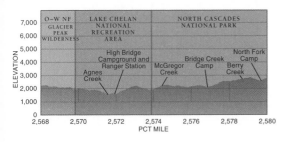

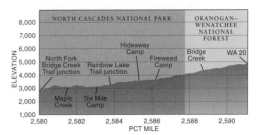

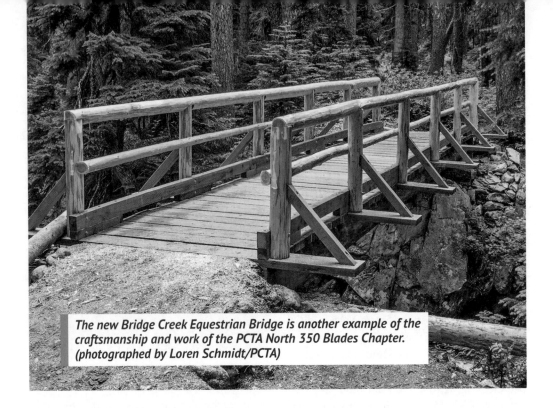

The new Bridge Creek Equestrian Bridge is another example of the craftsmanship and work of the PCTA North 350 Blades Chapter. (photographed by Loren Schmidt/PCTA)

dominates the Stehekin complex, providing good meals and accommodations. The old Golden West Lodge has been transformed into the National Park Service's Golden West Visitor Center, where you can get wilderness permits and information. Nearby are a public shower, a laundromat, and, in the Stehekin Ranger Station, the Stehekin Post Office (98852).

WILDLIFE You'll find camping 0.25 mile north of the complex at Purple Point Campground. It is possible, though very unlikely, that you'll encounter western rattlesnakes here, for they are quite common in the Stehekin area, though they become less common upcanyon. More likely, however, you'll meet black bears, which have become an increasing nuisance as they've grown bolder in recent years. You can expect to see them at any of the nine roadside campgrounds. Be sure you have your food and scented items protected in a bear-proof canister.

Many backpackers hiking from Stevens Pass through Glacier Peak Wilderness to High Bridge end their hike there and take the shuttle bus to Stehekin. They can then take one of three boats that ply between Stehekin and Chelan, a popular resort town at the far end of Lake Chelan. The slowest and cheapest boat takes about 4 hours; the faster and more expensive, about 2.5 hours. Round-trip rates are $41–$61.

The advantage of ending at Chelan rather than at Rainy Pass is that you are much closer to Stevens Pass, your starting point for this section. The drive from Stevens Pass to Chelan is 90 miles, but it is an additional 103 miles to Rainy Pass. For non-thru-hikers, that additional shuttle is not worth the generally viewless hike along the last stretch of this section.

To complete this stretch on the PCT from the Agnes Creek trailhead, walk down to the nearby bridge over the Stehekin River, immediately beyond which you'll find another trailhead past the outhouse at the High Bridge Ranger Station (2,571.9–1,611'). Take this trail, which starts initially east and then switchbacks up to a granitic bench with a trail junction (2,572.3–1,851'); it descends southeast to the Cascade Corral on Stehekin Valley Road. The PCT climbs north, topping a low bedrock ridge and reaching a junction at the west arm of swampy Howard Lake (2,573.2–2,180'), named for a pioneering miner who settled here.

SIDE TRIP From this junction, the McGregor Mountain Trail rigorously climbs about 7 switchbacking miles to the top of McGregor Mountain.

The PCT heads northwest, passing two seasonal creeklets on a mostly descending grade, and coinciding with a stretch of the Old Wagon Trail before climbing to McGregor Creek (2,574.4–2,204'). The ascent abates, and soon the trail fords Buzzard Creek (2,574.9–2,244') and, later, two-branched Canim Creek (2,575.5–2,160').

CAMPING In about 0.3 mile, you leave the Old Wagon Trail and make an undulating traverse that ends about 50 yards before Clear Creek, roughly opposite the Bridge Creek Ranger Station (2,576.8–2,101'). Just beyond it, you pass Bridge Creek Camp with its shelter. After a few more minutes of walking, you arrive at the PCT Bridge Creek trailhead (2,577.1–2,180'), located 240 yards southeast of FS 3505's crossing of Bridge Creek.

Back on a trail again, you climb a wandering path that passes a small lily-pad pond on a bench, winds to the edge of the Bridge Creek gorge, and climbs its slopes to jump-across Berry Creek (2,578.7–2708').

WILDLIFE Watching out for western toads, you climb a little higher on the slope before descending to an equestrian bridge above wild, roaring Bridge Creek (2,579.7–2,540').

CAMPING Climbing a few yards north of the bridge, you reach dusty, rustic North Fork Camp and a nearby toilet atop a rocky bluff that overlooks the junction of Bridge Creek with its north fork. The camp's resident landlords, golden-mantled ground squirrels, may exact "rent" from your backpack while you're not looking.

From this site, the trail switchbacks east up to a junction with the North Fork Bridge Creek Trail (2,580.0–2,815'), which climbs north. You climb east up a bushy, aromatic slope; reach a point several hundred feet above Bridge Creek; and take in gorgeous views below as you descend slightly to a saddle. Beyond it, the trail descends north to wide, alder-lined Maple Creek (2,581.6–3,097'), which a suspension bridge crosses 25 yards upstream. Be careful climbing the talus boulders to and from the bridge.

Now follow the level, relaxing path east to a 250-yard-long spur trail (2,583.1–3,134'), which descends southeast, steeply at first, through a meadow of tall cow parsnips, to Six Mile Camp, a well-furnished site designed with equestrians in mind. Not far beyond the spur trail, the

Rainbow Lake Trail (2,583.8–3,258') peels off from the PCT.

SIDE TRIP Just 330 yards down Rainbow Lake Trail is South Fork Camp beside Bridge Creek. The trail descends southeast and then climbs up South Fork Canyon to Pass 6,230, immediately west of domineering Bowan Mountain (7,895') and reaches Rainbow Lake south of the pass after 5 miles.

From the junction, the PCT continues east through alternating forest and brush cover and then reaches a junction with a 110-yard-long spur trail (2,585.3–3,512').

CAMPING This spur trail descends first southwest and then southeast to the loveliest Bridge Creek campsite: Hideaway Camp. Strictly for backpackers, this shady, creekside campsite has log stumps, a fire ring, and a nearby toilet.

Continuing east within earshot of the creek, the PCT leaves this junction and eventually turns northeast just before reaching a junction with Twisp Pass Trail 432 (2,586.2–3,632'). Ahead, while the old (pre-1990s) PCT veers right to drop and cross Bridge Creek, the newer PCT route angles uphill to the northeast. The trail contours in a lazy arc around the southeast flank of Frisco Mountain until turning due north (2,587.0–3,855'). On its drive north toward WA 20, the trail crosses three impressive avalanche chutes and their attendant streams. Bridge Creek remains your eastern handrail as you pass the confluence with State Creek from the east.

In about 1,000 feet, cross Bridge Creek (2,588.7–4,303') directly to the east, and then return to your northwestern heading. Now parallel Bridge Creek at a closer distance on your left as you arc from north to west to an important junction (2,589.6–4,514').

SIDE TRIP If you're not going on through Section L, you'll want to end your Section K hike here. Take a spur trail 70 yards northwest up to WA 20. From there, you walk 90 yards west on the highway to the PCT Bridge Creek Trailhead parking area for southbound hikers. This trailhead parking area is 70 yards east of where the highway crosses Bridge Creek and is 1.2 miles before the highway tops out at Rainy Pass.

Staying on the official PCT route, you take slightly longer, first crossing Bridge Creek immediately past the spur trail and then heading west, gradually up and away from the creek, to Rainy Lake's outlet creek (2,590.3–4,712'). From it, your path climbs gently north, levels off, and strikes a course through the soggy headwaters of Bridge Creek immediately before it ends beside WA 20 at the entrance to spacious Rainy Pass Picnic Site and Trailhead (2,591.1–4,855'). Here you'll find tables and toilets but no tap water. Rainy Lake Trail also starts south from here. Just across WA 20 from the picnic site's entrance road is short, north-curving FS 600, which goes to the PCT trailhead parking area and equestrian area for northbound trekkers (for Section L).

RESUPPLY ACCESS

About 22 miles east on WA 20, you'll find the small town of Mazama, with restaurants, lodging, a store, and an outdoors outfitter. For more information, see "Supplies" on page 298.

SECTION K

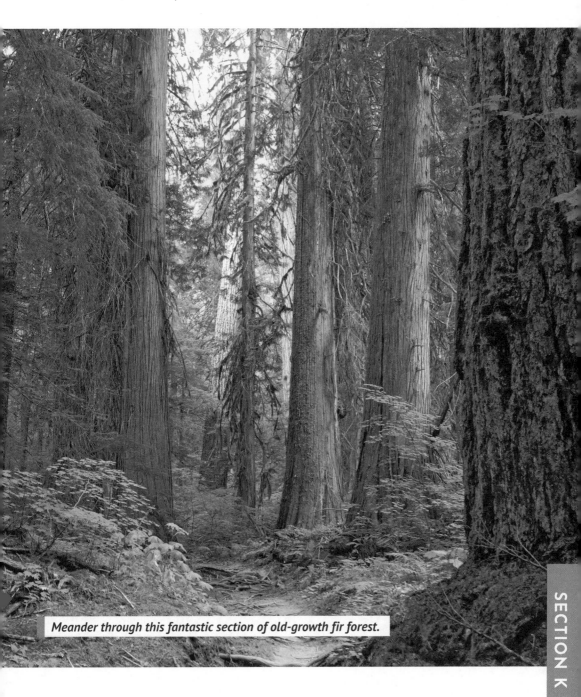

Meander through this fantastic section of old-growth fir forest.

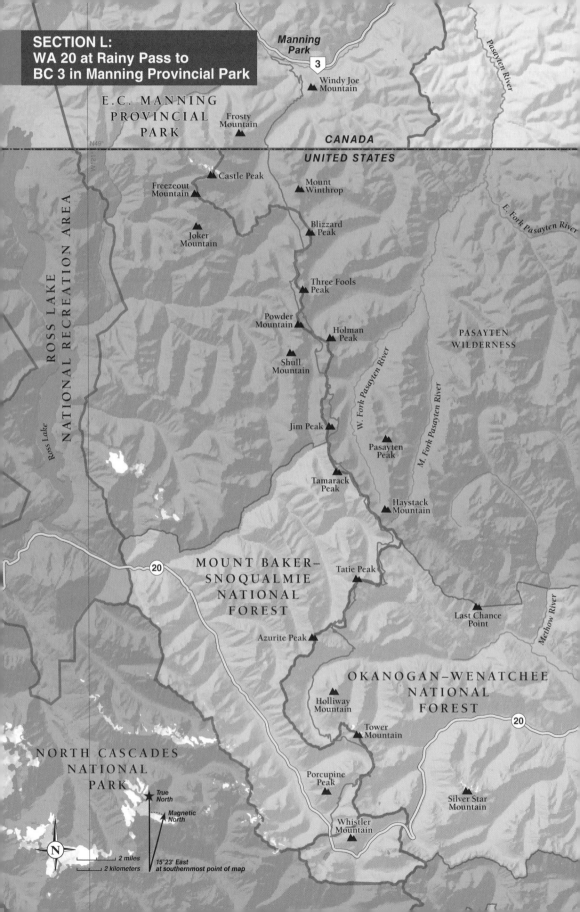

SECTION L:
WA 20 at Rainy Pass to
BC 3 in Manning Provincial Park

Manning
Park

3

Windy Joe
Mountain

E.C. MANNING
PROVINCIAL
PARK

Frosty
Mountain ▲

Pasayten River

CANADA
UNITED STATES

N 49°
W 121°

Castle Peak ▲

Mount
Winthrop ▲

E. Fork Pasayten River

Freezeout
Mountain ▲

Blizzard
Peak ▲

Joker
Mountain ▲

ROSS LAKE

Three Fools
Peak ▲

NATIONAL RECREATION AREA

Powder
Mountain ▲

Holman
Peak ▲

PASAYTEN
WILDERNESS

Shull
Mountain ▲

W. Fork Pasayten River

M. Fork Pasayten River

Ross Lake

Jim Peak ▲

Pasayten
Peak ▲

Tamarack
Peak ▲

Haystack
Mountain ▲

20

MOUNT BAKER–
SNOQUALMIE
NATIONAL
FOREST

Tatie Peak ▲

Last Chance
Point ▲

Methow River

Azurite Peak ▲

OKANOGAN–WENATCHEE
NATIONAL
FOREST

Holliway
Mountain ▲

20

NORTH CASCADES
NATIONAL
PARK

Tower
Mountain ▲

★ True
North

Porcupine
Peak ▲

Silver Star
Mountain ▲

Magnetic
North

Whistler
Mountain ▲

N

2 miles

2 kilometers

15°23' East
at southernmost point of map

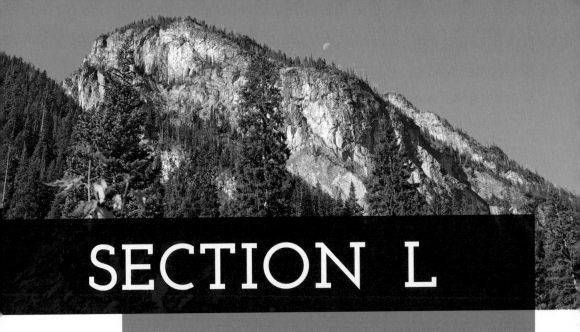

SECTION L

WA 20 at Rainy Pass to BC 3 in Manning Provincial Park

THE FINAL LEG OF THE PACIFIC CREST TRAIL (PCT) leads from the North Cascades Highway (WA 20) at Rainy Pass to E. C. Manning Provincial Park, British Columbia. In this relatively short trek, there is vehicle access only at Harts Pass (30 miles north), where gravel Forest Service Road 5400 crosses the crest to serve a turn-of-the-20th-century mining district.

In this entire section, the PCT is well east of much of the Cascade Range. To the west, Mount Baker, Mount Shuksan, and the Picket Range receive the brunt of any bad weather. Overall snow accumulation along the PCT route here is much less than it is at Mount Baker, and PCT hikers may enjoy sunshine when Puget Sound and the western mountains are cloud- and rain-bound. Nonetheless, until midsummer, hikers should be prepared for a snow-covered and icy trail. After the snow melts, the mosquitoes have a heyday, so the most pleasant month to hike this section is usually

Above: Morning vista from Brush Creek

September. Typically, the winter snows do not start in earnest until at least October (but beware the exception!).

Near Rainy Pass, the scenery is spectacular, and many mountains are crowned with craggy spires of Golden Horn granodiorite. Consequently, the PCT only occasionally follows the crest of the Cascades exactly: much of the mileage is in long traverses and river valleys. Even if backpackers were as surefooted and agile as mountain goats, they would not choose a route true to the divide. Then, as the intrusive rocks give way to lower Cretaceous graywackes, the terrain becomes hilly so the PCT can follow the crest more closely than before.

North of Harts Pass, the PCT offers a variety of scenery and terrain. High meadows; wooded slopes and valleys; and rugged, precipitous ridges make up the bulk of this section, which traverses the backbone of the 790-square-mile Pasayten Wilderness. In good weather, the views are frequently spectacular, particularly in the fall when larch, spruce, and scrub maple splash gold, green, and red across the slopes.

DECLINATION 15°23'E

USGS MAPS

Washington Pass, WA	Azurite Peak, WA (PCT barely enters map)
Slate Peak, WA	Shull Mountain, WA
Mount Arriva, WA	Castle Peak, WA
Pasayten Peak, WA	

POINTS ON THE TRAIL, SOUTH TO NORTH

	Mile	Elevation in feet	Latitude/Longitude
WA 20 at Rainy Pass	2,591.1	4,855	N48° 30' 53.2653" W120° 44' 01.9904"
Cutthroat Pass	2,596.4	6,837	N48° 33' 17.3547" W120° 42' 02.1164"
Methow Pass	2,601.8	6,593	N48° 34' 55.8942" W120° 43' 58.5157"
Glacier Pass	2,612.2	5,581	N48° 39' 51.4042" W120° 43' 51.3265"
Harts Pass	2,622.0	6,188	N48° 43' 16.0641" W120° 40' 11.9717"
Windy Pass	2,627.2	6,273	N48° 46' 16.7088" W120° 42' 42.7646"
Holman Pass	2,635.5	5,066	N48° 50' 25.0611" W120° 44' 14.3958"
Woody Pass	2,641.6	6,624	N48° 53' 06.9440" W120° 46' 02.6503"

POINTS ON THE TRAIL, SOUTH TO NORTH *(continued)*

	Mile	Elevation in feet	Latitude/Longitude
Hopkins Pass	2,646.5	6,140	N48° 55' 43.1736" W120° 45' 43.7394"
US–Canada border at Monument 78	2,652.6	4,258	N49° 00' 01.0274" W120° 48' 07.6382"
BC 3 in E. C. Manning Provincial Park	2,661.4	3,910	N49° 03' 46.1725" W120° 46' 57.6297"

CAMPSITES AND BIVY SITES

Mile	Elevation in feet	Latitude/Longitude	Number of tents	Feature	Notes
2,594.9	6,155	N48° 33' 08.2140" W120° 42' 32.6330"	2	Nearby stream	
2,600.9	6,241	N48° 35' 08.1701" W120° 43' 12.6126"	3	Nearby stream and spring	
2,601.8	6,593	N48° 34' 55.7561" W120° 43' 58.0826"	2	Methow Pass	Shady, flat spot near trail on left with good vista
2,606.6	4,384	N48° 37' 37.7507" W120° 45' 11.4929"	2	Methow River	
2,612.1	5,580	N48° 39' 48.1845" W120° 43' 52.3023"	4		Flat spot near trail on left in shade
2,612.2	5,581	N48° 39' 49.9880" W120° 43' 51.7812"	4	Equestrian friendly	Bivy on left and right
2,620.7	6,200	N48° 42' 33.2640" W120° 40' 26.7240"	14	Meadows Campground	0.5 mile off-trail; vault toilets, picnic table, fire ring
2,622.0	6,188	N48° 43' 15.7887" W120° 40' 12.7677"	5	Harts Pass Campground	Vault toilets, picnic table, fire ring, guard station
2,627.2	6,273	N48° 46' 19.1274" W120° 42' 45.4967"	2	Near Windy Pass	In shade on right
2,630.1	6,265	N48° 47' 38.0049" W120° 44' 09.6592"	3	Jim Pass	Flat spot near trail on left
2,630.2	6,289	N48° 47' 42.7259" W120° 44' 10.9174"	4	Jim Pass	Near trail on right
2,631.4	6,180	N48° 48' 27.4399" W120° 43' 27.4199"	2	Ridgecrest vista	Flat spot near trail on right
2,633.0	5,944	N48° 49' 16.3112" W120° 44' 03.4155"	4		Flat spot near trail on right
2,637.9	6,200	N48° 51' 29.2757" W120° 44' 36.9264"	>4		In trees below trail
2,646.2	6,254	N48° 55' 39.6702" W120° 45' 53.3400"	>4	Hopkins Lake	0.1 mile south of trail
2,648.9	5,460	N48° 57' 25.1903" W120° 46' 50.7899"	3	Castle Pass	A good spot to spend your last night in the wilderness
2,652.9	4,215	N49° 00' 09.9615" W120° 48' 14.1858"	>4	Monument 78 Backcountry Camp	Vault toilet, bear-proof box, corral
2,656.4	5,035	N49° 02' 11.7705" W120° 45' 47.5441"	4	Pacific Crest Backcountry Camp	Vault toilet, fire ring, bear-proof box

SUPPLIES

No supply points are found until northbound hikers reach trail's end, in E. C. Manning Provincial Park. In it, just west of the trailhead, you'll find Manning Park Resort (604-668-5922, manningpark .com/resort), with food and lodging, and the park headquarters, where you can get information.

Greyhound bus service is no longer available to and from Vancouver, British Columbia, and there is no public transit available from E. C. Manning Provincial Park. The closest town with public transit is Hope, British Columbia. Via Rail Canada has a train line from Hope to Vancouver once a day with a stop in Chilliwack. BC Transit oversees a number of small regional transit systems with buses from Hope to Agassiz to Chilliwack to Abbotsford, where there is a local line that goes to within a couple hundred feet of the US border crossing (or walk a mile from where the bus from Chilliwack stops). After you cross the US border on foot into the town of Sumas, Washington, Whatcom Transportation Authority has a bus line to Bellingham, which has Greyhound and Amtrak connections in addition to the airport. Alternatively, Canadian Craft Charters has a shuttle service with a fixed rate for up to 14 people from Manning Park to Vancouver. E. C. Manning Provincial Park maintains a list of resources for PCT hikers on its website.

SPECIAL CONCERNS

Very early- and very late-season hikers should be ready for treacherous, precipitous snow slopes, avalanche hazards, and dangerously exposed hiking along parts of this PCT section. It is also wise to acquaint yourself with the border-crossing information in chapter 2 on page 14 to avoid unpleasant hassles associated with US and Canadian customs and immigration regulations.

WA 20 AT RAINY PASS TO BC 3 IN MANNING PROVINCIAL PARK

>>>THE ROUTE

A large, off-road rest area equipped with picnic tables and vault toilets stands west of WA 20 at Rainy Pass. The northbound PCT continues east of the highway and follows the driveway entrance to the 0.25-mile-long eastern parking lot. Ample trailhead parking parallels the shoulder of the road. Nearby toilets are similar to those on the sunset side of the highway.

At the north end of the parking lot (2,591.4–4,882'), you enter Douglas-fir forest and begin climbing north. One creek draining Cutthroat Peak (8,050') cascades across the path even in September and October. Numerous other streams are of nuisance value early in the season but typically dry up by late August. The grade levels as the trail nears Porcupine Creek (2,593.1–5,299') and bridges it. Then you turn northeast to parallel it and resume the ascent.

A pair of switchbacks lifts the path away from the streambed and guides you onto a steep, open slope where avalanches sweeping down from Peaks 7,004 and 7,762 may threaten May and June hikers. After traversing higher to contour around the headwaters bowl of Porcupine Creek, you switchback up the steep, glacier-formed basin wall.

| PLANTS | Deciduous larches, the poetic tamaracks, add foreground

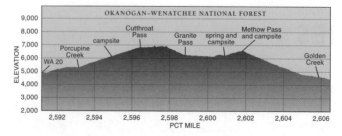

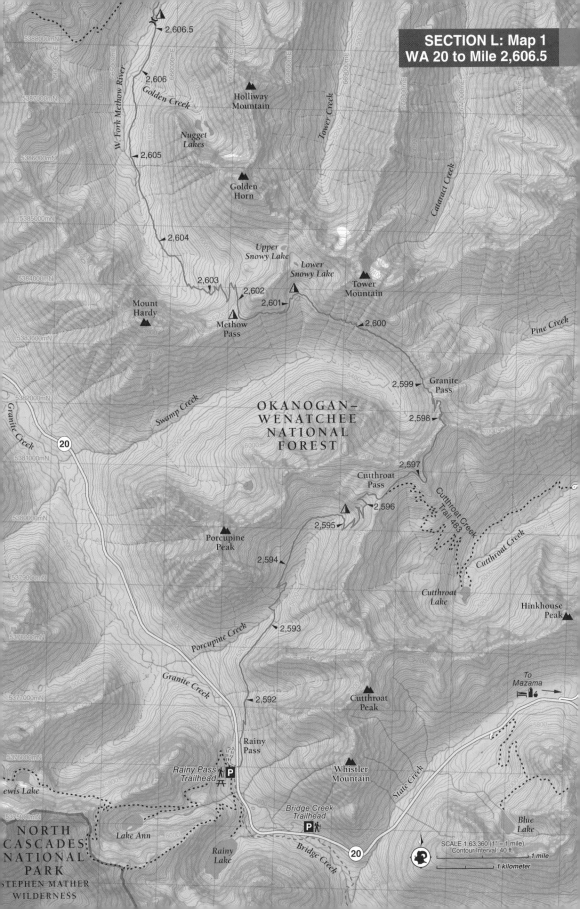

△ 2,606.5

W. Fork Methow River

2,606

Golden Creek

Holliway
Mountain

Tower Creek

Cataract Creek

Nugget
Lakes

2,605

Golden
Horn

2,604

Upper
Snowy Lake

Lower
Snowy Lake

Pine Creek

2,603

2,602

△ Tower
Mountain

2,601

△

Mount
Hardy

2,600

△
Methow
Pass

Swamp Creek

2,599 Granite
Pass

2,598

OKANOGAN–
WENATCHEE
NATIONAL
FOREST

2,597

Granite Creek

20

Cutthroat
Pass

2,596

2,595 ▸

Cutthroat Creek Trail 483

Porcupine
Peak

2,594

Cutthroat Creek

Porcupine Creek

2,593

Cutthroat
Lake

Hinkhouse
Peak ▲

Granite Creek

2,592

To
Mazama

Cutthroat
Peak

Rainy
Pass

State Creek

Rainy Pass
Trailhead P

Whistler
Mountain

Lewis Lake

Bridge Creek
Trailhead P

Blue
Lake

NORTH
CASCADES
NATIONAL
PARK

Lake Ann

Rainy
Lake

Bridge Creek

20

SCALE 1:63,360 (1" = 1 mile)
Contour Interval: 40 ft.

STEPHEN MATHER
WILDERNESS

1 mile

1 kilometer

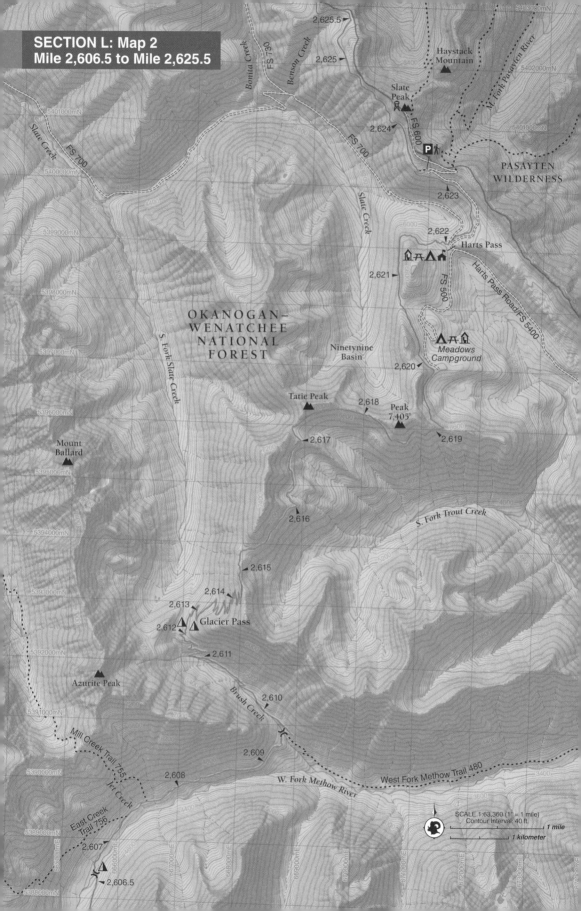

2,625.5

2,625

Haystack
Mountain

Bonita Creek

Benson Creek

FS 730

Slate
Peak

2,624

FS 600

FS 700

M. Fork Pasayten River

P

PASAYTEN
WILDERNESS

Slate Creek

FS 700

2,623

Slate Creek

FS 700

2,622

Harts Pass

2,621

FS 500

Harts Pass Road/FS 5400

OKANOGAN–
WENATCHEE
NATIONAL
FOREST

Ninetynine
Basin

Meadows
Campground

2,620

S. Fork Slate Creek

Tatie Peak

2,618

Peak
7,405'

2,617

2,619

Mount
Ballard

2,616

S. Fork Trout Creek

2,615

2,614

2,613

Glacier Pass

2,612

2,611

Azurite Peak

Brush Creek

2,610

Mill Creek Trail 755

2,609

West Fork Methow Trail 480

2,608

W. Fork Methow River

Jet Creek

East Creek Trail 756

2,607

SCALE 1:63,360 (1" = 1 mile)
Contour Interval: 40 ft.

1 mile

1 kilometer

2,606.5

to the rugged panorama unfolding before you. Black Peak (8,970') and Corteo Peak (8,100') across the highway front the more distant North Cascades. Scrub huckleberry and heather compose the basic ground cover that "springtime" (July) flowers eloquently embroider.

CAMPING You pass campsites that are inviting, though lacking late-season water (2,594.9–6,155'), as the PCT levels west of grassy, granitic Cutthroat Pass (2,596.4–6,837'). Here, Cutthroat Creek Trail 483 forks east to begin its descent to Cutthroat Lake (4,935'), visible in the valley below. Liberty Bell Mountain (7,720'), a favorite rock climbing destination, peeks above the ridge across the lake.

Head northeast to arc around two bowls, contouring across steep scree slopes beneath precipitous cliffs. Before leaving the second cirque, you choose the upper and more traveled of two trails; the lower trail dead-ends on the ridge 100 yards ahead. Climbing slightly, you reach a crest and pause to enjoy a picturesque view of Tower Mountain (8,444').

The route continues north, balancing precariously across a precipice before executing several short, tight switchbacks down the rugged north ridge. Avoiding the rock walls above Granite Pass, you descend south to zigzag above beautiful, glacier-carved Swamp Creek valley. Then, at Granite Pass (2,598.8–6,263'), you reach flat ground and are welcomed into a sheltered area. Don't expect convenient late-season water here.

CAMPING From the pass, the PCT makes a long traverse of the open, lower slopes of Tower Mountain on the way to Methow Pass (pronounced MET-how). Scrub subalpine fir, western white pine, mountain ash, and heather provide little protection for sun-beaten or windswept walkers. Upon reaching the bowl below the Snowy Lakes, you lose precious elevation as the trail drops into an idyllic park where a small spring, a bubbling stream, grassy flower lands, larch, and spruce all recommend this campsite (2,600.9–6,241'). Avoid degrading the spring or stream areas. Set your tent on surfaces that are more durable than the flowers and grasses. Shed your pack, don your sweater, and settle in. Firewood in this delicate alpine valley is in limited supply, and it is better left unburned. A cross trail from the campsite heads north, up-valley, to Upper and Lower Snowy Lakes in a higher cirque.

CAMPING From the camp, a pair of switchbacks helps you climb out of the bowl to set up the approach to Methow Pass (2,601.8–6,593') and a bivy site large enough for two tents. Like most high-elevation bivy sites, Methow Pass is waterless when it is not swampy. Views of Mount Arriva (8,215') and Fisher Peak (8,050') are the last you'll have of the mountains west of Granite Creek. Mount Hardy (7,197'), just west of the pass, and Golden Horn (8,366), to the north, will stay with you during the trek down the valley of the Methow River's West Fork.

Leaving Methow Pass to the north, you now zigzag into the valley, cross a few infant streams, and then straighten to parallel the West Fork of the Methow. From here, at sunset, Golden Horn glows spectacularly against the deep blue-black of the eastern sky.

CAMPING Take a long and slight-but-steady downgrade to Golden Creek (2,605.9–4,584'). Nimbly rock-hopping

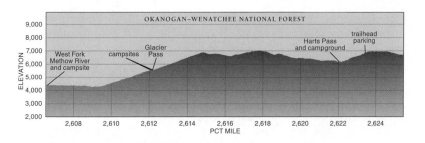

the stream, you have only a short stint before bridging the West Fork Methow River (2,606.6–4,384'). A signed camp by the wooden bridge on the east bank is the best trailside camp between here and Brush Creek. Within 200 yards, the level path enters the first of several avalanche paths.

At a PCT mileage sign, the trail merges onto the route of the old Cascade Crest Trail (now East Creek Trail 756) (2,607.4–4,380').

SIDE TRIP Westbound, this overgrown trail climbs out of the Methow Valley via Mebee Pass to descend along East Creek, pass Gold Hill Mine, and meet Granite Creek and WA 20.

The PCT, bending east and crossing a tributary of the West Fork Methow River, reaches a junction with Mill Creek Trail 755 (2,607.6–4,380'), which looks like a rocky streambed in

the grass of the clearing. Almost immediately, you cross another tributary, signed Jet Creek, which is dry in late season.

GEOLOGY From here, the trail continues east. The scree fields change in character and composition as the trail heads east out of the granodiorite body and into a zone of lower Cretaceous graywackes ("muddy" sandstones), conglomerates, argillites, and shales.

Then the trail turns northeast to enter the mouth of beaver-inhabited Brush Creek's canyon. You cross Brush Creek on a bridge and, in 50 yards, meet West Fork Methow Trail 480 (2,609.5–4,305'). Here the PCT zigs once and starts climbing in earnest along steep, brushy Brush Creek. Enjoy the scenery of this fairly hospitable and picturesque valley, and, high in the west, some small glaciers cling between the rugged upper cliffs of Azurite Peak (8,400').

CAMPING A few switchbacks ease the grade of the final climb to Glacier Pass (2,612.2–5,581'), where some small

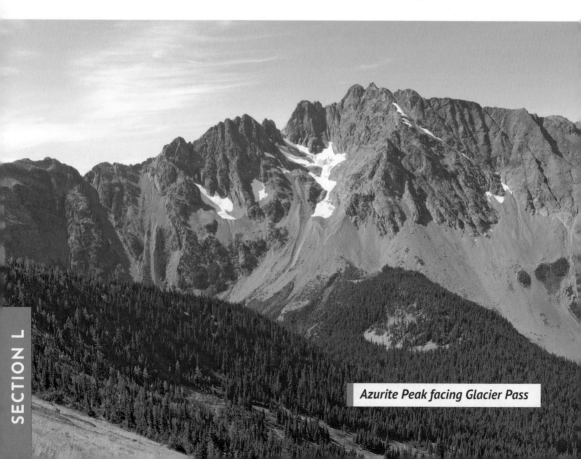

Azurite Peak facing Glacier Pass

campsites without nearby late-season water are found in the forest-sheltered gap. Two trails, the first heading north and the second trending west, are separated by 100 PCT trail yards.

PLANTS Now you gear down for a long, zigzagging climb to a grassy pass. Dwindling scrub subalpine fir, spruce, and larch accompany the trail up the slope.

Pausing for breath, you appreciate the view of three little lakes nestled near the head of South Fork Slate Creek's glacial valley, as well as the broadening panorama of the North Cascades. At last the trail tops off the climb and descends slightly along the ridge into an alpine-garden pass (2,614.8–6,866') above South Fork Trout Creek.

Here, the trail begins a long traverse northeast. Beyond the first ridge you round, you will find a spot to relax (2,616.1–6,600'). Continuing, you climb to a windy, scenic pass on the southwest shoulder of Tatie Peak (7,386'). As the trail contours around the peak, it passes stratified outcrops of alternating shale and conglomerate and then approaches a knife-edge saddle above Ninetynine Basin, beyond which the Slate Peak Lookout Tower is prominent. A descending traverse guides you around Peak 7,405 through a gap in a side ridge. Both Harts Pass Road/FS 5400 and the remains of the Brown Bear Mine house can be seen from here.

Angling down, the trail passes below the sites of the mine tunnels—not obvious from the trail—and approaches dirt FS 500. Twenty yards short of the road (2,619.8–6,550'), PCT emblems guide you onto a newer stretch of trail that avoids that road. In 150 yards, you cross the jeep-trail access to the Brown Bear tunnels and then continue to traverse above FS 500. A trail from the road joins the PCT as it approaches and threads a minor gap (2,620.7–6,363'). This trail descends briefly to the environs of Meadows Campground, where you can find a vault toilet and plenty of downed timber but no water.

CAMPING The PCT heads north along a steep hillside before turning

to go down to Harts Pass (2,622.0–6,188'). An infrequently manned U.S. Forest Service guard station, on the east side of Harts Pass Road/FS 5400 across from a trailhead parking lot, sometimes has a backcountry register for hikers to sign. The campground here provides shelter among the trees, picnic tables, and vault toilets but no water. A small seasonal stream crosses the trail 0.4 mile north of the pass.

SIDE TRIP The small community of Mazama is about 13 miles east on FS 5400. Also at the pass, a road branches east-northeast from FS 5400 to parallel the PCT for 1.3 miles before switchbacking up to Slate Peak Lookout.

HISTORY The Slate Creek mining district was a relatively rich mining area in the state of Washington. Boom camps were fairly populated in the early 1890s until word of the Klondike bonanza lured all the miners away. Del Hart, who owned some mines near Slate Creek, commissioned Charles H. Ballard in 1895 to survey a road from Mazama to the mining area. The pass through which the road was routed now bears Hart's name. Today, the road is a favorite summer-recreation route and one of the best access roads to Pasayten Wilderness, which you'll soon enter. Gold, silver, copper, lead, and zinc are among the metals whose ores were mined in the Slate Creek District. An interesting side note to the history of this area is that the first hydroelectric power plant in the high Cascades was installed here. O. B. Brown designed, paid for, and supervised construction of the 350-kilowatt plant that he located on the South Fork of Slate Creek.

From the PCT crossing of FS 5400, a scant 35 yards north-northwest of the pass proper, you proceed east-northeast through partly open spruce-fir woods, paralleling a U.S. Forest Service road about 100 feet below it. Beyond a meadow, the trail switchbacks up onto a small shoulder where you come to a junction (2,623.4–6,852') with a spur trail to the road; it is about 0.1 mile east-southeast down this spur to a parking area with a vault toilet.

Continuing west-northwest on the PCT, you ascend gradually past scattered Lyall larches, common on this small shoulder. Soon the shoulder gives out, leaving the trail hanging on the side of Slate Peak, with spectacular views down the Slate Creek valley, which is dominated by Mount Baker (10,778') and other peaks to the west.

Passing occasional outcrops of gray and green slate, you descend gradually to the pass (2,625.6–6,700') just above Benson Creek. Still on the west side of the divide, the trail climbs around an arm and descends past Buffalo Pass (2,626.3–6,557') to Windy Pass (2,627.2–6,273'), from which a trail crosses the PCT to descend south-southwest to Indiana Basin. In about 35 yards, you pass a sign heralding your entrance into Pasayten Wilderness.

The PCT continues north–northwest, leading out of true-to-its-name Windy Pass and around to the northeast cirque of Tamarack Peak (7,290'), clad in tamarack (larch). After crossing a small basin with water, the trail switchbacks up to and over an arm of Tamarack Peak, descends the open north cirque, and finally traverses the northwest arm of the mountain to Foggy Pass (2,629.4–6,182').

From this pass, the PCT | **CAMPING** | crosses to the west side of the divide for a brief, wooded hike to Jim Pass (2,630.1–6,265'), where you'll find several good campsites on either side of the trail. Then, back

on the east side of the divide, the PCT traverses around Jim Peak (7,033') to the rocky shoulder called Devils Backbone (2,631.4–6,180'), where you'll find another good site with a view.

Descending into the north cirque of Jim Peak, the PCT crosses the head of Shaw Creek and ascends gradually. About 1 mile farther, the route begins a plunge down switchbacks to a junction with Pacific Northwest Trail 752 and Holman Creek Trail 472A at Holman Pass (2,635.5–5,066'). This pass is heavily wooded, and wildlife abounds in the vicinity.

WATER ACCESS

CAMPING Climb northwest out of Holman Pass, crossing the outlet stream from Goat Lakes in about a mile, and switchback up a grassy knoll to a few bivy sites scattered among the trees (2,637.9–6,200').

From here, the trail traverses up the steep, grassy slopes bounding Canyon Creek to top a narrow crest about 300 yards southeast of a minor gap, Rock Pass (2,639.0–6,502'). The trail now makes a switchback east, often through snow, and then takes a descending route northwest. It soon levels off, and then, from a crossing of a tributary of Rock Creek, switchbacks briefly up to a junction with Rock Creek Trail 473 (2,641.1–6,353'), which descends Rock Creek canyon about 7 miles east to the Pasayten River. Keeping high on the PCT, you curve counterclockwise up to misnamed, rock-strewn Woody Pass (2,641.6–6,624').

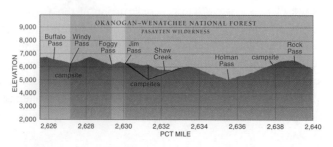

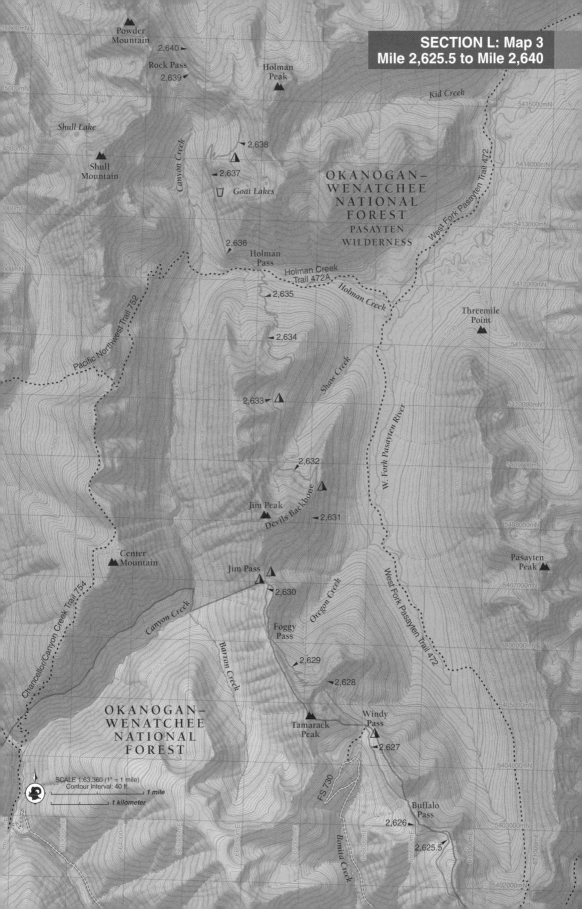

Powder
Mountain

2,640

Rock Pass
2,639

Holman
Peak

Kid Creek

Shull Lake

2,638

Shull
Mountain

2,637

Goat Lakes

OKANOGAN–
WENATCHEE
NATIONAL
FOREST
PASAYTEN
WILDERNESS

Canyon Creek

West Fork Pasayten Trail 472

2,636

Holman
Pass

Holman Creek
Trail 472A

2,635

Holman Creek

Threemile
Point

2,634

Pacific Northwest Trail 752

Shaw Creek

2,633

W. Fork Pasayten River

2,632

Jim Peak

Devils Backbone

2,631

Center
Mountain

Pasayten
Peak

Jim Pass

2,630

Oregon Creek

West Fork Pasayten Trail 472

Chancellor/Canyon Creek Trail 754

Canyon Creek

Foggy
Pass

Barron Creek

2,629

2,628

OKANOGAN–
WENATCHEE
NATIONAL
FOREST

Tamarack
Peak

Windy
Pass

2,627

SCALE 1:63,360 (1" = 1 mile)
Contour Interval: 40 ft

1 mile

1 kilometer

FS 730

Buffalo
Pass

2,626

2,625.5

Bonita Creek

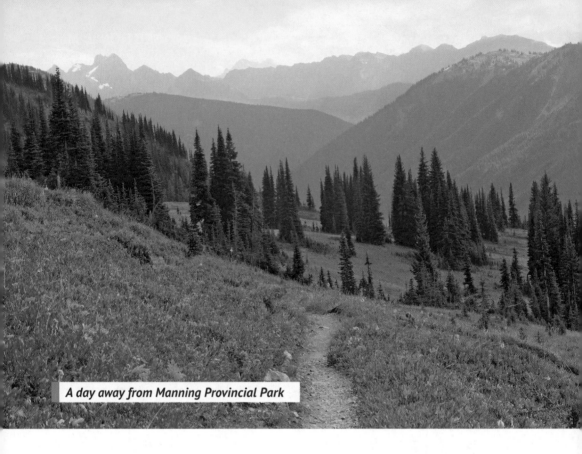

A day away from Manning Provincial Park

From here, you traverse open slopes with a few wooded fingers—the least spectacular side of Three Fools Peak (7,930')—until the trail rounds the south arm of the cirque and begins to climb steadily as it traverses the grassy headwall of the cirque. Shortly after, you arc north, climb through occasional stands of scrub conifers, and then a short switchback eases you up to the crest of Lakeview Ridge, on which a short spur trail takes you to an enticing view of a lake 1,000 feet below and the valley of Chuchuwanteen Creek beyond. The PCT continues along the crest for a short distance, then is forced west just long enough to switchback once more before climbing to an unnamed summit (2,644.8–7,126') on Lakeview Ridge.

VIEWS From here, at the highest PCT point in Washington, you have views on all sides, weather permitting: to the south, the very rugged Three Fools Peak; to the north, your first glimpse of Hopkins Lake; and farther north and west, the rugged Cascades of Washington and Canada.

Now heading down toward Hopkins Pass, the trail sticks to the ridgecrest most of the time until it is forced by Peak 6,873 on the ridge to pass east of that peak. Then the route switchbacks around the north side of the amphitheater for which Hopkins Lake is the stage.

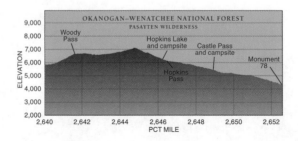

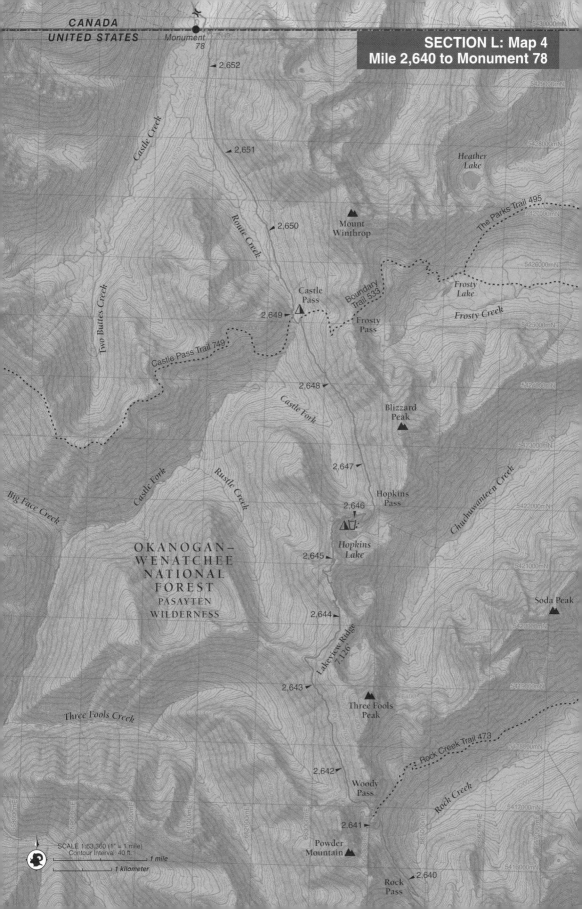

CANADA
UNITED STATES

Monument 78

2,652

2,651

Castle Creek

2,650

Route Creek

Mount Winthrop

Heather Lake

The Parks Trail 495

Frosty Lake

Two Buttes Creek

Castle Pass

2,649

Boundary Trail 533

Frosty Pass

Frosty Creek

Castle Pass Trail 749

2,648

Castle Fork

Blizzard Peak

Chuchuwanteen Creek

Big Face Creek

Castle Fork

Rustle Creek

2,647

Hopkins Pass

2,646

Castle Fork

OKANOGAN–
WENATCHEE
NATIONAL
FOREST
PASAYTEN
WILDERNESS

Hopkins Lake

2,645

2,644

Soda Peak

Lakeview Ridge
7,126

2,643

Three Fools Peak

Three Fools Creek

Rock Creek Trail 473

2,642

Woody Pass

Rock Creek

2,641

SCALE 1:63,360 (1" = 1 mile)
Contour Interval: 40 ft.

1 mile

1 kilometer

Powder Mountain

Rock Pass

2,640

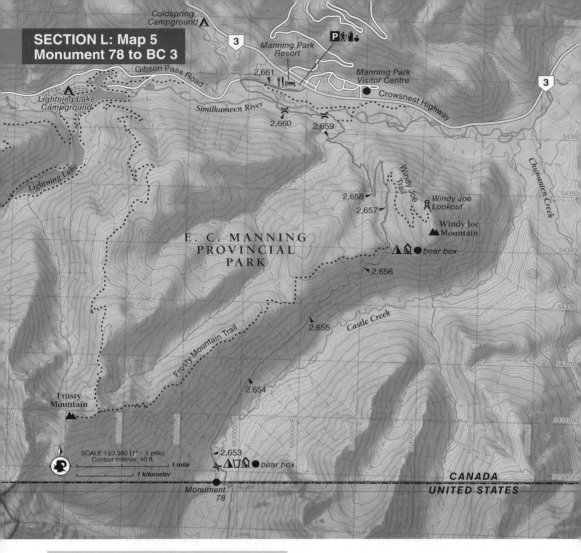

E. C. MANNING
PROVINCIAL
PARK

WATER ACCESS

CAMPING Several short switch-backs and two longer ones bring you down nearly to the level of the lake, where a trail (2,646.2–6,254') to dependable campsites at Hopkins Lake (6,171') takes off to the southwest. Preserve the lake's visibility for all hikers by camping no closer than 200 feet to the shore.

The trail then continues almost east for a few hundred yards to Hopkins Pass (2,646.5–6,140'). The PCT continues north-northwest

from Hopkins Pass, traversing the mostly wooded west slopes of Blizzard Peak (7,622'). After a mile, you reach a stream and its clearing, then reenter woods and continue the traverse about 0.4 mile before starting a gradual descent toward Castle Pass.

CAMPING Shortly before the pass, you see Frosty Pass Trail on the right; one minute later you join Boundary Trail

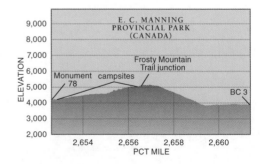

533, turn sharply left, and follow it around a small hummock to Castle Pass (2,648.9–5,460'). Here, you might want to have lunch in the sunshine of a small, open area or spend your last night in the wilderness at one of several campsites before reaching civilization at trail's end.

TRAIL INFO The Boundary Trail is a component of the Pacific Northwest National Scenic Trail (PNNST). The PNNST is colocated with the PCT for about 15 miles from Holman Pass north to Castle Pass.

After meandering north down 0.25 mile of lush alpine gardens, the PCT becomes firmly established on the east slope of the Route Creek watershed. You cross two seasonal streams and two avalanche paths, one from the east and one from the west. Continuing the traverse, you come to two reliable streams in about a mile and then leave the woods for more-open slopes with rounded granite outcrops.

TRAIL INFO After passing two more streams, you finally pound down the last four switchbacks to Monument 78, a survey monument maintained by the International Boundary Commission on the United States–Canada border (2,652.6–4,258'). The monument is a scaled-down version of the Washington Monument. Of more significance for hikers are the inscribed wooden posts beside it. One marks this spot as the northern terminus of the United States' Pacific Crest National Scenic Trail. Ahead, in Canada, it is merely the Pacific Crest Trail. Another displays the mileage from Canada to Mexico as 2,650. This measurement may have fluctuated over the years, but thanks to GPS use, the accuracy has increased, and Halfmile's published measurements have standardized the mileages for all hikers. Every decade since the trail's inception has seen reroutes—with the attendant mileage changes—and more reroutes and realignments are being planned for, worked on, and completed every hiking season. In 2017 a realignment in Northern California lengthened the trail by 2.5 miles. There may be more miles to come.

WATER ACCESS

CAMPING Plunging into the dense, wet, valley-bottom woods, you quickly reach, just 0.25 mile into Canada, trailside campsites (with a bear-proof box, fire ring, and vault toilet) followed by a bridge across seasonally raging Castle Creek (2,652.9–4,215'). *Beware:* At press time this bridge was in dangerously terrible shape. However, it is scheduled for replacement during the summer of 2021.

CAMPING Still in the woods, the trail winds through a dense spruce–fir forest and soon begins a mostly viewless climb steadily but gently northeast. As the path climbs, you plod up a short switchback leg, cross a few ravines, jump a few creeklets, and arrive at the southwest base of Windy Joe Mountain (2,656.4–5,035'). Here, you'll find the PCT's northernmost campsite, with a bear-proof box and toilet, about 4 miles from the Canadian trailhead.

The PCT soon turns north and climbs briefly to a saddle and a junction with the Frosty Mountain Trail (2,656.5–5,110'), which starts to climb southwest.

From here, the PCT makes an undulating traverse north across Windy Joe Mountain's west slopes. Soon you hear the traffic on Canada's main east–west thoroughfare, BC 3, cutting a swath through the dense forest on the unseen, deep canyon floor below you. A convenient sign instructs hikers to follow Windy Joe pathway north to a hairpin turn on the closed Windy Joe Trail (2,657.5–5,220'). You may have encountered mountain bikes on the PCT at various spots along your journey, and you may encounter them here. Whereas in the United

States they are banned, here in Canada, along the Windy Joe Trail, they are allowed. On this trail—a closed road—you descend first north and then south, down to a creek crossing. You immediately recross the creek, descend 0.5 mile, and then cross it for the last time.

The moderately descending route soon winds down gentler slopes 0.6 mile northwest to a crossing of a larger creek, and, just beyond it, you reach a junction (2,659.3–4,100'). Through much of the 1990s, the PCT headed northeast to a BC 3 trailhead at Beaver Pond, but too much flooding of the bottomlands of the Similkameen River made this route often boggy and impassable. A better route now exists, one that crosses only its major tributary, Little Muddy Creek. On a mostly gentle descent west, you go almost a mile to bridge that creek (2,660.2–3,855'). Head northwest about 0.5 mile to a trailhead parking area and the MAN-NING PARK sign (2,661.4–3,910'). *Congratulations on completing your trek!*

This trailhead is along Gibson Pass Road immediately west of the Similkameen River.

RESUPPLY ACCESS

West, Gibson Pass Road goes about 2 miles to Lightning Lake Campground, in the popular Lightning Lake area. East, the road goes about 0.7 mile to BC 3, where you'll find Manning Park Resort. You may want to stay there to shower and get a warm meal. The accommodations are tempting, but they are beyond the budget of many backpackers. From the resort, economy-minded backpackers can trek 1.25 miles west on BC 3 to Coldspring Campground.

Currently, there's no scheduled bus service from Manning Park to Vancouver, but you can book a private shuttle bus through Canadian Craft Charters (vancouvershuttle hire.com) or schedule a pickup in Manning Provincial Park with Mountain Man Mike's Bus Service (mountainmanmikes.ca), which runs from Kaslo to Vancouver. Hikers can also return to Harts Pass to hitch out and avoid the border crossing.

We hope you have arrived in good spirits and in good health. And we also hope that your hike through Section L was, despite the odds, warm, dry, and insect-free.

If you've hiked all or most of the way from Mexico to Canada, please contact us at pct .wildernesspress.com and tell us about your experiences and about the usefulness of these guidebooks. The comments we received from your predecessors helped make this edition more useful for PCT trekkers. Safe journeys on all your trails.

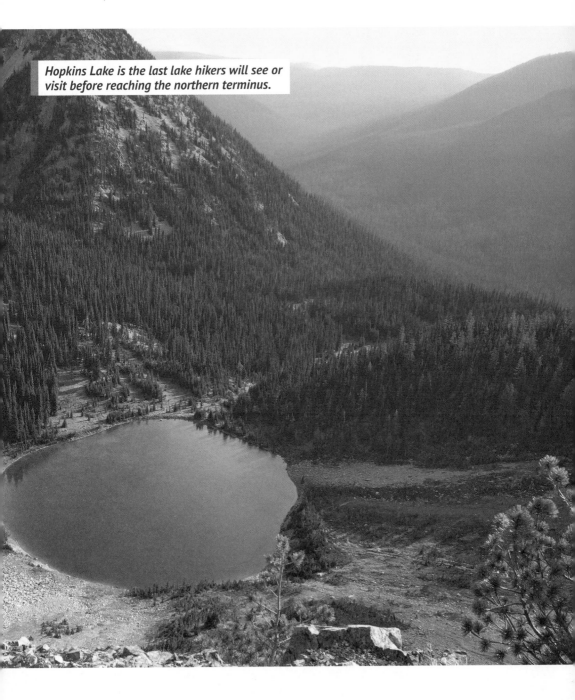

Hopkins Lake is the last lake hikers will see or visit before reaching the northern terminus.

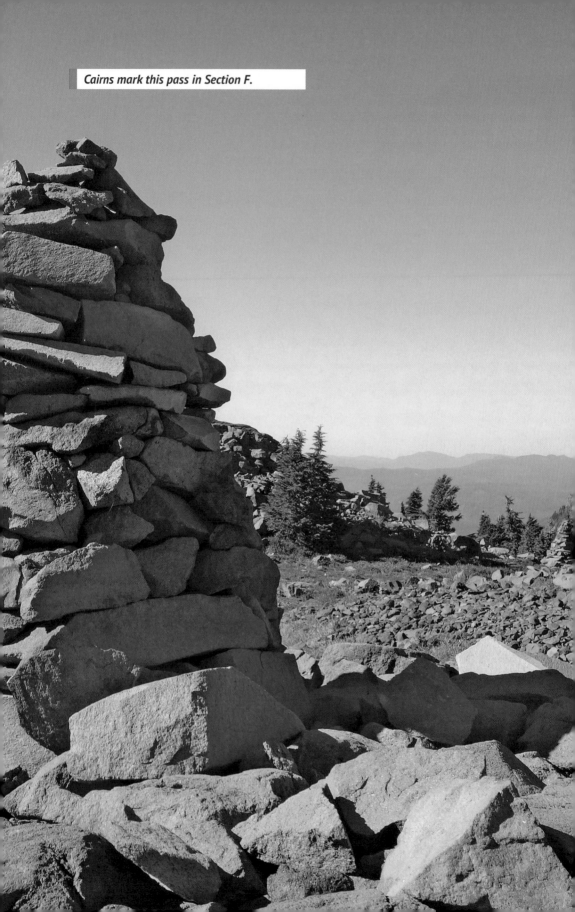

Cairns mark this pass in Section F.

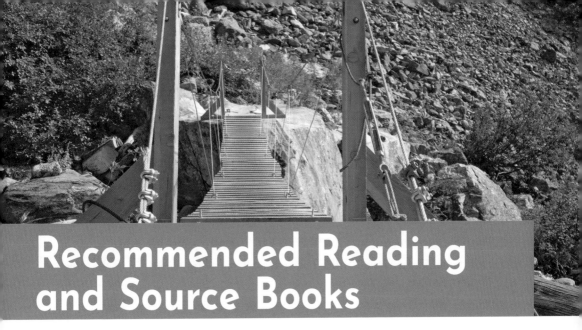

Recommended Reading and Source Books

Note: An asterisk (*) indicates an out-of-print book.

PACIFIC CREST TRAIL (PCT)

Berger, Karen, and Daniel R. Smith. *The Pacific Crest Trail: A Hiker's Companion.* 2nd ed. New York: The Countryman Press, 2014.

Bodnar, Paul. *Pocket PCT: Complete Data and Town Guide.* 4th ed. Scotts Valley, CA: CreateSpace Independent Publishing, 2016.

Clarke, Clinton C. *The Pacific Crest Trailway.* Pasadena, CA: The Pacific Crest Trail System Conference, 1945.*

Davis, Zach, and Carly Moree. *Pacific Crest Trials: A Psychological and Emotional Guide to Successfully Thru-Hiking the Pacific Crest Trail.* Golden, CO: Pacific Crest Trials, 2016.

Egbert, Barbara. *Zero Days: The Real-Life Adventure of Captain Bligh, Nellie Bly, and 10-Year-Old Scrambler on the Pacific Crest Trail.* Berkeley: Wilderness Press, 2008.

Gerald, Paul. *Day & Section Hikes, Pacific Crest Trail: Oregon.* 3rd ed. Birmingham, AL: Wilderness Press, 2019.

Go, Benedict. *Pacific Crest Trail Data Book.* 6th ed. Birmingham, AL: Wilderness Press, 2020.

Green, David. *A Pacific Crest Odyssey: Walking the Trail from Mexico to Canada.* Berkeley: Wilderness Press, 1979.*

Harris, David. *Day & Section Hikes, Pacific Crest Trail: Southern California.* Birmingham, AL: Wilderness Press, 2012.

Hazard, Joseph T. *Pacific Crest Trails.* Seattle: Superior Publishing Co., 1946.*

Jardine, Ray. *The Pacific Crest Trail Hiker's Handbook.* 2nd ed. Arizona City, AZ: AdventureLore Books, 1996.*

Above: For a safe, stable journey over Maple Creek in Section K

Larabee, Mark, and Barney Scout Mann. *The Pacific Crest Trail: Exploring America's Wilderness Trail*. New York: Rizzoli, 2016.

Lautner, Wendy. *Day & Section Hikes, Pacific Crest Trail: Northern California*. Berkeley: Wilderness Press, 2010.

Mann, Barney Scout. *Journeys North: The Pacific Crest Trail*. Seattle: Mountaineers Books, 2020.

McDonnell, Jackie. *Yogi's Pacific Crest Trail Handbook*. rev. ed. Inyokern, CA: Yogi's Books, 2019.

Ross, Cindy. *Journey on the Crest: Walking 2,600 Miles from Mexico to Canada*. Seattle: Mountaineers Books, 1987.

Ryback, Eric. *The High Adventure of Eric Ryback*. San Francisco: Chronicle Books, 1971.*

Schaefer, Adrienne. *Day & Section Hikes, Pacific Crest Trail: Washington*. 2nd ed. Birmingham, AL: Wilderness Press, 2017.

Strayed, Cheryl. *Wild: From Lost to Found on the Pacific Crest Trail*. New York: Vintage Books, 2013.

BACKPACKING, PACKING, AND MOUNTAINEERING

Back Country Horsemen of Montana. *Back Country Horsemen's Guidebook*. 5th ed. Columbia Falls, MT: Back Country Horsemen of Montana, 2019. bchmt.org/documents/Guide_Book_FINAL2019.pdf.

Back, Joe. *Horses, Hitches, and Rocky Trails*. 1987. Reprint, Denver: Johnson Books, 2018.

Beckey, Fred. *Cascade Alpine Guide, Climbing & High Routes, Volume 1: Columbia River to Stevens Pass*. 3rd ed. Seattle, Mountaineers Books, 2000.

———. *Cascade Alpine Guide, Climbing & High Routes, Volume 2: Stevens Pass to Rainy Pass*. 3rd ed. Seattle: Mountaineers Books, 2003.

———. *Cascade Alpine Guide, Climbing & High Routes, Volume 3: Rainy Pass to Fraser River*. 3rd ed. Seattle: Mountaineers Books, 2008.

Beffort, Brian. *Joy of Backpacking*. Berkeley: Wilderness Press, 2007.

Brame, Rich, and David Cole. *NOLS Soft Paths: Enjoying the Wilderness Without Harming It*. 4th ed. Mechanicsburg, PA: Stackpole Books, 2011.

Brame, Susan C., and Chad Henderson. *NOLS Wilderness Ethics*. rev. ed. Mechanicsburg, PA: Stackpole Books, 2005.

Elser, Smoke, and Bill Brown. *Packin' In on Mules and Horses*. Missoula, MT: Mountain Press, 1980.

Gonzales, Laurence. *Deep Survival: Who Lives, Who Dies and Why*. 2003. Reprinted with a new introduction by the author. New York: W. W. Norton & Co., 2017.

Gookin, John, and Tom Reed. *NOLS Bear Essentials*. Mechanicsburg, PA: Stackpole Books, 2009.

Harvey, Mark. *The National Outdoor Leadership School's Wilderness Guide*. New York: Simon & Schuster, 1999.

Hinch, Stephen. *Outdoor Navigation with GPS.* 3rd ed. Berkeley: Wilderness Press, 2010.

Letham, Lawrence. *GPS Made Easy: Using Global Positioning Systems in the Outdoors.* 5th ed. Seattle: Mountaineers Books, 2008.

Light, Richard A. *Backpacking the Light Way.* Birmingham, AL: Menasha Ridge Press, 2015.

March, Laurie Ann. *A Fork in the Trail: Mouthwatering Meals and Tempting Treats for the Backcountry.* Berkeley: Wilderness Press, 2008.

The Mountaineers. *Mountaineering: The Freedom of the Hills.* 9th ed. Seattle: Mountaineers Books, 2017.

Powers, Phil. *NOLS Wilderness Mountaineering.* 3rd ed. Mechanicsburg, PA: Stackpole Books, 2008.

Schimelpfenig, Tod. *NOLS Wilderness Medicine.* 6th ed. Mechanicsburg, PA: Stackpole Books, 2016.

Tilton, Buck, and John Gookin. *NOLS Winter Camping.* Mechanicsburg, PA: Stackpole Books, 2005.

Trantham, Gene, and Darran Wells. *NOLS Wilderness Navigation.* 3rd ed. Mechanicsburg, PA: Stackpole Books, 2018.

Tremper, Bruce. *Avalanche Essentials: A Step-by-Step System for Safety and Survival.* Seattle: Mountaineers Books, 2013.

Wilkerson, James A., ed. *Hypothermia, Frostbite, and Other Cold Injuries.* 2nd ed. Seattle: Mountaineers Books, 2006.

———. *Medicine for Mountaineering & Other Wilderness Activities.* 6th ed. Seattle: Mountaineers Books, 2010.

HISTORY

Bentley, Judy. *Hiking Washington's History.* Seattle: University of Washington Press, 2015.

Buck, Rinker. *The Oregon Trail: A New American Journey.* Reprint ed. New York: Simon & Schuster, 2016.

Hayes, Derek. *Historical Atlas of Washington and Oregon.* Berkeley: University of California Press, 2011.

Jepsen, David J., and David J. Norberg. *Contested Boundaries: A New Pacific Northwest History.* Hoboken, NJ: Wiley-Blackwell, 2017.

Molenaar, Dee. *The Challenge of Rainier: A Record of the Explorations and Ascents, Triumphs, and Tragedies on the Northwest's Greatest Mountain.* 4th ed. Seattle: Mountaineers Books, 2011.

GEOLOGY

Haugerud, Ralph, and Rowland Tabor. *Geology of the North Cascades: A Mountain Mosaic.* Seattle: Mountaineers Books, 1999.

Harris, Stephen L. *Fire Mountains of the West: The Cascade and Mono Lake Volcanoes*. 3rd ed. Missoula, MT: Mountain Press, 2005.

Lynch, Dan R., and Bob Lynch. *Rocks & Minerals of Washington & Oregon*. Cambridge, MN: Adventure Publications, 2012.

McPhee, John. *Annals of the Former World*. New York: Farrar, Straus and Giroux, 1998.

Miller, Marli B. *Roadside Geology of Oregon*. 2nd ed. Missoula, MT: Mountain Press, 2014.

Miller, Marli B., and Darrel S. Cowan. *Roadside Geology of Washington*. 2nd ed. Missoula, MT: Mountain Press, 2017.

Tucker, Dave. *Geology Underfoot in Western Washington*. Missoula, MT: Mountain Press, 2015.

BIOLOGY

Moskowitz, David. *Wildlife of the Pacific Northwest*. Portland: Timber Press, 2010.

Murie, Olaus J., and Mark Elbroch. *Peterson Field Guide to Animal Tracks*. 3rd ed. Boston: Houghton Mifflin Harcourt, 2005.

Poppele, Jonathan. *Animal Tracks of the Northwest*. Cambridge, MN: Adventure Publications, 2017.

Sibley, David Allen. *The Sibley Guide to Birds*. 2nd ed. New York: Alfred A. Knopf, 2014.

Tekiela, Stan. *Birds of Oregon Field Guide*. Cambridge, MN: Adventure Publications, 2001.

———. *Birds of the Northwest*. Cambridge, MN: Adventure Publications, 2017.

———. *Birds of Washington Field Guide*. Cambridge, MN: Adventure Publications, 2001.

Whitney, Stephen R., Robert Cocuzzo, and Rob Sandelin. *Field Guide to the Cascades and Olympics*. 2nd ed. Seattle: Mountaineers Books, 2004.

BOTANY

Arno, Stephen. *Northwest Trees: Identifying and Understanding the Region's Native Trees*. 2nd ed. Seattle: Mountaineers Books, 2020.

Derig, Betty B., and Margaret C. Fuller. *Wild Berries of the West*. Missoula, MT: Mountain Press, 2001.

Little, Elbert L. *National Audubon Society Field Guide to North American Trees: Western Region*. New York: Alfred A. Knopf, 1980.

Miller, George. *Wildflowers of the Pacific Northwest*. Cambridge, MN: Adventure Publications, 2019.

Underhill, J. E. *Sagebrush Wildflowers*. Blaine, WA: Hancock House, 1986.

Watts, Tom. *Pacific Coast Tree Finder*. Rochester, NY: Nature Study Guild Publishers, 2004.

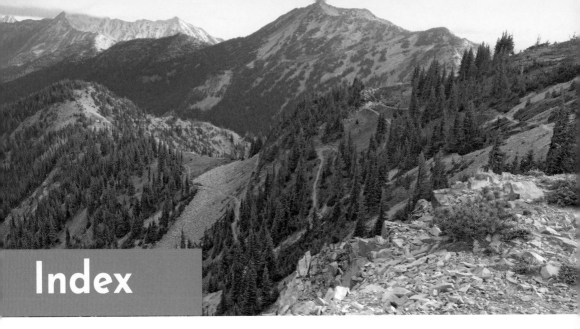

Index

Above: Three more hours for reflection, just south of the Canadian border

Taking care of the Pacific Crest Trail is a full-time effort.

The Pacific Crest Trail Association's mission is to protect, preserve and promote the trail as a resource for hikers and equestrians and for the value that wild lands provide to all people.

Through a formal partnership with the U.S. Forest Service, our nonprofit membership organization is the primary caretaker of this 2,650-mile National Scenic Trail as it winds through the American West's most beautiful landscapes.

Each year, PCTA volunteers and paid staff members clear downed trees and repair washed out tread. We monitor threats to the trail and speak up on its behalf. We tell the trail's story in print and online. And we advocate for federal support by visiting our elected leaders in Washington, D.C.

All this effort safeguards the experiences and solitude people deserve when they venture into the wild.

Please help preserve this national treasure for future generations by joining the PCTA.

Your $35 annual membership will ensure that this trail will never end.

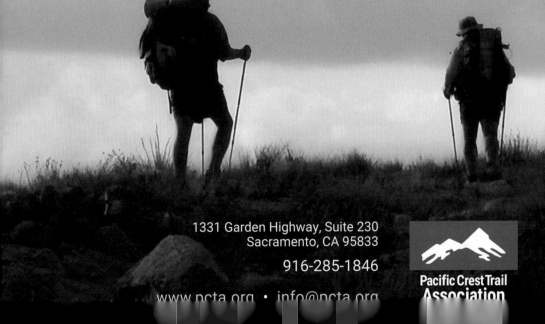

1331 Garden Highway, Suite 230
Sacramento, CA 95833

916-285-1846

www.pcta.org • info@pcta.org

Pacific Crest Trail Association

ABOUT THE AUTHORS

Since he was 6 years old, **Jordan Summers** has had more fun sleeping on rock, snow, and dirt than any one person should be allowed— spending absurd amounts of time in mountains, forests, canyons, and deserts. Jordan's newest guidebooks, *Pacific Crest Trail: Northern California* and *Pacific Crest Trail: Oregon & Washington,* are the result of his 4,000-plus miles trekking this national treasure.

Jordan's passion for the outdoors and love for the Sierra Nevada range combined to propel his motivation in writing guidebooks: "to help hikers of all abilities get out there, have a great time out there, Leave No Trace there, and come home safely from there." Jordan is an alumnus of the National Outdoor Leadership School (NOLS), a Leave No Trace trainer, and a NOLS Wilderness Medicine Wilderness First Responder. He lives in the Sierra Nevada foothill town of Pioneer, California, and is a volunteer for the Tahoe Rim Trail Association and the Pacific Crest Trail Association.

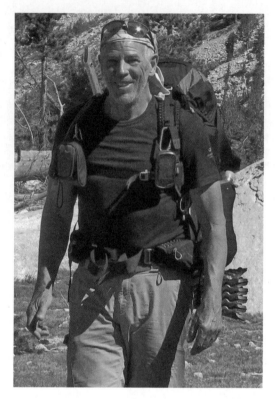

Wilderness Press would also like to acknowledge the contributions of **Jeffrey P. Schaffer** and **Andy Selters**, whose text from many prior editions was revised by Jordan Summers for this edition.